THE
HEALTHY
HOUSE

THE HEALTHY HOUSE

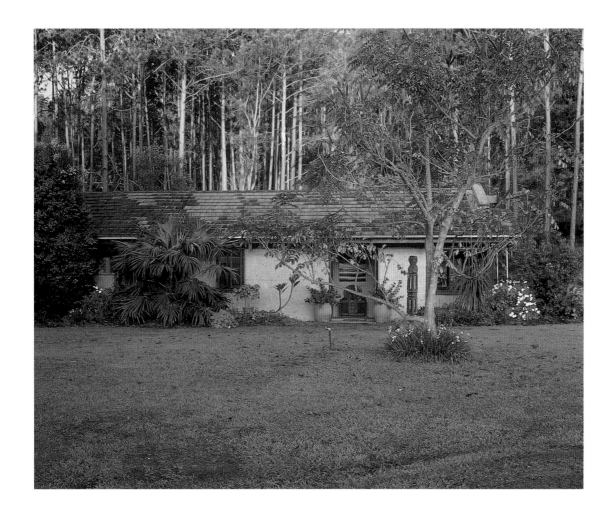

Sydney and Joan Baggs

HarperCollins*Publishers*

Dedicated to the memory of author and journalist
Vicki Peterson, a victim of 20th-century syndrome
and
to our grandchildren:
Adam, Katheryn, Anthony, Alexandra and Georgia
who, with all the other grandchildren of this planet,
will carry our hopes for a more loving and cleaner world into
the 21st century

HarperCollins*Publishers*

First published in Australia in 1996
by HarperCollins*Publishers*
ACN 009 913 517
A member of the HarperCollins*Publishers* (Australia) Pty Limited Group

Copyright © Sydney Baggs and Joan Baggs 1996

HarperCollins*Publishers*
25 Ryde Road, Pymble, Sydney NSW 2073, Australia
1160 Battery Street, San Francisco, California 94111-1213, USA
Hazelton Lanes, 55 Avenue Road, Suite 2900, Toronto, Ontario M5R 3L2
and 1995 Markham Road, Scarborough, Ontario M1B 5M8 Canada
31 View Road, Glenfield, Auckland 10, New Zealand
77-85 Fulham Palace Road, London W6 8JB, United Kingdom
10 East 53rd Street, New York NY 10032, USA

National Library of Australia Cataloguing-in-Publication data:

Baggs, Sydney A., 1930-.
   The healthy house: the Gaian approach to creating a safe,
   healthy and environmentally friendly home.
   Bibliography.
   Includes index.
   ISBN 07322 56682
   1. Dwellings - Environmental aspects. 2. Architecture - Human factors.
   3. Gaia hypothesis. 4. Architecture, Domestic.
   5. Landscape design - Environmental aspects.
   I. Baggs, Joan C. (Joan Constance), 1930- . II. Title.
728.047

Illustrations by Sydney Baggs

Printed in Hong Kong
987654321 96 97 98 99

CONSULTING ARCHITECTS
(RESOURCES LIST)
USA: CAROL VENOLIA
UK: DAVID PEARSON

THE AUTHORS WOULD LIKE TO ACKNOWLEDGE:

Vanessa Mickan's persevering, tolerant and nothing short of brilliant editing, and Kerry Klinner's careful interpretation of the exacting needs of graphics and extremely creative approach to the overall design

PHOTOGRAPHS:

Page 1: Healthy house, Coromandel, New Zealand (Architects: J. Schulze and F. Poursoltan; Photograph: F. Poursoltan). Page 3: Rammed-earth house, Queensland, Aust. (Architect: D. Oliver, Greenway Architects; Photograph: D. Oliver). Page 5: Entrance court to low-allergy, earth-sheltered house in bushland on Central Coast of NSW, Aust. (Architects: E.C.A. Space Design Pty Ltd). Page 6: Environmental Education Centre, Worcestershire, UK (Architects: Technical Services Department, Hereford and Worcester County Council; Photograph: A. Carew-Cox). Page 7: Dining room of 'Bidri Park', NSW, Aust. (Architect: C. Pattinson, Arcoessence; Photograph: C. Pattinson)

Preface

back in 1979 when we spent six months in the United States researching earth-sheltered buildings, we met a young couple who were travelling throughout America searching for somewhere safe and unpolluted to raise their family. They had set out from their home in Oak Ridge, Tennessee, where the headquarters for the World War 2 atomic energy program, the Manhattan Project, had been situated. After months of searching they had not found one unspoilt place, and decided to return to Oak Ridge, despite the fact that a nuclear research facility and two uranium processing plants are currently located there. The disillusioned husband referred to the way that humanity was 'fouling its nest' — and the seeds for this book were sown. *The Healthy House* is directed not only to those with health problems caused by modern ways of life, but also to those who are concerned about the despoilation of our planet.

Over the past decade or so, while we have been researching the material for this book, public interest in the potential of living environments to harm our health has quickened and attitudes have changed. People are far more concerned with the health effects of the buildings in which they live and work. Now, people not only have less money to waste on theories and experiments but they appear more anxious and even more physically stressed than they were 10 years ago. Many have serious problems with their environments, such as one woman who was advised to leave her home of 40 years because of the deterioration in her health when the wind blew fumes, to which she was sensitive, into her home from a new marina across the bay. We are constantly receiving queries from such people, seeking healthy

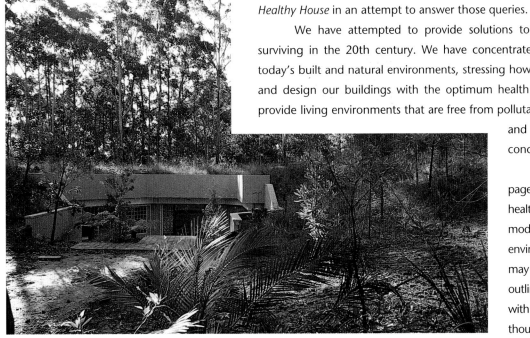

alternatives. Frustrated by our inability to advise everyone individually, we have written *The Healthy House* in an attempt to answer those queries.

We have attempted to provide solutions to many of the problems of living and surviving in the 20th century. We have concentrated on aspects of living and working in today's built and natural environments, stressing how we can choose suitable, non-toxic sites and design our buildings with the optimum health of inhabitants in mind. The aim is to provide living environments that are free from pollutants, are in tune with the needs, feelings and spiritual aspirations of the family, and in concert with the nature around us.

We hope that a journey through these pages will result in the restoration of your health if it is failing because of exposure to modern pollutants, and in the creation of an environment in which you and your family may grow in body, mind and spirit. The ideas outlined here will help you integrate more fully with all life on the planet, surely the aim of all thoughtful and concerned human beings.

Contents

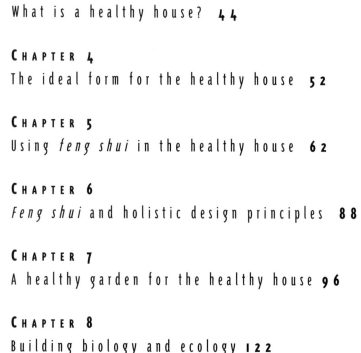

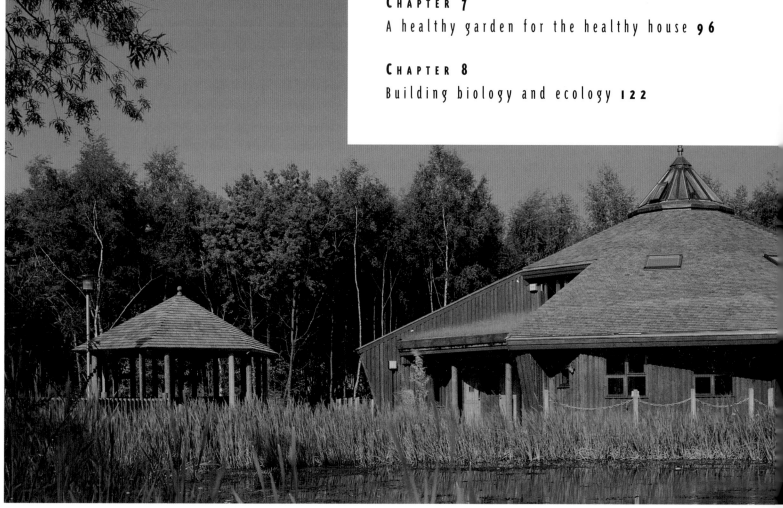

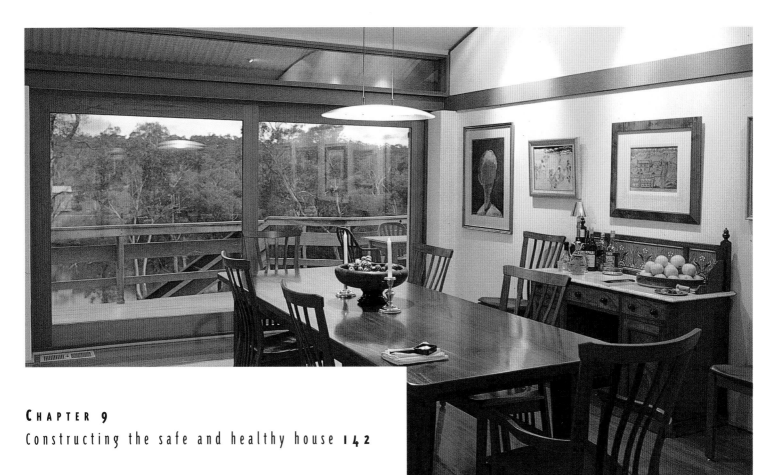

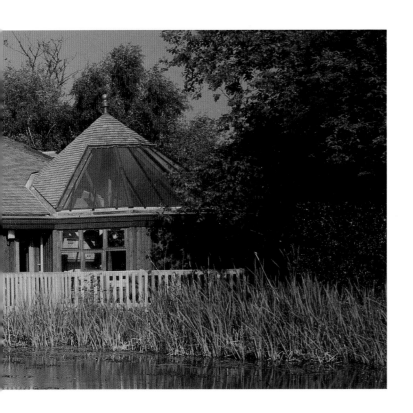

Introduction

the building industry has caused many problems in the past which are only now surfacing in some of today's health problems. Many people suffer symptoms which could be categorised as part of a 20th century 'malaise'. The upsurge in these illnesses seems to have begun with the invention of long-chain molecule plastics, glues and laminates, and certain types of electrical equipment.

The results of exposure to environments filled with such inventions have been described by environmental medical practitioners in terms such as Serotonin Irritation Syndrome (SIS), General Adaptation Syndrome (GAS), and Chronic Fatigue Syndrome (CFS) or Myalgic Encephalomyelitis (ME). Many people suffer a range of allergic symptoms, such as migraine, stomach cramps, asthma, eczema and joint and muscle pain. Sometimes this leads to Multiple Chemical Sensitivity (MCS) or Total Allergy Syndrome.

They may not acknowledge it, but generations of architects, engineers and builders have specified and installed various chemical-based and mineral products and electrical and building-construction systems that have only recently been suspected, and in some cases proven, to have endangered the health and happiness of those using their buildings. Outgassed toxic chemicals, aerosols, radioactive and mineral pollutants — as well as electrical and magnetic fields — have become an integral part of the built environment. They are time-bombs waiting for a level of toxicity or cumulative radiation

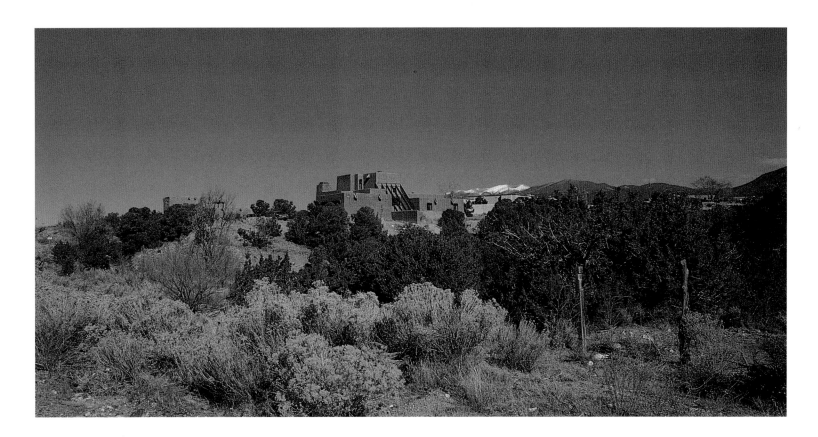

to build up within the body of an individual until it exceeds their tolerance threshold, causing symptoms of debilitation and ill health. Chronic disease results when the individual's immune system finally fails.

Yet there is hope. Such a situation can usually be corrected when the person is shown the real cause of their health problems, and that there are alternatives to the customary methods of building design and construction. The human body is wonderfully regenerative, cells being replaced many times during a life span. No matter what your age, attempt to heal those cells now. Give your body a better environment as free from toxins and electromagnetic pollution as possible. Supply it with the best nutrients and minerals you can afford and surround it with the beneficial life fields of nature. Cell by cell, it will replace the *you* of today with a new *you* in the years to come.

At first, the task of finding economical and practical solutions to correct all the mistakes of the past may seem insurmountable, but persevere. As you read, you may obtain ideas that will enable you to rejuvenate yourself and change your living environment, creating a safer, healthier lifestyle for you and your family. You will be able to repair some of the damage of the past, look forward to an improved quality of life in the future, and perhaps enjoy a longer, healthier and more creative life. In *The Healthy House* we have assembled an arsenal of strategies from which to choose, many of which challenge the preconceptions that are currently held by the majority of designers, architects and engineers.

Our purpose is not to set out the whole plan for a healthy life. We aim to indicate what may be wrong with present buildings and lifestyles and how they can be corrected. We hope to encourage the general public to become more knowledgeable and critical of the environments created for them in the past by members of the building profession. Attitudes seem to be changing but trained professionals, mostly through ignorance, have settled in the past for less than the standards necessary to ensure the health of a building's occupants. On the whole, the medical profession has also been ignorant of the potential dangers of using the wrong sorts of building materials in hospitals and nursing homes. However, with the recent growth of information on the subject of healthy buildings and healthy lifestyles, there is no longer any excuse for the continuation of practices that damage our environment and health. As our level of awareness increases, we have a right to assume that the professionals upon whom we depend will also be knowledgeable. Ignorance or neglect can produce results that rob people of their health.

Above: Adobe building, Santa Fe, USA

Previous page: The Eco-house, Bandon, Cork, UK (Architect: P. Leech, Photograph: P. Leech)

ABOUT THIS BOOK

Some of the topics discussed in *The Healthy House* are inherently complicated. In simplifying them, we have endeavoured to follow the advice of Albert Einstein: 'the goal for writing [is that] "everything should be made as simple as possible, but not one bit simpler"' (Mygind 1986). Many of the ideas we have outlined are being taught in Germany by the Institute fur Baubiologie™ und Oikologie under Doctor Schneider, in New Zealand by the Building Biology and Ecology Institute under Reinhard Kanuka-Fuchs, and in the United States and Scandinavia.

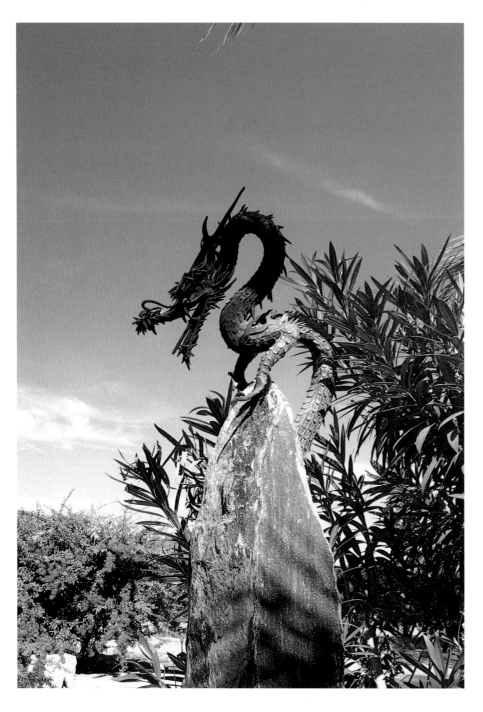

East entrance of the garden at Taliesen West, outside Phoenix, USA (Architect: Frank Lloyd Wright)

We address the issues of how the average person can modify their old house or flat to make it healthier — or if the opportunity arises to escape an old, polluted environment, how to choose a healthy district and site and design a health-promoting, low-allergy house. We look at how to avoid creating a 'sick' building by carefully considering the materials used in its construction, including the interior furnishings, fitments and finishes. We outline the principles of the Chinese practice of *feng shui*, and how it can help us design a healthy building. The importance of a building's solar access is discussed, in relation to temperature modification for energy efficiency and comfortable living. Because a healthy house should also have a healthy garden, we examine how you can create low-allergy, non-toxic, healthy landscaping around your building.

A lifestyle based on caring for all living things and understanding and cooperating with natural systems is described in the final chapter. Integral to this lifestyle is a gentle architecture that treads lightly upon the Earth, making it possible for urban populations to live and work in sunlit, health-promoting buildings which are part of their parks and gardens.

The appendices at the back of the book contain information which expands on technical concepts raised in particular chapters. The resources list will help you find the products and services necessary in your quest for personal health and fulfilment. A comprehensive glossary has also been provided for ease of reference.

SCIENCE, PARASCIENCE AND PROTOSCIENCE

The information contained in this book has been classified into three main types — science, parascience and protoscience — according to the way in which that information has been arrived at.

Science, as we know it today, is based upon a strict process. A scientist develops a hypothesis to explain a particular phenomenon; experiments are undertaken in attempts to prove that the hypothesis is incorrect. Only after innumerable experiments have shown no exceptions to the hypothesis does it become a theory, and after replication by many experimenters, a natural law.

Protoscience, on the other hand, refers to original, primal or ancient knowledge. It suggests covert, esoteric meanings that can sometimes enlighten the enquirer better than contemporary science is able to. Pythagoras' description of the elements of the universe is one example of this type of knowledge.

Parascience (from the Greek, *para*: beside, near by, along with) has its roots in both science and protoscience. It involves not only the controlled experimental procedures of science, but also the mysticism and occultism of protoscience. Many of the activities of parascience are subjective or intuitive and are difficult to measure. For example, dowsing (using a divining rod or other device to find underground water, minerals or areas of geomagnetism) is almost totally subjective and results can only be quantified with scientific instruments in a small percentage of cases, yet skilled dowsers often astound with their capabilities.

Parascience is a developing area of research. While it first produced only anecdotal evidence, parascience is rapidly entering the realm of controlled scientific experimentation and in many instances is part of the arsenal of complementary medicine practitioners. The science of tomorrow, parascience, will be characterised by intuitive leaps across disciplines, the hallmark of great scientists like Tesla, Galileo and Newton.

In *The Healthy House*, we have linked the science of the past, present and perhaps even the future into an instrument for changing your life if you should so desire. These steps are only the beginning of a lifetime of challenges for those who have courage and care enough to think about the effects of everything they do.

This can be a new and interesting journey in exciting times.

Adobe residence, Sante Fe, New Mexico, USA (Architect/builder: J. McGowan)

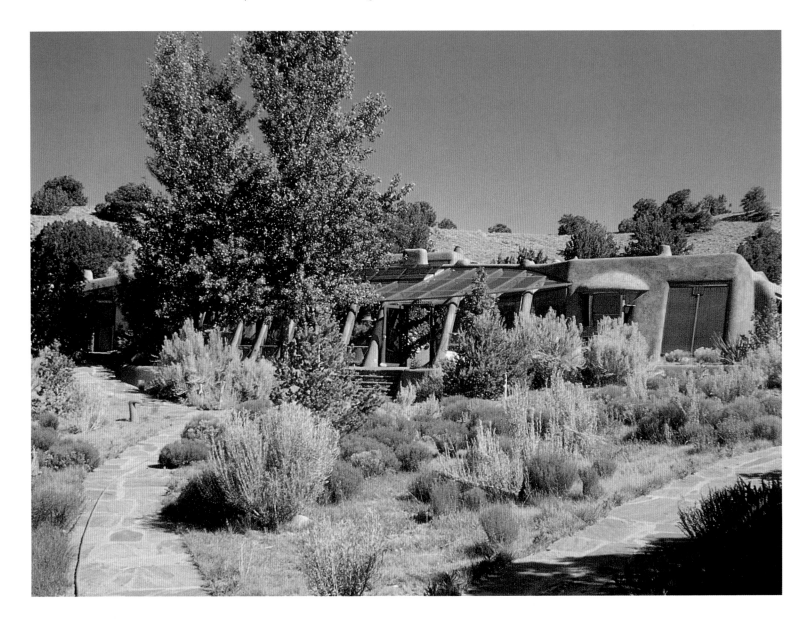

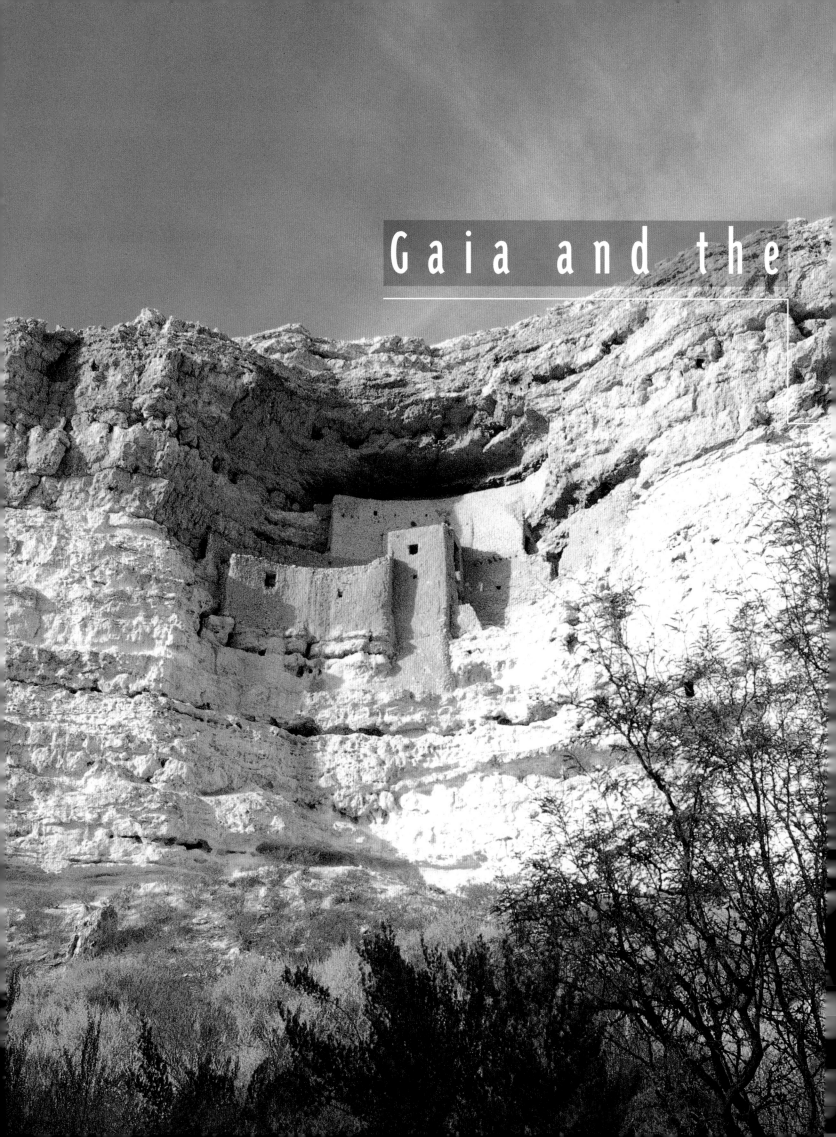

Gaia and the

five elements

No matter how deeply scientists delve into nature, and no matter how subtle their measurements, the nature of 'being' eludes them. As we examine the world of subatomic particles, boundaries merge and the universality of all matter and living things becomes evident. The hidden life vibrant in every atom and the hidden light shining in every creature is the paradigm of this age.

. . . the universe is sustained by an act of such stupendous and ineffable creativity that it simply cannot be [asked] if the part is creating the whole or the whole is creating the part because the part is the whole (Talbot 1991).

At the scale of the subatomic particle, there are no boundaries between your hand and the table upon which it rests. The quanta of energy of hand and table interpenetrate and some of the qualities of each are shared at the physical subatomic level — some would say at the level of even more subtle energy states.

Just as we share our atomic particles with all the world with which we come in contact, in a more general sense, nature and humanity share a common field of energy interaction. Nature's life fields interact intimately with our own. Hence, by creating toxic conditions we harm ourselves as well as the environment.

As an integral part of the vibrant, whirling world of energy, we are, in a strictly physical sense, only differentiated from other things because the energy field of every person or thing is held in place by some type of biological force-field, similar in effect to the magnetic field that holds iron filings in a specific three-dimensional pattern. In a physical sense, we are *one* with nature.

THE GAIA HYPOTHESIS

In describing the interrelationship between the planet and its life forms, Doctor James Lovelock (1979) used the term Gaia, the name of the ancient Greek goddess of the Earth. A poetic title, it is not intended to imply a feminine goddess in human form, but to identify the sentient entity that is the totality of our planet's components and systems, all its living things together. Lovelock began formulating his theory while working on the Mars space probe for NASA with Professor Lynn Margulis. Since then they, and others, have compiled a vast amount of data to support the Gaia hypothesis.

Lovelock proposes that all life on Earth has a symbiotic relationship with the planet. The balance between living organisms and the planet's systems is maintained so precisely that the multiplicity of all living things may be considered as one great organism, in the same way that all the cells of your body go together to make up 'you'. A change in any one part of the system produces follow-on effects throughout the web of life which makes up the greater organism.

As we are in such close contact with all life on the planet, should we not surround ourselves with health-promoting environments? The intimate inter-relationship of all life forms and non-living objects at the subatomic level is the basis for how and why we should care for ourselves and all living things, including our planet. The choices of gentle, non-polluting practices of food selection, cooking, cleaning and clothing the body, housing, furnishing the home and developing the landscape around it, are all direct pathways towards the goal of caring for the Earth. We are our environment (and vice versa) at a very fundamental level.

The Earth and its atmosphere can best be considered as a living entity with the equivalent of senses, energy cycles, and feedback and control mechanisms that have the capacity to interact and maintain the balance and stability of the planet in an intelligently functioning web of interrelatedness.

The Gaia hypothesis is a metaphor for a self-regulating world system. Thermodynamic and chemical equilibriums are sustained despite the changes over time in the gases of the atmosphere and the physical location of the Earth in the solar system. For example, since life first appeared on this planet, radiation from the sun has increased by over 30 per cent, yet temperature balance has been maintained on Earth. The planet revolves around the sun's uncontrolled radiant heat, yet the geological record shows that the Earth has maintained a relatively constant range of mean surface temperatures throughout the period in which life has been evolving, in much the same way as the human organism maintains a steady temperature regardless of its environment. Despite massive changes in the composition of the atmosphere and varying output of energy from the sun, it has never been either too hot or too cold on Earth for life to survive. The Earth and its life forms may be likened to a giant system that uses feedback controls to maintain equilibrium. Feedback control can be observed in such things as air conditioning systems, where an automatic thermostat maintains a certain air temperature regardless of outside factors. Such self-regulation is observable in a wide variety of environmental aspects too, such as the chemical composition of the atmosphere, salt content of the oceans and the distribution of trace elements in plants and animals.

Gaia is not just like an organism — it is an organism, with properties and capacities that cannot be predicted by observing its individual parts. It is greater than the sum of its parts. Doctor Kit Pedler (1979) explained the outcome of his years of studying the 'beautifully integrated' human body.

The Kirlian photograph is an image of an individual's health aura, or corona discharge. Photograph: Graydon H. Rixon, Auragraphic Energy Research Centre

I saw how . . . each part, each organ and network functioned as a self-repairing and stable complex with its own apparent boundary . . . The body, in reality, is a microcosm of Gaia. Just as animals relate to the plants, and cycles of stability in the biosphere maintain the continuum of life among the species, so do the organs of the body all interrelate to create a stable whole. But just as the body is mortal so may Gaia be.

If the living world is organised into many levels of structures, there must also be many levels of mind. In human beings, there is a type of 'mind-ordering' evident in the organisation of tissues, cells and organs, while the brain has its own neural pathways which have evolved over millions of years. Taken together, they can be considered as the multi-level, human mind of which a person is only partly conscious. Individual minds are part of larger social and cultural 'minds' — part of the planetary mental ecological system, the 'mind' of Gaia. Some think that the system continues to the level of a cosmic or universal mind (Blavatsky 1950).

An understanding of the functioning of Gaia cannot be attained by studying it according to the separate disciplines of the scientific specialist fields. Communication across disciplines is needed to try and obtain an overview of the system as a whole.

INTEGRATING HOME AND LIFESTYLE WITH GAIA

If humanity is to continue in the future, we must learn a new way of life that can be sustained over the coming centuries. The old ways of the advanced industrial nations — high per capita food consumption, energy use and waste-heat production — are no longer acceptable.

Not only do we need to control population growth throughout the world but we must also develop energy-efficient technologies with minimal waste production. This would result in a sustainable society profoundly different from the status quo. How can such a society be attained? The Gaia concept guides us towards a solution. Considering the Earth as a living organism, amongst the systems and organs that allow it to maintain its stability are its climate, nutrients, waste and mineral cycles and the feedback control systems inherent in all of them. Human beings may be seen as individual 'cells' in the body of the Earth organism.

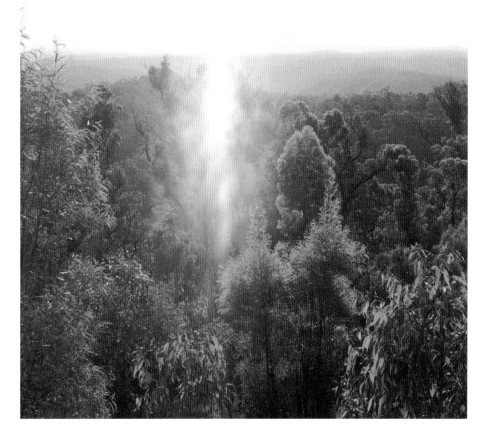

A sustainable society can be built by preserving all those functions of Gaia that, by adjusting to change, maintain stability. Think of human society as the nervous system of the Earth organism. We take information from the environment, process it and make decisions in response to it. If we were to become creative in our processing and not just reactive, human society could function as the brain of the organism. As the brain manages the body, so humanity could manage the planet. The brain has two choices. It could recklessly control the body, profligately using it for amusement and gratification, at the expense of its health. Or, it could frugally administer the body, conserving its energy and making decisions that result in good health.

This authenticated and unaltered photograph shows the great *Deva of Light* that appeared on a sunless day in 1993 at a sacred Aboriginal women's site on the mountain *Yango* in New South Wales, Australia. The light emitted by the image onto the surrounding vegetation indicates that it is not the result of a rogue reflection in the camera lens. Photograph: Neena Scott

In the past, humanity has chosen the profligate mode, abusing the resources of the planet. However, attitudes are gradually changing, with many choosing to adopt a nurturing mode, managing the Earth for the good of all its biota. To do this we must first learn to manage our own lives. To manage society '. . . we need to start with ourselves' (Schumacher 1973). We need to utilise our intelligence and knowledge of environmental science, and avoid the frontier mentality that 'there is always more where that came from'. There is not.

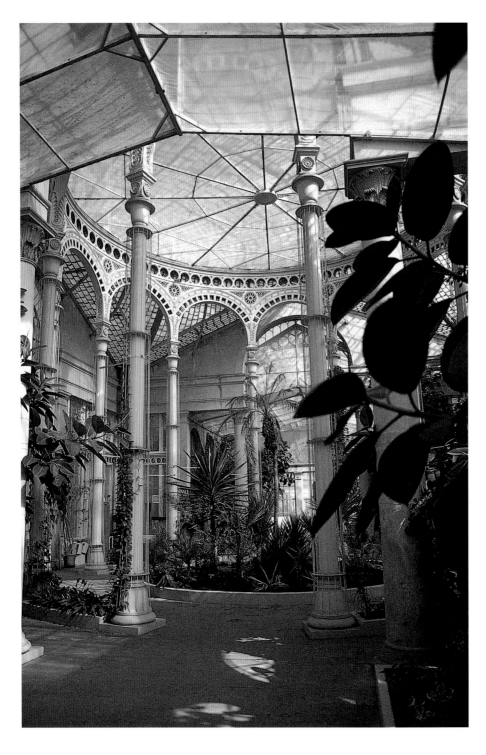

The principles of solar design were correctly implemented for plants (but not for people) in the Conservatory of Syon House, England

If, as individuals, we learn to manage our lives, families, homes and work in such a way that they optimise health, beauty and conservation of the Earth's resources, the practices we institute can be extrapolated to society at large. It may take generations to achieve a post-industrial age of living in consonance with Gaia. It will require a vast effort in the scientific study of organisms and ecosystems at all levels. Such a study is not just ecology, it is human ecology, for if we wish to remain on this planet, our present parasitical role must be reversed so that we become a useful part of the total planetary ecosystem.

The basics of environmental science need to be communicated to all, particularly politicians and economists for whom an understanding of the principles of Gaian management is necessary if they are to make sensible decisions. Once people have taken responsibility for ordering their lives, motivation and knowledge will move to action, but time is our shortest resource. For millennia we have aimed to increase our ability to control and use nature. For human evolution to continue, it is now time to operate not in control of, but in cooperation and harmony with Gaia. Time is running out for us to become responsible stewards, caring for and attending to all of nature as part of ourselves. If we do not, the outcome is probably unthinkable to many — humanity could be dispensable and other life forms may evolve to fulfil our current role.

THE FIVE ELEMENTS OF GAIA

All life on Earth depends upon the viability of Gaia's ecological systems. These, in turn, depend upon the ongoing quality of what the classical Greeks isolated as the elements of nature: fire, earth, air, water and ether (or aether). Humanity's role is to act as the organising mental body of Gaia, to nurture and protect her health.

While modern science recognises 105 elements, each with its own physical and chemical characteristics, we can gain much by setting aside our modern notions for the moment, and reconsidering the protoscientific explanation given by the Greeks of the elements of the physical world. In the 6th century BC, Pythagoras taught that the world of matter was composed of five elements, to each of which he ascribed a particular solid shape. The Earth was composed of a cubiform elemental particle (the most stable, regular solid); fire was tetrahedral (the simplest, regular solid, hence the lightest); water particles were icosahedral (because they are complex and heavy); while air, intermediate to fire and water, was octahedral. The fifth element, ether, was an interpenetrating substance which was both common solvent and common denominator of them all. It was symbolised by the 12-sided solid, the dodecahedron.

The solids symbolically represent the physical matter of our three-dimensional world. These particular shapes were chosen because of their ability to completely fill a three-dimensional space, leaving no voids. Just as cubes can be stacked together to leave no gaps, each of the other shapes also packs together to fill a three-dimensional area, with no space left over.

In the 5th century BC, Hippocrates based a medical system on these elements, which influenced Indian, Arabic, Islamic, Graeco-Arabic and Western medicine. In the 4th century BC, Aristotle explained that the original elements were linked through their properties of hot and cold, dry or humid. Heat and dryness equalled fire, heat and humidity air, cold and dryness earth while cold and humidity equated to water.

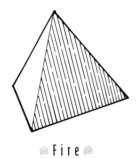

Fire

The element of fire is a potent symbol to cultures all over the world. As Prometheus' gift from heaven, it represents the rational, analytical mind which can, through reason, burn away accumulated superstition. To the early Christian, it symbolised the fire of the Holy Spirit, manifesting itself in its lowest form as sexual union and procreation, and in its highest form as spiritual union with the divine, creative principle — the third aspect of the Holy Trinity, the Holy Spirit (Van der Leeuw 1976). To the Gnostic, the Fire of Creation, or the Holy Spirit, is the great purifier, burning away our connection with the lower aspects of human nature and leading us to higher levels of spiritual consciousness.

In Hindu philosophy, fire symbolises kundalini, the 'serpent-fire' coiled in the base of the spine. This central creative energy in the human body symbolises the divine transmutation of sexual energy into spiritual energy.

At a basic level, fire represents the hearth: the warmth and comfort necessary for life. For us, the fundamental fire of life is the sun, which sustains all organisms on Earth. Fire has been used by human beings for at least 750,000 years when it was first recorded in Vallonet Cave on the Mediterranean coast.

FIRE, THE SUN AND SOLAR ENERGY

The sun's energy drives the photosynthesis of plants. Plant photosynthesis and respiration maintain the balance of oxygen and carbon dioxide in the atmosphere, necessary for our survival. The sun also enables our bodies to synthesise vitamin D by acting on the oils of our skin. Without vitamin D the body cannot assimilate calcium, phosphorus and other minerals, resulting in rickets, tooth decay, osteoporosis and retarded growth in children as well as muscular weakness and premature aging. The sun also contributes to some of the stellar cosmic radiation which arrives on Earth.

Most of the energy supplied to modern industry and our homes is derived from oil, petroleum, coal and natural gas, which are finite resources. In most cases some environmental damage is caused in the production of that energy. Solar

Solar collectors at White Cliffs, NSW, Australia

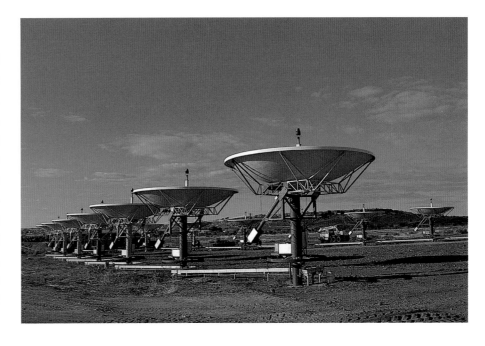

power is an ethical alternative which contributes to the healthy lifestyle.

The use of solar energy has a long history. The solar orientation of buildings was discussed by Socrates, Aristotle, Vitruvius and others. Solar building design was employed in ancient Greece, China and Asia Minor and by the Anasazi and Sinagua Indians in America.

In 1803 Humphrey Repton (in his *Observations on the Theory and Practice of Landscape Gardening*) wrote:

'I have frequently smiled at the incongruity of Grecian architecture applied to buildings in this country whenever I have passed the beautiful Corinthian portico to the north of the mansion house . . . such a portico toward the north is a striking instance of the false application of a beautiful model' (Butti and Perlin 1961).

A visit to such a mansion in winter would make this misapplication of design principles very clear. If fires were not roaring day and night people inside the building would be freezing while outside in the solar conservatory, plants and trees would be well cared for.

While for many years the principles of solar energy design have been ignored in favour of fossil fuels and nuclear power, in the past two decades progress in solar collection for water heating and photovoltaic electricity generation has been significant. In Australia, research has been stimulated by the telecommunication industry's use of outback, autonomous relay stations and experiments in solar generation of electricity and water heating have been undertaken at White Cliffs, New South Wales. Worldwide, universities are developing improved technology for the photovoltaic cell as well as for solar collection devices. Some architects incorporate passive-solar design principles (utilising photovoltaics, solar hot water collectors and sun control louvres) with the ultimate in energy conservation strategies, the earth-sheltered building (Baggs, et al 1991).

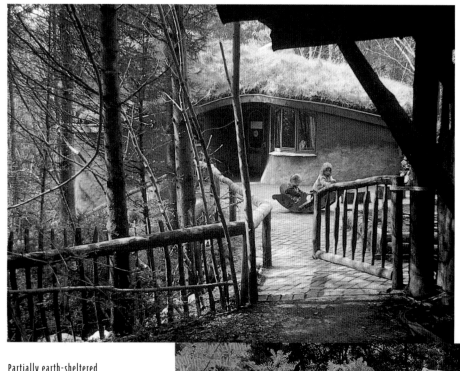

A healthy building constructed of earth from the site. The Nant-y-Curm kindergarten at Ty-Curdd Bach in Wales, UK (Architects: Christopher Day Associates; Photograph: C. Day)

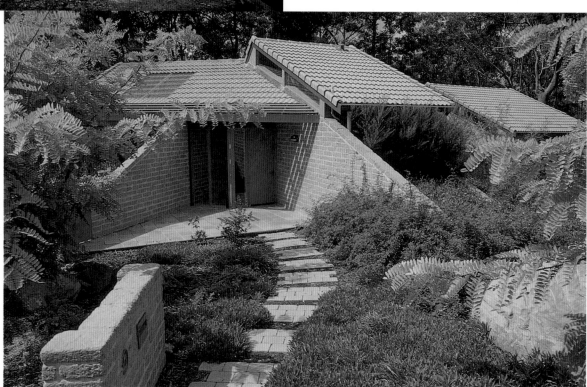

Partially earth-sheltered building with solar collector for water heating incorporating glass tiles in same profile as roof tiles (top left). Sun-control louvres determine the amount and degree of penetration of winter and summer sun (Architects: D. and S. Baggs; Landscape Architect: S. Baggs)

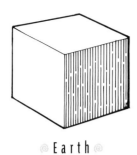

Earth

Soil is a very precious resource which is being wasted all over the world. It originates from the rock that makes up the Earth's crust, a mixture of granite, sedimentary and metamorphic rock. Over a period of 200 to 1200 years, depending on the type of parent rock, only a mere 2.5 centimetres (1 inch) of topsoil will form.

Daily heating and cooling (which causes rock to fragment where temperatures vary widely) and water entering cracks, cause rock to break down into soil. Roots of small plants, shrubs and trees grow into small cracks in the rock, fracturing it and extracting inorganic nutrients, minerals and chemicals from deep soil layers and rock fissures. The leaves and branches of these plants eventually fall, and with the help of fungi and other organisms, they become part of the soil itself. A variety of small creatures and insects participate in soil formation by decomposing the 'cement' holding sedimentary rock particles together, or actually gnawing away at soft rock. Lichens break down rock by secreting carbonic acid, capturing soil, dust, seeds, excrement and dead plant matter.

HOW SOIL AND ROCK AFFECT OUR HEALTH

Radioactivity

Soil and ground water, through natural processes, sometimes generate radioactive pollutants which can affect health. Uranium, occurring naturally in soil and rock, breaks down over millions of years to reach a stable state as lead. About half-way along uranium's decay chain, an element known as radon$_{222}$ forms. One of radon's airborne daughter products, which has a half-life of around 20 minutes, emits radiation which is hazardous when inhaled. The effect is cumulative over time and may represent the few per cent of cases of environmental lung cancer currently unaccounted for. The release of radon and other radioactive compounds is more pronounced in areas of geological faulting or where certain rocks, such as granite, occur. (See Chapters 2 and 10.)

Soil deficiencies

Many soils in the world are deficient in phosphorus, nitrogen and the trace elements copper, zinc and molybdenum. Australia is well-known for its gross deficiencies of trace elements over thousands of square kilometres. Most deficiencies are counteracted artificially with fertilisers but some experts suspect that something is lacking in the quality of vegetation produced on chemically fertilised soils. Well may we ask why fruit and vegetables grown organically without fertiliser, herbicides and pesticides taste so much better than those grown with chemicals.

Soil abuse

The most serious problem of all is that of soil that has been rendered totally useless by the dumping of toxic chemicals or their leaching into the ground water. Other forms of soil abuse arise from leaking storage tanks or pipelines and old stock-drenching sites.

Soil pH

The degree of acidity and alkalinity in soils (as well as their mineral element content) has a marked effect on plant growth, and hence on the availability of those nutrients upon which our health depends. If the pH is too low (acidic) the physical condition of clay soils becomes poor because of their loss of crumb structure. The separated colloidal clay particles then pack tightly together and may also be washed into the subsoil where they form an impervious layer called a hardpan. Due to the formation of insoluble compounds in acidic soil, the availability of essential mineral elements can also be affected.

An earth-sheltered adobe healthy house in Santa Fe, U.S.A. (Architect: D. Wright)

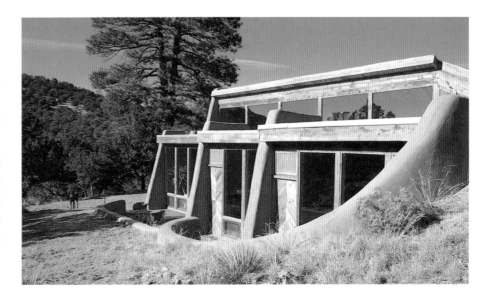

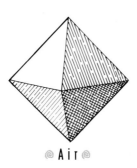

◎ Air ◎

Originally the Earth was surrounded not by the atmosphere we know today, but by sulphurous gases and methane. Oxygen formed firstly as a result of ultraviolet light turning water molecules into hydrogen and oxygen. Photosynthesising organisms evolved, and as a result of their respiration, additional oxygen was produced. Plants and animals are now mutually dependent upon each other for their survival; animals need the respired oxygen from plants, and plants need the carbon dioxide that animals respire. All living organisms are in balance with the oceans and atmosphere and Gaia maintains this equilibrium with astounding accuracy.

AIR POLLUTION

NATURAL AIR POLLUTION

Nature pollutes the air in many ways without our help. Sulphur oxides and particulates from forest fires and volcanoes, dust from wind storms, the hydrocarbons and pollens of plants that live on the methane and the hydrogen sulphide given off by decaying vegetation, viruses and dust from soil, the salt particulates of seas, carbon monoxide, carbon dioxide and oxides of nitrogen all result in various degrees of air pollution.

HUMAN AIR POLLUTION

The atmosphere is a gift from nature which costs us nothing and requires only that we care for its quality. Gaia provides the natural processes that renew the atmosphere and generates the winds that sweep away noxious fumes generated by industry and transportation. Yet today, haze, smog and acid rain prevail over our cities. Humanity generates pollutants in such concentrations that this ultimate environmental amenity may become the ultimate environmental obscenity. While water can be locked up as ice, and soil as rock, air must be kept circulating if plants and animals are to survive. It is the ubiquitous, interconnecting medium upon which mobile, energy-burning animals depend, while an atmosphere with cloud cover and ozone shields them from destructive solar rays.

Air is a reusable resource provided the ocean and land vegetation that produces its oxygen content are allowed to coexist. It is gentle and life-sustaining unless it is abused by humanity; it can be moved in immense volumes by climatic events, causing havoc and destruction, reaching across borders and continents.

The major primary human air pollutants are carbon monoxide, sulphur oxides, oxides of nitrogen, lead, hydrocarbons, photochemical oxidants, particulates and radiation. When these pollutants react with sunlight, moisture or other primary

The Pratatu Doi Tong temple, northern Thailand, a shelter of the element Air, open to air and forest

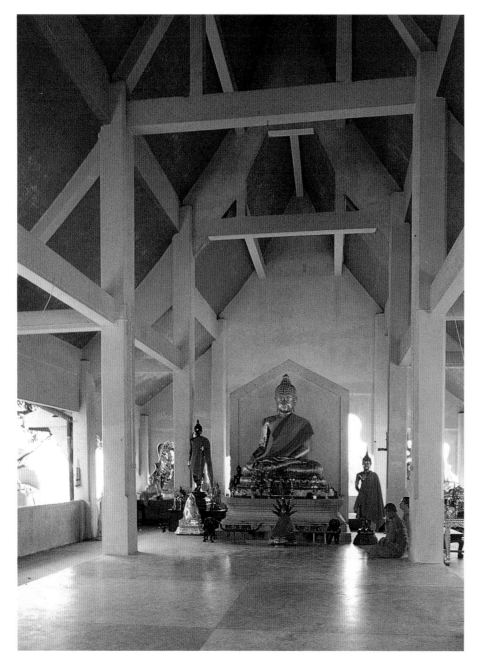

pollutants they may become secondary pollutants. For example, sulphur dioxide reacts with oxygen and water to produce sulphuric acid that falls as acid rain.

The effects of air pollution can be serious, with one in 10 people 'atopic', that is, inherently liable to develop allergies (Ferguson 1987). The aged, infirm, the very young, and those with lung problems are most at risk.

INDOOR AIR POLLUTION

In the United States, the Environmental Protection Agency has identified 1000 pollutants that occur indoors, 60 of which can cause cancer. In Massachusetts, a special commission has stated that it is probable that half the illnesses in that state could be ascribed to exposure to indoor pollution (Gilbert 1992).

A typical Australian who lived to 80 years of age would have spent around 49 years inside buildings; if that person did not work outside of the home, they would have spent around 58 years indoors (Delpech 1992). The building of healthy houses, free from indoor pollution and causing as little damage to the atmosphere as possible, is paramount to maintaining the health of occupants and the balance of life on this planet.

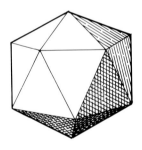

◎ Water ◎

Every drop of water has been here since the beginning of the Earth. Apart from the small amounts lost in the debris of craft sent into deep space, it will remain here, polluted or unpolluted, until the planet's end. All that varies is where it is found: on or beneath the Earth's surface, in organisms, or in the atmosphere.

Water circulates in complex pathways and therefore needs to be conserved and its purity protected.

Some 97 per cent of all water is sea water which covers three-quarters of the Earth's surface. Of the remaining 3 per cent, 2.94 per cent is captured in the ice caps and at inaccessible depths in the Earth. This leaves only 0.06 per cent of all the water in the world as usable fresh water (Myers 1985).

CONTAMINATED WATER

Throughout the world water is being contaminated in a variety of ways, diminishing the amount of fresh, healthy water available.

DISEASE

Water, the ultimate sustaining element of life, kills some 25 million people in developing nations each year. Sixty per cent of these are children. Their scarce water supplies are used over and over, becoming a breeding ground for pathogens and disease carriers, resulting in outbreaks of diarrhoeal infections, dysentery, salmonella, typhoid and cholera. The situation is made worse by the dumping of waste products in rivers and oceans.

ACID RAIN

Factories emit sulphur and oxides of nitrogen which dissolve in atmospheric moisture; when it rains, the droplets can be 1000 times more acidic than natural rain (Myers 1985). Australia and Brazil are in the early stages of developing acid rain, while countries such as Scandinavia, Central Europe and parts of North America have been scourged by its effects. The Black Forest of Germany has lost one-third of its trees, and lakes by the thousands are in the process of becoming lifeless.

Once acid rain enters the ground, the acidified water leaches plant nutrients out of the soil and activates cadmium, mercury, arsenic and other heavy metals which enter the water supply. Rain can also carry pollution from pesticides and herbicides.

Figure 1.1: Hydrological cycle measured in cubic kilometres per year (1 km³=0.244 mile³) (after Ehrlich and Ehrlich 1972)

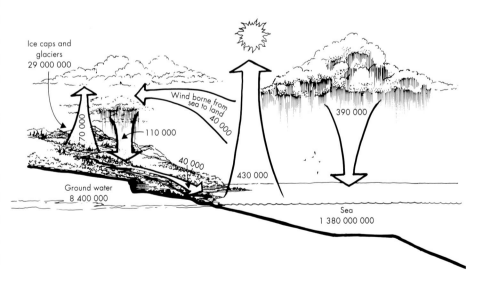

Ice caps and glaciers
29 000 000

Wind borne from sea to land
40 000

70 000

110 000

40 000

430 000

390 000

Ground water
8 400 000

Sea
1 380 000 000

PESTICIDES AND HERBICIDES

Agricultural practices cause pesticide and herbicide neurotoxins to run off into ground water and drinking supplies. Research has been slow and scientists do not yet understand how humans are affected by these neurotoxins. Many of the synthetic organic chemicals used in the past on agricultural land such as heptachlor, DDT, lindane, aldrin, dieldrin and chlordane, show up in laboratory tests of drinking water. Many of these are carcinogens and possible causes of birth defects.

NUTRIENTS IN RUN-OFF

Phosphorus and nitrogen from fertilisers and sewage effluent are washed by rain and irrigation into the soil and into streams by erosion. These nutrients feed algae in the streams, the worst being blue-green (cyanobacteria) algae which can cause serious illness. Algae have caused terrible problems in Australian inland river systems particularly the Murray-Darling. Usually copper sulphate is added to the water to kill algae but this causes them to release toxins.

PROCESSES AFFECTING WATER QUALITY

SOIL DEGRADATION

The removal of too much vegetation and injudicious irrigation can cause soil erosion and salinisation. Eroded soil runs off into streams, polluting the water supply. Ground water affected by salinity can be unusable for plants, causing desert conditions.

ADDITIVES

Chemical compounds added purposely to our water supplies can also cause problems. Chlorine, used to disinfect water, has been linked to heart disease, the formation of arterial plaque, bladder cancer, bowel and stomach cancer, reduced intake of vitamins C and E by the body, and birth abnormalities. Fluoride, added to water to prevent dental caries, has been linked to cancer, allergies, and kidney and heart disease.

THE 'SPIN' IN HEALTHY WATER: PARASCIENCE

Living water contains a vortex imparted by the Earth's geomagnetic field. This vortex energises the life-energy field in living organisms (Hardy and Killick 1987). Without this 'spin', water may cause disruption to the body's bioelectric field and to its ability to absorb minerals.

To be so energised, water has to complete its full hydrological cycle. This only occurs when vegetation allows rain to enter deeply into the earth. When rain penetrates deep into the soil it initially cools, but as it penetrates deeper it passes through a zone of constant temperature and gradually begins to warm from the geothermal effect. As its temperature increases, its relative density lessens and hence it begins to rise back towards the surface. As it rises, its molecules bond with metals and salts. It is also vaporised to some degree and the oxygen and hydrogen in the water molecules become separated. The damp hydrogen gas forces its way to the surface in a spinning vortex with tremendous pressure. Thus carbon dioxide is released for the deeper drainage basins. At the same time surrounding salts are dissolved and carried away with the gas to be deposited again in layers near the vegetation (Alexandersson 1982).

Nutrition is released to vegetation in a continuous cycle. This cycle is disrupted when vegetation is stripped from the land so that the ground surface is warmed by the sun. Rain falls on the warm ground, heats up and runs off instead of soaking deep into the soil. Thus the water is not energised by its 'spin' pattern and minerals are not properly raised to the surface to be absorbed by vegetation.

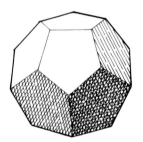

⊚ Ether ⊚

Ether (or aether) is the sea of radiation and energy which creates the necessary conditions for the life, health and demise of all organisms. It could be said to embrace the geoenergetic, electromagnetic, electrostatic and gravitational forces exerted upon us by the Earth, the sun and other planets.

Aristotle considered ether to be interpenetrating, omnipresent and the basis of all of the other elements. It is the universal substance, the vital essence known as *akasha* in the Hindu *Vedas* and as the *monoke* of Shinto. Vitalism proposes that ether forms the basis of all matter. It is perhaps even the enigmatic earthly and heavenly *ch'i* considered by eastern *feng shui* to be the force governing the biological processes of all living things.

THE ELECTRICAL AND MAGNETIC BACKGROUND TO LIFE

The Earth acts as a giant magnet with opposing poles at the north and south. Its geomagnetic field (GMF) changes constantly, mostly due to the effects of solar radiation. The sun emits cosmic rays which form a solar wind, a torrent of radiation which bombards the Earth. The solar wind is made up of positively and negatively charged particles which separate when they hit the Earth's magnetic field. The negative particles are deflected to one side of the Earth and the positive particles to the opposite side. Some particles are trapped in the Van Allen Belts located 1–5000 kilometres (620 –3200 miles) and 15–25,000 kilometres (9320–15,500 miles) above the surface of the planet (see Figure 1.2).

The solar wind fluctuates according to the cycle of sunspot activity. At the peak of the cycle, which averages around 11 years, solar flares explode from sunspots, sending clouds of charged particles into the solar wind, resulting in geomagnetic storms on Earth. The solar wind also fluctuates on a 27-day cycle due to the rotation of the sun.

Magnetic storms caused by the sun's activities can result in the heating of the outer layers of the Earth's atmosphere, causing satellites to alter or fall out of orbit, power line surges which sometimes make equipment fail, the corrosion of long pipelines due to the presence of electrical currents, and the unusual occurrence of aurorae (luminous atmospheric electrical events) at high latitudes near the poles.

GLOBAL ENERGY GRIDS AND LEY LINES: PARASCIENCE

It has been postulated that the Earth's GMF follows certain patterns.

LEY LINES

It is believed that ley lines are paths of ionising radiation. Ultrasonic and atomic radiation has been shown to be emitted from ley line zones at specific times of the day and year (Robins 1985). Their frequencies are the same as the harmonic wave patterns created by thought. It is believed that ancient monolithic stone monuments were located along these lines and that, being related to

the beta frequency of the brain, they may have been used as lines of communication.

THE EARTH GRID AND THE EARTH NET

Two German medical practitioners, Hartmann and Curry, have characterised the Earth's GMF as being bundled in strips which cover the globe. The Hartmann global Earth Grid consists of a series of strips running from north to south, intersected by other strips running from east to west (Hartmann 1976). These lines follow the lines of force of the Earth's magnetic field and may be caused by 'interactions between the Earth's liquid core and the atmosphere . . . influenced by the sun's and the moon's gravitational fields' (Mackay 1992). The lines may also be influenced by the amount of interference and turbulence present in the local environment.

The Curry Net has wider bands running northeast to southwest and northwest to southeast which consist of 'standing waves', extending out from the Earth's centre (Bachler 1980). Cosmic microwaves 'charge the widths of the bands . . . the grids alter infrared radiation from the Earth and affect the Earth's magnetic field' (Mackay 1992).

THE COSMIC ENERGY SHADOW

The location of the Hartmann Earth Grid shifts throughout the year in relation to the stronger Curry Net. Doctor Joseph Oberbach calls this effect the Cosmic Energy Shadow and argues that it is due to the interaction of the lower and upper Van Allen Belts which surround the Earth (Oberbach 1980). Ionised

Figure 1.2: Interaction of Earth's magnetic field with the solar wind and the interplanetary magnetic field. (After: Smith and Best 1989; Eastland 1990)

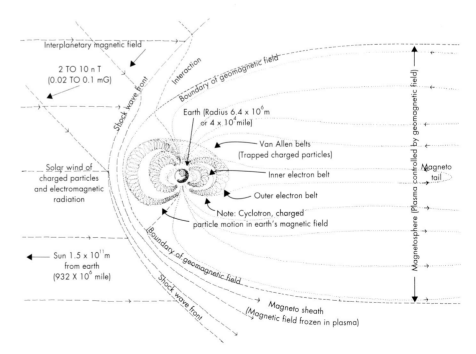

particles from the solar wind hit these belts and, due to the Earth's rotation and the movements of the sun and moon, the aggregation of those particles changes shape and energy. These changes result in the shifting of energy grids on Earth.

HOW DO CHANGES IN THE GEOMAGNETIC FIELD AFFECT LIVING ORGANISMS ON THE EARTH?

Since human cells first began their evolution they have been bathed in a vast sea of radiation, comprised of the Earth's electromagnetic and electrostatic fields and its ionosphere, as well as the incoming electromagnetic energies from outer space, the sun, moon and major planets. The effects of the Earth's GMF, and disturbances to it, are integral to the human experience, from conception to death. Covert and all-pervading, the GMF influences every one of the body's cells, fluids and biological rhythms. As our cells contain magnetite, we are prone to disorientation when changes occur in the GMF around us. The Earth's GMF peaks at about 8–12 Hertz. This happens to be the frequency of the alpha state of the human brain in a condition of quiet contemplation or sleep. It follows that our bodies and brains are in resonance with the GMF and that variations in this field may, and sometimes do, biologically 'change' us. Doctor W. Stark from Switzerland has suggested that the field seems to act as a 'pacemaker' to the brain (Soyka and Edmonds 1978).

Geopathogenic areas and 'geostress'

As well as the influences of the sun and other planets, the Earth's GMF can also be affected by ground water movement. Faults in the Earth's crust can increase neutron radiation from the core of the Earth; these neutrons may be slowed down by the presence of underground water and become low-energy, thermal neutrons which can cause cell degeneration in organisms. The friction produced by the flow of water in underground channels formed by sand and gravel beds can also induce electromagnetic fields.

Microwave radiation from a 'spring line' or subterranean stream and thermal neutrons brings about a concentration of the thermal neutrons and a similar effect with geological faulting. This effect is exaggerated when a geological fault is combined with a spring line and the global radiation grid.

Zones that are capable of causing ill health due to their GMF are referred to as geopathogenic (Schneider 1988). Geopathology refers to influences originating from the soil that cause illness.

Geomagnetic field disturbances have been linked to cardiovascular diseases, and to changes in the central nervous system, the morphology and functioning of internal organs, and the physiological and biochemical processes of animals. They can affect blood clotting times and exacerbate the effects of other illnesses.

By exposing us to changes in the GMF, building over, or close to, geomagnetic anomalies like geological faulting can affect our health. This applies even when the anomalies are deep below the surface of the Earth. The deterioration in health associated with living in such a zone has been termed 'geopathogenic stress' (or 'geopathic stress'). The GMF of a site can be measured in a number of ways (see Chapter 2).

ARTIFICIAL ELECTROMAGNETIC FIELDS

Not only are we affected by solar storms in the vast geomagnetic 'sea' that we inhabit, but we also create our own mini-storms with electronic devices. The effects of ionising radiation, such as X-rays, gamma and ultraviolet rays, are well known. Such radiation can break down the chemical bonds of our cells and even rearrange the particles of our atoms, and can kill instantly or cause cancer. However we can also be affected by non-ionising radiation such as that from radio, television, microwaves (emitted by CB radios, electrical security systems, telephone relays, computer terminals, sonar and satellites) and by extremely low frequency (ELF) radiation which occurs around power lines (50–60 Hertz) and electrical appliances.

This non-ionising radiation which we are surrounded by in modern life has been linked to leukaemia, brain tumours and chronic fatigue syndrome. Some people are allergic to certain artificial magnetic fields and may have reactions which are extreme, even disabling.

POSITIVE AND NEGATIVE IONS

Ions are molecules or atoms in the air around us that carry an extra negative or positive electrical charge. Each molecule of air consists of a core of positively charged protons surrounded by negatively charged electrons. When an electron is displaced from an air molecule, the molecule is left with a positive charge, forming a posion. When the displaced electron attaches itself to another molecule, that molecule becomes negatively charged, forming a negion. This process is due to nuclear radiation emitted by certain materials within the Earth's rocks and soil (radon); cosmic radiation from outer space; lightning; short-wave and ultraviolet radiation; and frictional electrical charges from the movement of sand and dust through dry air or waterfalls, fast-moving streams and heavy rain.

In general terms an excess of posions is not good for organisms while an excess of negions appears to have a beneficial effect. The radiation given out by rocks and soil produces equal numbers of both posions and negions, however an excess of posions can develop due to the friction caused by: certain weather patterns; different layers of air in the atmosphere moving at different speeds; movements of air over the ground; sand or dirt carried in the airstream; and the movement of high and low air pressure cells. Friction causes the negions to attach themselves to particles of dust, pollution or moisture and lose their charge, resulting in an excess of posions.

In clean mountain places where sunlight is plentiful and there are no dust storms, the build-up of ions from rocks and geological anomalies produces high levels of both types of ions. Because of the clean air the negions are not 'consumed' by dust. Waterfalls and cascades alongside trees full of moisture result in air with a dominance of negions because posions attach themselves to large water molecules and lose their charge while negions attach themselves to smaller molecules which we breathe in; sea spray can have the same effect. The discharge of electricity in lightning also counteracts a posion build-up.

Being in air that contains a greater number of negions than posions makes us feel vigorous, while an excess of posions can make us feel edgy (for instance, before a thunderstorm), or even result in nausea, extreme headaches or depression. Ion formation, and thus human health and wellbeing, is affected by geographical factors which govern the dominant type of ions which will be formed. When siting a house, negion-forming conditions should be sought, a high incidence of thunderstorms, the presence of waterfalls and streams and the absence of dry winds.

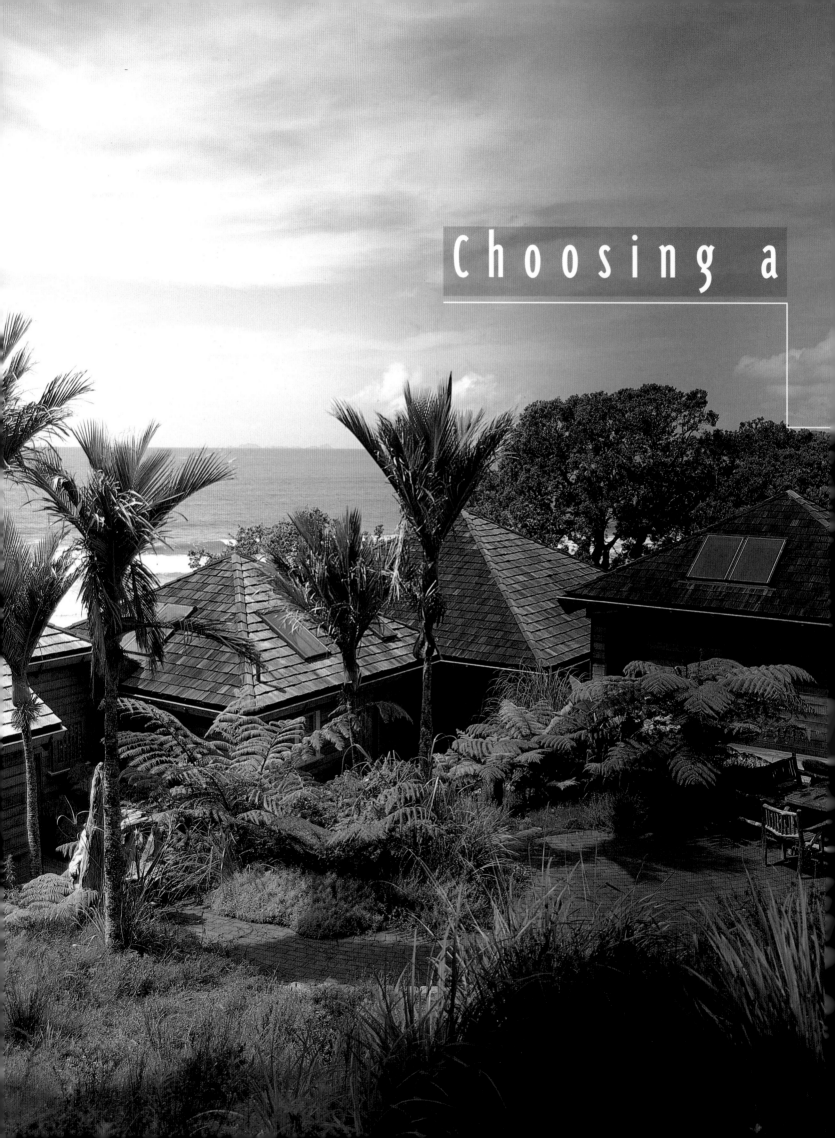

Choosing a

healthy location

In choosing the ideal healthy location, you need to follow several steps. First, decide what is the most beneficial region in your country of choice. The next step is to choose an area within that region, and finally, a street or a particular site within that area.

Choose the location of your house carefully as the health of you and your family will depend upon the choices you make early in the planning process. Undertake thorough research so you are fully equipped to make the right decision.

THE HEALTHY CLIMATE

◎ Anthropogeography ◎

The anthropogeographers of earlier decades studied the effects of a person's geographical location upon their physical and mental health. Anthropogeographers insisted that for human beings to be in peak condition, they should live in temperate climates with regular thunderstorm activity. Ellsworth Huntington (1947) hypothesised that the great civilisations of the past arose between the latitudes of 20 degrees north and 20 degrees south of the equator, where temperatures are mild and thunderstorms occur frequently.

The conditions before and after a thunderstorm were shown by Huntington to produce increased brain activity and a feeling of wellbeing due to the increased number of negions and decreased number of posions in the air. He argued that to be as happy and healthy as possible, we should live in places where thunderstorms occur frequently and where the temperature rarely falls below 16 degrees Celsius (61 degrees Fahrenheit), with a noonday yearly average of 24 degrees Celsius (75 degrees Fahrenheit).

Biometeorology

'One day I wake up depressed, the next I'm happy, but nothing has changed in my life or circumstances to explain the difference in feelings.' How many times have you heard a statement such as this? Doctor Jim Rotton, a social psychologist from Florida International University, estimates that about one-fifth of the populace has similar experiences to this, caused by changes in the weather (Leviton 1988). The study of the causal links between atmospheric changes and the biological responses of human beings is called biometeorology. Climate can affect our health in many ways, with all individuals responding differently to meteorological conditions.

Depression is more prevalent in countries where the daylight hours are short, causing Seasonal Affective Disorder (SAD) — this can also be experienced by those who work night shifts. Extending the period of 'sunlight' by 6 hours per day using bright lights alleviates symptoms by stimulating melatonin, a light-sensitive pineal gland hormone (Soyka and Edmonds 1978). Temperature can also affect mood and behaviour. Doctor Craig Andersen has reported a clear correlation between violent behaviour and temperatures above 30 degrees Celsius (86 degrees Fahrenheit) in all geographic regions (Leviton 1988).

Diseases can have a climatic distribution when the bacteria and viruses that cause them thrive in certain climates but not others, for example, poliomyelitis becomes more deadly as it moves away from the equator and diseases such as malaria, yellow fever and dysentery are more prevalent in hot, humid climates where carrier-mosquitoes breed.

With rheumatism, the influence of a cold, damp climate is obvious (there are five times more sufferers in the northern United States than in the south). A link has also been found between rheumatism and stormy regions and areas of impermeable clay soils. To lessen your susceptibility to the health problems covered here, you should ideally live in a sunny, warm (but not hot), dry climate with stimulating cool nights. Avoid clay soils, and igneous and granitic rock outcrops.

Will future climatic change affect health?

Sudden shifts in climate occurred at the end of the last Ice Age all around the world. Even in the last interglacial period a series of temperature fluctuations occurred which lasted from decades to centuries. The conclusion reached by researchers who have studied geological samples in New Mexico and Greenland is that our recent climate stability is an exception rather than a rule (Hecht 1993).

Global warming due to the greenhouse effect could change the stability we have taken for granted. Firm data on warming are difficult to obtain but according to R. Kemp of the Australian Bureau of Meteorology, 'there appears to have been more warm years globally [and that temperatures in] the last 10 years have been higher than the last 40 years'. Most climate models predict that in the future the weather will be warmer in winter during the night as one moves away from the equator (Pearce 1992). Changes in rain patterns will occur, for example, in Australia there will be more rain in coastal regions and less in the interior of the continent.

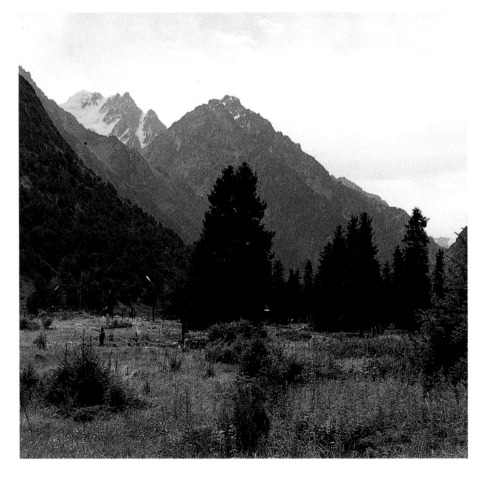

This could result in the spread of several diseases. Andrew Haines, professor of primary health care at University College, London, predicts possible serious outbreaks of mosquito-borne and parasitic diseases for Australia (Pearce 1992). With a rise in temperature, malaria may migrate into regions where natural immunity is absent. This happened in Madagascar in the 1980s where 50 per cent of those infected died, according to D. Warhurst, London School of Hygiene and Tropical Medicine (Pearce 1992). An unpublished report from the British Government's Public Health Laboratory Service claims that 'malaria and even the plague, could soon be stalking Europe once more' (Pearce 1992). Yellow fever, schistosomiasis (from snails in contaminated water) and other tropical diseases could spread worldwide. According to the report, they will come in partnership with new animal diseases and crop pests as well as deadly bacteria, viruses, rats and flies. Brown rats can carry disease just as effectively as black rats carried the bubonic plague during the Middle Ages. One theory is that the 14th century plague commenced with massive flooding in China which drove the black rats into Europe. Ominously there has been a massive increase in Britain's rat population (Pearce 1992).

What preventative measures can be taken to protect health if such changes occur? The Engineers' Institute of Australia has already predicted that bridges, dams, drainage systems and ocean-front protection will have to be redesigned. If you are considering purchasing waterfront property, it would be wise to remember that the site should be at least one metre (3 feet 3 inches) above the highest surge wave in the worst cyclone to date. Such cyclones will probably increase in frequency and intensity and the prudent will stay well above sea level so that even a tidal wave will not reach their site.

Should sea levels rise, marshes and river deltas will reach much further inland than they do at present. To avoid these potentially tropical disease-prone regions, it would be wise to choose a site around the 200 metres (656 feet) contour (above sea level) on a map. Because of the increased rainfall, new land will need to be carefully graded to drain so that breeding conditions for pests like tsetse flies (sleeping sickness carriers) or mosquitoes (yellow fever and malaria carriers) are eliminated (Pearce 1992).

THE EFFECT OF ROCKS AND SOILS ON HEALTH

Biogeology

Some rocks have more radioactivity than others and when they break down to form soil, or enter the soil through geological faults, radioactive radon gases are released and can then be breathed into the lungs. Excess radon may be a cause of cancer. Radioactivity is most commonly found in igneous (volcanic) rock such as basalt or metamorphic rock like granite.

The presence of igneous rocks, which have a higher than average incidence of radon, may be linked to the incidence of stomach cancer. Igneous rocks are often responsible for the scenic quality of an area and it may be that, in order to benefit from a scenic view, you decide to seal your building against radon ingress.

In general, sedimentary rocks such as sandstone and limestone contain low levels of radon, except where age-old igneous rocks have weathered away to form the clay soils overlaying sedimentary rock. The presence of soil moisture seems to increase radon release from the damp, underfloor spaces of buildings built on these clays. Leichhardt in Sydney, Australia, has twice as many asthma sufferers as neighbouring suburbs and three times the national average in the 45 to 64 year age group (Curson and Siciliano 1992). As factors such as food additives, dust mite, the incidence of colds and viral infections and pollens would be similar in nearby suburbs, a significant factor may be that Leichhardt is situated on deep clay deposits near Brickfield Hill, a historic source of clay for brick-making. In another study, the people of west Paris, whose houses are built on limestone and sand, were found to have a low incidence of cancer while the incidence was high in the south, where the houses are built on clay (Gauquelin 1980).

Geomagnetic field anomalies

The Earth also affects our bodies through the extremely low frequency (ELF) component of its geomagnetic field (GMF). Disruptions to the GMF are greater where there is geological faulting and fissures have formed in the Earth's crust, releasing greater levels of radioactive gas from radon. Underground water can also increase the amount of radon released. This can have serious health consequences.

Geomagnetic field anomalies can also cause crop yields to diminish (Gauquelin 1980). Where localised anomalies prevail, one often finds that even minor raised levels of geomagnetic activity can produce twisted and distorted branching, vulnerability to disease and even plant death (Tietze 1988). Germination and seed growth is greatest when seeds are oriented to the poles of the Earth. Magnetotropism, as it is called, can affect sex determination and symmetry in plants, and the quantity of sap in plant cells increases as the GMF rises in strength.

CHOOSING A HEALTHY AREA IN WHICH TO LIVE

So far we have considered the large-scale effect of climate and geology on the health of inhabitants to help decide on a favoured region. We now sharpen our focus and search for a more specific area within the chosen region.

⊛ Maps to use ⊛

For the processes described, specific types of maps are needed. First obtain a general map showing roads and towns. You may use a map with a scale of 1:1,000,000 or any map normally used for tourism. This allows you to work in very broad terms to locate an area. Then go to a good map supplier and ask for a topographic map (or topomap), the scales of which vary from 1:10,000 to 1:1,000,000. In general terms, the map you use can be the same type of map once used by the military, at a scale of 1:63,366 (1 inch:1 mile). Consult your telephone directory for sales outlets for these maps. Topomaps are produced in Australia by the National Mapping Authority and the various state governments. At the scales of 1:10,000 and 1:250,000, they will show all major buildings.

You will also need an orthophoto map. In general, these maps of major cities are produced at scales large enough to show contours overlaid on an aerial photo of the district (with all buildings).

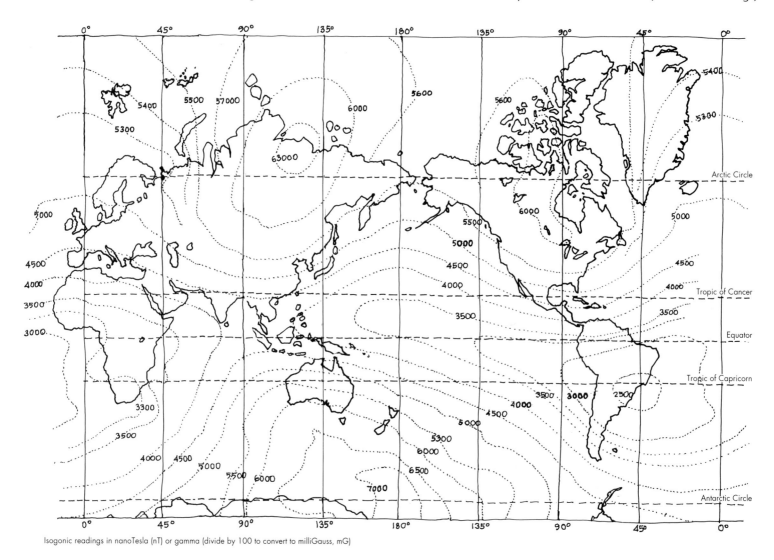

Isogonic readings in nanoTesla (nT) or gamma (divide by 100 to convert to milliGauss, mG)

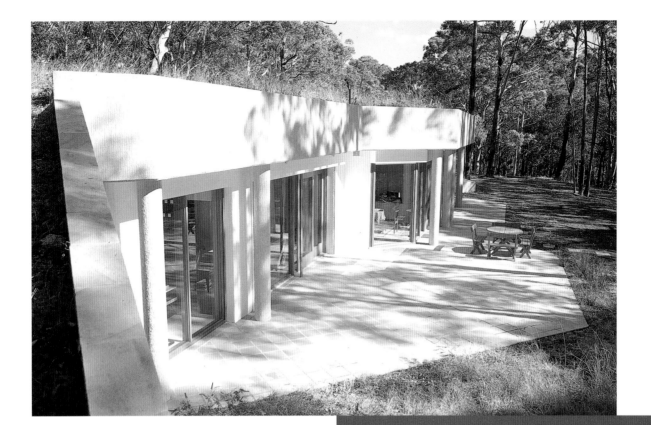

Earth-sheltered low-allergy house at McMasters Beach, NSW, Australia. Very efficient sound-attenuation by deep earth-cover for all but low-frequency vibration. (Architects: ECA Space Design Pty Ltd)

Commencing with these special maps of inner urban areas and moving further away from the city centre, the scale broadens.

◎ Choosing a healthy area by sound, sight and smell ◎

In choosing a healthy place to site your house, be guided in the first stage by your senses of hearing, sight and smell. The most orderly way to proceed is to mark on a map various areas and corridors that are affected by electromagnetic fields, odours, smog and visual pollution.

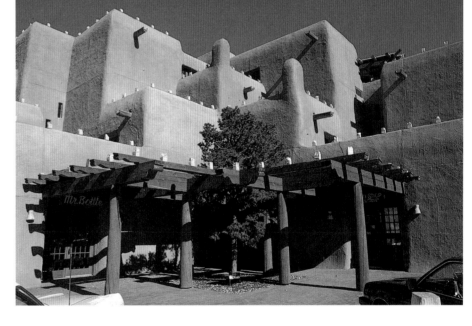

◎ Noise factors ◎

We are extremely vulnerable to sound and it has considerable effects on our feelings, thoughts and bodily wellbeing. If sounds are discordant, erratic or too loud, they are experienced as noise. Noise is measured on a logarithmic scale of sound pressure, known as decibels (dBA). A noise level of say 70dBA is 100 per cent louder than a noise level of 60dBA; a level of 63dBA is 30 per cent louder than 60dBA, and so on.

ROAD TRAFFIC

Ideally a portable, sound-pressure level meter should be used to measure noise (see Resources List). However if it is not possible to measure noise levels, it is still possible to draw lines on your selected map to indicate zones of influence using, say, a 300 metre wide area (1000 feet) each side of railway tracks and main vehicular routes. This makes the noise corridor 600 metres wide (2000 feet) overall if the source of sound is visible. In relation to a route containing mainly cars, the acceptable noise level limits for housing estates are: 63dBA on a still, fine day at 150 metres (490 feet) from the road; about 60dBA at 500 metres (1640 feet); and 55dBA at 600 metres (2000 feet).

Adobe construction in Santa Fe, New Mexico. Thick earth walls provide excellent sound-attenuation for most frequencies

Figure 2.2: Noise attenuation
contours around a single 90dBA
source of industrial noise: 55dBA
at a distance of 1000 m (5280
ft), 50dbA at 1700 m (5577 ft)
and 45dBA at 3100 m (10,170 ft)

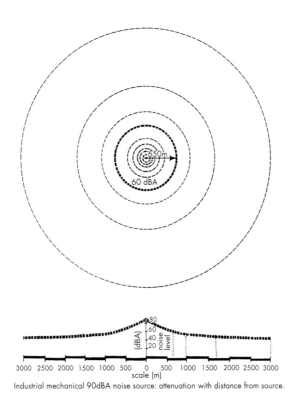

Industrial mechanical 90dBA noise source: attenuation with distance from source.

an apparent drop in impact if the source of the noise is not visible — this may partly be a psychological effect.

To measure noise levels associated with the type of trains used in your region, hire or buy a sound level meter (see Resources List). The measurements you take will permit you to determine the width of the noise corridor to suit the type of house you have in mind. Plot this corridor on your map as a zone limited by the 63 dBA sound level. If a road underpass of an old design (steel, not concrete) happens to be within noise-impact distance, the noise level rises significantly and the noise corridor needs to be widened around it.

The effects of noise on people depends on their sensitivity, the length of time over which they are exposed, and the level of noise. If noise rises and falls it is not as objectionable as continuous noise. If two people a few metres apart are speaking at normal levels, what is said is around 95 per cent intelligible if the ambient noise does not rise above certain levels, 60dBA for ordinary noise and 65dBA for aircraft noise (US Environment Protection Agency 1974). See Table 2.1 for typical levels.

In general people can fall asleep with a steady noise level of not more than 25–30dBA, but an intermittent noise of 50dBA will awaken them. Some 97 per cent of the population do not suffer hearing loss from continuous noise if levels are kept below 70dBA (Federal Airports Corporation 1990).

OTHER SOURCES OF NOISE

Find out any future plans concerning projected airport developments from your national airport authority, then check where future airstrips may be located in relation to your area and predictions of noise levels for stationary, ascending, descending and low-altitude aircraft.

The data shown in Figure 2.2 (page 34) could be taken as very approximately representative of all but the heaviest industries as well as of sports ovals with night lighting. If you plot all sources of noise on a map of the area in contours, you will be able to see which areas are not exposed to excessive levels of mechanical noise, that is, areas below 60dBA.

An interesting point to be considered is the link between noise level and weather. If a temperature inversion occurs (as often happens in coastal regions) noise levels increase. Hence any noise footprint should be overestimated to allow for this effect.

Table 2.1 shows typical sound levels within a house compared to the Australian Standard AS2107–1987 and how a house designed to control sound can significantly lower these typical levels. Such a house could be earth-sheltered or have thick earth-walls, as efficient noise attenuation depends only on the density and mass of the intervening material between the noise and you. The best sound attenuator is lead (not the low-density 'insulating' materials often promoted for 'sound-proofing') and a thick earth cover to a building is the next best. If you are constructing an earth-sheltered or sound-insulated building, you can draw a narrower corridor on the area plan.

RAILWAYS

As well as the effect of rogue electromagnetic fields from electric railway lines, there may be a noise impact on an area if the railway line is in view. The noise level is increased where a third rail is used to carry the electrical current, as in the United Kingdom. There is

Table 2.1: Sound levels in a
typical house (in dBA) compared
to a house designed to
counteract noise*

ROOM	TYPICAL HOUSE	STANDARD**	HOUSE DESIGNED TO COUNTERACT NOISE
Lounge	45	35	30
Kitchen	42	35	32
Family Room	46	35	32
Bedroom	43	30	25

* Adapted from New South Wales State Pollution Control Commission 1991; **AS2107–1987

@ Visual factors @

Considering that the portion of the brain which responds to visual stimuli is larger than those portions receiving information from the other senses, it is understandable how much we rely on the visual quality of an area for enjoyment of it. Visual quality is very subjective. What is attractive to one person may not be so appealing to someone else. Even professional opinion is confused and methods of assessment abound for measuring visual quality. Very few of these methods involve consultation about individual preferences, but utilise procedures that depend on abstract measurement. Survey your family members for their opinions about the visual quality of the site.

@ Odour factors @

The nose is the first line of defence in the detection of pollution problems. It is a subtle and sensitive detector, particularly of formaldehyde and hydrocarbon emissions.

Unhealthy (and hence allergenic) air can be transported by circulation from distant sites where unpleasant smells are generated. Prevailing winds are a critical consideration if a garbage tip or main highway is upwind from the land, for instance. To analyse the winds in your area, you can construct a wind rose diagram. The information needed to construct such a diagram can be obtained from the meteorological station nearest to the area in which you are considering purchasing. The meterological station can tell you the number of times per year that the wind in your area blows from a given direction. You then draw an ordinary compass diagram on your orthophoto map, showing north, south, east and west. Now, with your ruler passing through the intersection of the

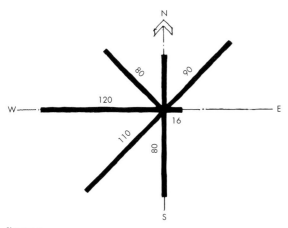

Figure 2.3

compass points, draw a line away from the centre of the compass, towards the direction of the wind. You may have winds occurring 80 times per year from the south, 120 from the west, 90 from the northeast, 50 from the north, 80 from the northwest and 116 from the southwest. Choose an appropriate scale, say, 1 centimetre (½ inch) equals 10 occurrences. Now you can draw a wind rose diagram as in Figure 2.3.

A more complex wind rose diagram than this can be drawn based on the seasonal occurrences of the various winds (see Figure 2.4). If this information is not available from either your bureau of meteorology or from a climatic atlas, it can be collected as part of a daily record. It takes a full cycle of seasons to measure the wind velocity and direction yourself using a hand-held anemometer (see Resources List).

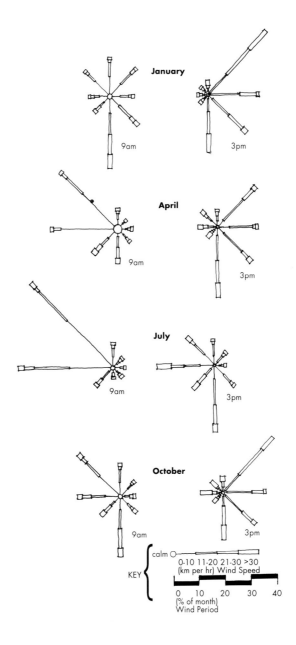

Figure 2.4: Wind rose diagrams for the same location as Figure 2.3 showing morning and afternoon conditions for the four seasons. A more comprehensive diagram than Figure 2.3, it includes wind speed and the proportions of the month on which a particular wind direction occurred. The circle at the centre of each rose has an area proportional to the number of calm days. (Redrawn from Australian Bureau of Meteorology 1991)

Figure 2.3: Constructing a simple wind rose diagram to record how often wind blows from certain directions over one year (this does not take the wind speed into consideration)

Wind analysis should precede the design of a building and its garden, and will make it easy to determine the potential impact of noxious odours from adjoining districts. Hopefully sources of odours such as industrial or waste dumps may also be determined from the map.

AIRPORT ODOURS: HARBINGERS OF TROUBLE

The constituents of exhaust gases emitted by aircraft engines are the unburnt or partially burnt hydrocarbons, oxides of nitrogen, carbon monoxide, smoke particulates and sulphur dioxide from aircraft fuel. The aircraft engine is least efficient when taxiing on the tarmac. At this stage very high levels of hydrocarbons and carbon monoxide are emitted. In addition, particulates increase by two to three times normal levels. In 1988, aircraft movements and operations at Kingsford-Smith Airport in Sydney, Australia, resulted in the emissions shown in Tables 2.2, 2.3 and 2.4.

The quantity of noxious material that can be transported by winds from Sydney airport to adjoining districts amounts to some 18 tonnes (17.94 tons) every day. Enquire at the local airport authority about flight paths in your area and mark them on your map. Avoid sites beneath and windward of such pollution zones.

Doctor Meecham of the University of California conducted a survey of the incidence of disease and death in two socially equivalent areas, one of which was located beneath flight paths. He found that in the area beneath flight paths, the incidence of death was 20 per cent higher, with heart attack and strokes 20 per cent higher and sclerosis of the liver 140 per cent higher than those in the area away from the flight paths.

INDUSTRIAL EMISSIONS

Areas can be affected when stack emissions from industrial areas are carried by the wind. Give careful consideration to your wind rose diagram if there are industries within several kilometres of the chosen area.

A WORD OF WARNING: TOXIC WASTE

It is sometimes claimed that sites in the vicinity of a toxic waste dump are safe because the dump has been sealed and will not leach into adjoining areas due to the clay content of the soil (Cook 1993). If you wish to build a healthy house you will avoid such areas, whether the land has been treated or not. Quite

EMISSIONS	TONNES (TONS) PER DAY	TYPE OF ODOUR
Hydrocarbons	0.464 (0.46)	Distinctive petrol or kerosene odour
Oxides of nitrogen	36.677 (36.1)	Pungent odour when more than 0.5 ppm. (Nitrogen oxide is odourless.)
Carbon monoxide	7.245 (7.13)	Odourless but dangerous at high concentrations
Particulate matter	1.075 (1.06)	Reduces clarity of air
Sulphur dioxide	2.773 (2.72)	Pungent sulphurous odour when above 20–30ppm concentration. Dangerous at high concentrations
Total	18.782 (18.484)	

* Federal Airports Corporation 1990

Table 2.2: Combined daily emissions from Sydney Airport*

EMISSION	KG (LB) PER HOUR
Total hydrocarbons	0.64 (1.41)
Oxides of nitrogen	8.8 (19.4)
Carbon monoxide	9.2 (20.28)
Particulate matter	0.7 (1.54)
Sulphur dioxide	1.3 (2.87)
Total	20.64 (45.5)

* Federal Airports Corporation 1990

Table 2.3: Emissions on landing approach for a Boeing 737-200*

EMISSION	KG (LB) PER HOUR
Total hydrocarbons	0.18 (0.40)
Oxides of nitrogen	56.0 (123.46)
Carbon monoxide	3.6 (7.94)
Particulate matter	1.2 (2.65)
Sulphur dioxide	3.6 (7.94)
Total	64.58 (142.39)

* Federal Airports Corporation 1990

Table 2.4: Emissions during climb for a Boeing 737-200*

possibly your senses will not be able to detect contamination. If you have the slightest suspicion, research the incidence of stillbirths or genetic deformities in humans or animals in the area over the last few years. Compare this information with local or state records and err on the conservative side in making your final decision.

It is absolutely essential to check the history of any area under consideration. Avoid areas contaminated by wastes arising from medical, dental, veterinary and pharmaceutical activities or scientific research. Hazardous radioactive conditions can also exist when an area has been used in the past to house certain manufacturing industries, such as in Hunters Hill, a suburb of Sydney, Australia. All the radioactive soil had to be removed from the affected area before the land was fit for housing purposes. To avoid buying a contaminated site, have the soil and ground water tested with a radiation monitor (see Resources List).

CHOOSING A HEALTHY SITE WITHIN THE SELECTED AREA

You have selected a healthy area in which to live, now you need to locate a particular site where you can construct a healthy home. There is no substitute for familiarising yourself with the area, street by street if necessary. At this stage, it may be helpful to read Chapter 5: *Using feng shui in the healthy house* as it may assist in your selection of a particular site in a street. If the principles of *feng shui* appeal to you, you can use them in deciding what side of the street your house should be located and the appropriate street number. Then consult the current chapter so you can conduct detailed site surveys. If *feng shui* is not for you, use the current chapter alone to help isolate a healthy site. As investment in property is one of the most important decisions to be made in life, it is well worth the effort.

A safe and stable site: geotechnical considerations

IDENTIFYING EXPANSIVE CLAYS

For the sake of stability, buildings should not be constructed on highly expansive clay soils, which increase significantly in volume when affected by moisture. The following characteristics are generally, but not always, indicators of expansive clays (US Department of Energy 1981). Under dry soil conditions, expansive clays are very difficult to penetrate with a mattock or spade; the soil is very hard, almost rock-like. In some cases, one cannot break off a small piece with the fingers. If it does break, it snaps like a biscuit and cannot be powdered in the fingers. Usually it has a slightly shiny surface where the spade has cut into it, and if there are any surface irregularities (such as tyre tracks), they cannot be removed by pressing with one's shoe. Cracks occur in a reasonably regular pattern.

When wet, such a soil becomes gluey and will build up on tyres and shoe soles. The soil can be easily moulded into a ball or bolus by squeezing in the hand. The resultant 'snake' can be squeezed out between the fingers without breaking until it is quite long. Hands will have almost invisible powdery clay on them when dry. A shovel will easily penetrate this soil when wet, and it will leave a very smooth, shiny surface.

SUBSIDENCE

Subsidence of the land surface can occur quite suddenly in old mining areas when mines cave in, or in limestone areas when a cave system collapses because of the chemical action of water on the limestone. It can also occur gradually due to mining activities, or the pumping of water or other liquids out of the ground. Areas in which both types of subsidence occur should be avoided; at least check with the governmental authority that controls mines in the area.

CREEP

Slow and continuous soil movement is called 'creep'. Its presence is marked by slanted fence posts or curved tree growth (with the convex side of the trunk pointing downhill). Although its action is little understood it can occur at all angles above approximately 1:14 (4 degrees) of slope. Probably caused by the effects of gravity and seasonal swellings and shrinkage, this type of failure is dangerous because it can trigger a landslide. Its progress can be slowed by the installation of drainage. By controlling the soil's moisture content, drainage increases soil strength. Creep is often evidence of the existence of expansive clays. Extensive cracking of paths and streets can indicate the presence of this problem.

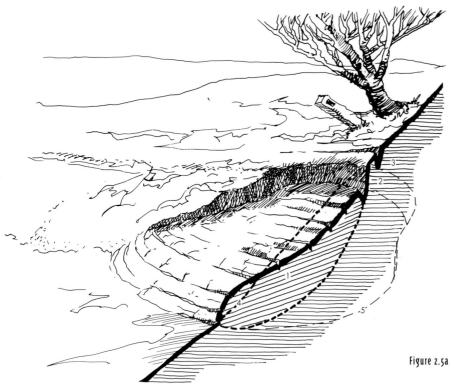

Figure 2.5a

1. Rotational slide
2. Scarp formed by slide
3. Tension cracking at crown
4. Bulge at toe
5. Outline of failure (without section)

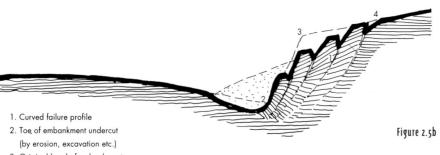

Figure 2.5b

1. Curved failure profile
2. Toe of embankment undercut
   (by erosion, excavation etc.)
3. Original head of embankment
4. Tension cracking at crown

Figure 2.5(a): Section through a
rotational slide on a hillside
(note curved shape in plan)

(b): Failure of toe of
embankment when a drain is cut
to divert stormwater run-off

LANDSLIDE

Look for signs of creep and 'lumpy' topography on a slope. If these indicators are present, such a hillside may be unstable over long periods. Each slide is unique and difficult to classify, but the following is a guide (Sowers 1979):

ROTATIONAL SLIDES

These occur in clays and other homogeneous soils that are deep with non-continuous planes of weakness and may be recognised by the slip-circle type of failure shown in Figure 2.5(a).

LINEAR SHEAR SLIDES

These are quite definite in appearance as they occur along clearly defined sloping planes. Small crescent-shaped areas of soil may break loose at the top of the slope and wave-like bulges of mud form at the bottom. The slide can retrogress uphill away from the bottom, each time leaving a steep, stepped slope which is likely to fail again.

Weathered shales and other rocks can be triggered to slide by the expansion of material exposed by excavation, or by an earlier slide. A whole hillside can move even when separate tests on the stability of the slope indicated adequate safety. A difficult situation arises when a weak sloping stratum of, say, clay or weathered shale overlays sloping strata of harder rock. Such cases have been known to fail on quite flat slopes when rainfall has penetrated the top seams because of the stripping of protective vegetation or an excavation cut has destabilised the bottom of an embankment.

FLOW SLIDES

If a cohesionless soil is loose and saturated, it is particularly vulnerable to flowslide. Pile driving at the shoreline of a body of water can trigger a slide on a nearby hillside. An explosion can also trigger a slide in a pile of mine tailings, a stockpile of coal or some types of industrial waste. Flow slides occur when a soil or rock mass suddenly loses its strength and behaves like a liquid, flowing downhill.

EXCAVATION

Land excavation must be undertaken with great consideration for the stability of the resulting slope or embankment. When stability is lost, a large, intact earth mass may shift, the surface becomes distorted and finally the mass breaks up. This may happen suddenly, or cracks may form gradually and settlements occur well ahead of the final failure. It can occur when an embankment of any age has been cut or in soil that is sensitive to rotational slides.

Figure 2.5(a) indicates one of the most common types of failure. It can be recognised by its ovoid shape, resembling half an egg (small end uphill). The 'scarp' is the uphill curved limit of the slide. Its presence can precipitate another rotational slide (as before, this process can retrogress uphill) and rain can cause a viscous flow downhill. When enough of these minor areas of rotational slide have occurred, a failure surface may form and a major landslide results.

While water is a principal cause, there is always a combination of contributory factors. When clay soil absorbs water, it expands and loses strength. Water also hastens the structural breakdown of loose or honeycombed soil that often accompanies seismic shock. Soil stress can also result from external loading applied to the ground by buildings or a body of water, or excavation of part of an existing slope. The presence of tilted trees and bulges or visible signs of soil instability are warnings that must be heeded. You can have these problems treated under the supervision of a geotechnical engineer before building, but it is better to avoid problem sites completely.

The angle of cut or fill of an excavation or embankment can also cause problems. In considering a site, it is wise to keep in mind that even a reasonably small angle of slope can develop a base failure if a soft stratum occurs over a harder base such as shale.

If a table drain has been excavated to divert water around an excavation, unless the drain is lined with sods, sleepers or paving slabs, drain blockage and failure at the foot of the cutting can occur, even when the soil has a reasonably high coefficient of internal friction. (This is the angle of the mound that the soil forms naturally when it is dry. The steepness of the angle depends upon the soil particles' resistance to sliding.)

When a soil has no cohesion and is homogeneous, for example sand, sliding may occur parallel to the face of the slope. This type of slide is triggered when the slope angle is above the angle of internal friction of the sand. The angle of internal friction can be gauged by pouring the sand through a funnel onto a level surface. As this can change with the texture of sand/silt, or clayey sand, this 'funnel test' is useful to perform on-site to determine the absolute maximum embankment or cutting angle for sandy soils.

Open cuts for constructing a building in reasonably stable soils can be 1:2 (approximately 27 degrees) for most conditions and 1:14 (approximately 4 degrees) for weak soils. If the depth of a proposed excavation is extreme, find a place away from the site of the building and construct a cut that is so steep it fails. You can then observe the type of failure likely to occur in the site's soil.

If a soil slope is unstable, a condition of high soil stress can be alleviated by lowering the slope angle or by using one of the standard retaining wall designs which can be detailed by a consultant. It is wise to relieve water pressure in the cracks of a cohesive soil by using surface drains running horizontally along, and driven into, the face of the slope. A diversion table-drain should be used at the head of the slope. Similarly, the strength of soils that are only slightly cohesive or even cohesionless, can be increased using surface and horizontal face drains.

A safe site: bush, forest and grass fires

The survival chances of any building exposed to fire depend upon its design and construction, but its location in relation to the surrounding valleys, hills and plains and the proximity of vegetation are also important factors.

The species of vegetation around a house govern the quantity of bushfire fuel available, how quickly it will ignite and at what rate it will release heat. (For a list of tree species that are fire resistant, see Appendix H.) Ignition occurs because of the natural heat produced by composting; lightning strikes; glass acting as a magnifier of the sun's rays; arson; campfires; discarded cigarettes or matches; and sparks from electrical power lines, machinery, engines and equipment.

In the southern hemisphere, northern and eastern slopes (southern and western slopes in the northern hemisphere) are more exposed to the extremes of the sun. Slopes that face drying winds or are shielded from moisture-laden winds are more prone to catching fire as dry fuel is more abundant than on less exposed slopes. Low humidity, drying winds and high temperatures all make fuel more prone to ignition.

Radiant heat ahead of a fire front can pass through unprotected windows (sometimes without breaking them) and ignite furniture and furnishings within a building. Such a conflagration ignites the roof which then collapses. In typical circumstances, burning debris carried by the wind seems to be the main problem. Debris can continue to be deposited for hours while the front itself can pass within minutes. Combustible material can pile up against such ignitable materials as fences, timber-lined walls, timber windows and doors, and sub-floor areas. It can accumulate in gutters, on timber decks, pergolas and window sills, in gaps left in combustible wall sheetings, windows, doors, etc. It is important to close windows if a fire alert has been announced. Once windows are broken, burning embers can penetrate the interior, igniting anything combustible.

Fuel availability, the slope of the land, wind speed and aspect affect the intensity of radiant heat. Radiant heat intensity is directly dependent on the distance from the flame. For instance, the radiant heat intensity of a fire 100 metres (328 feet) away is four times greater than that of one which is 200 metres (656 feet) away (Ramsay and Dawkins 1993).

Wind is of critical importance in determining the vulnerability of a building to bushfire. Check with local residents on the directions of past fires and prevailing winds and position vulnerable windows, doors and openings away from those directions.

When looking at a site in the forest or bushland, consider whether it could be at risk from bushfire. Find out from neighbours and the local fire brigade the frequency of fires in the area. If you want to minimise the fire risk, not only must you consider climate, the presence of ground fuel and canopy cover, but also the ground slope. On ground that slopes at greater than a 10 degree angle, the rate at which a fire spreads can double; on slopes of greater than a 20 degree angle, the rate doubles again. To minimise fire danger the best site is one on relatively level ground or a gentle slope. The highest risk occurs toward the upper areas of sloping ground, or on a ridge.

Avoid sites in subdivisions with cul-de-sacs as they are difficult for fire-fighting vehicles to access. Check that the access roads are wide enough for fire-fighting equipment. Make sure that access roads to 'battle-axe' sites have a clearance for vehicles at least 4 metres (13 feet) wide.

A safe site: soil and ground water pollution

When considering a new building site you should purchase pH measuring equipment and check the pH of the soil. Note whether the pH is very high (higher than 8.0–8.5) or very low (less than 5.5–5.0). While soil pH in the mid-range (5.0–8.0) probably can be modified to nearer pH 7.0 by certain horticultural practices, when above 8.0–8.5 it is too alkaline and below 5.0, too acidic. This can be an indicator of a pollution problem, either natural or artificial.

AGRICULTURAL LAND-MANAGEMENT PRACTICES

If a previous landowner has over-irrigated, removed too many trees or poorly drained the soil, the water table may have risen. If the water table is too near the surface, acidic conditions prevail, and roots can 'drown' through lack of oxygen in the soil. These lands are usually swampy and boggy; a further indication is the type of vegetation occurring. In Australia, even when surface water may be absent, an abundance of the *Melaleuca* species indicates acidic, waterlogged conditions. In North America, aspen groves and the ubiquitous *Juncea* species are indicators of high water tables.

Some treatments use lime or epsom salts to neutralise the acidic condition of the soil that has formed because of the anaerobic (lacking oxygen) conditions, but it is best to avoid such sites unless the land can be easily drained.

A safe site: geomagnetic fields

HIGH-TENSION POWER LINES

Do not purchase a site anywhere near high-tension power lines, steel towers or transformers. If you have children, check that the schools they would attend are also not located near such structures. Take care to check with local power supply authorities for future power service easements in your area.

MICROWAVE ANTENNAE, TOWERS AND POLES

The landscape of most countries is being peppered with antennae or tower structures to transmit radio, television and telephone information. It should be noted that the effects of microwave radiation are little understood.

Carefully locate all such installations on your map of the area, noting the directions that dish antennae face. Join these locations with lines drawn on your map. It would be wise to avoid property that is crossed by your lines.

As television transmission operates on the microwave band, you should try to determine the facing direction of the antennae on any nearby television transmission towers so that you can avoid them. If the direction of the antennae is indeterminate, do not purchase a property closer than 2 kilometres (1 mile, 350 yards) from a television tower.

Site Survey and Analysis

Much of the site information you gather from the following processes can be recorded on a set of overlay survey plans using clear sheets of film, preferably acetate. You will already have obtained some of the necessary information during your area survey. Your on-site surveys are best made by competent professionals, but by undertaking research at a local library and taking some measurements yourself, you can produce approximate results.

THE SITE SURVEY AND BASE PLAN

The land and topographic surveys need to be obtained first as they form the base plan of the site. On this plan, record slopes and rock outcrops as well as other features such as fences, poles, etc. Your land surveyor should be asked to show ground contour lines on this plan. (A contour line joins points of equal height or depth.)

GEOLOGICAL SURVEY PLAN

The site should have test holes drilled in locations chosen by a professional consultant. The resultant geological survey will show a contour plan of the geology of the upper strata of the site, together with a core-drilling analysis and report covering the selected locations. At this stage the water table levels, if any, are recorded, together with any other data on presence and rate of flow of other ground waters. This information is included on a transparent overlay of the same scale as the base plan.

SOILS SURVEY PLAN

The soils present on the site are mapped in conjunction with a soils analysis and report (which include pH, nitrogen, phosphorus and potassium content and tests for the presence of salts). These can be carried out on samples supplied by you to a soils laboratory. Contact your agricultural department for advice pertinent to your locality. Record this information on a set of overlay plans, one for each major type of soil horizon. (The soil horizon is the place where the colour and texture of the soil changes significantly.)

On small sites there will probably only be one or two soil types, but large sites may contain several. The soils survey should record all low-lying land, and all the different soil types. Soil texture should be analysed to determine how much sand, silt and clay it contains as these factors affect soil drainage which impacts on the health both of plants and the building's occupants. By recording the extent of different types of soil on your site plan, it will be easier to choose a location for your garden (where soils are around pH7), a good site for a 'borrow pit' (to make earth bricks or blocks), and the best place for your building. For example, an area of continuous and solid rock with shallow, infertile soil would be a suitable foundation for a building. See Chapter 9 for a simple procedure for analysing soil texture.

CATCHMENT AREA AND DRAINAGE PLAN

Although arid-region sites only experience occasional run-off, when it does occur it is usually extreme in its quantity, duration and sheet-erosion effects. The plotting of the extent of the catchment area (which should be drawn as a small-scale plan separate to your overlays) and the analysis of slope and run-off gives a clear indication of where flooding could occur during heavy rainfall.

It is necessary to study the site in heavy rain and note where the main drainage flow-lines occur, as well as the location of interrupted drainage. Your house should be sited away from areas where surface drainage is focused.

SLOPE AND ASPECT ANALYSIS PLAN

Following on from the previous survey, if you have a large site, an analysis should be made of topographical slopes and their relationship to the position of the summer and winter sun. This analysis has an important bearing on the optimal siting of the dwelling for energy effectiveness and on the design of the house and garden. If the site is small or fairly flat this need not take the form of a plan, but rather a guide to siting the building.

Slopes facing in a direction that ranges between 15 degrees east or west of the sun's direction at noon are satisfactory for the principal facade of an energy-efficient building designed on passive-solar design principles.

As indicated in Figure 2.6, slopes are categorised on the basis of the direction they face (their aspect). For optimal efficiency, the angular extremities of the plane facing north in the southern hemisphere (south in the northern hemisphere)

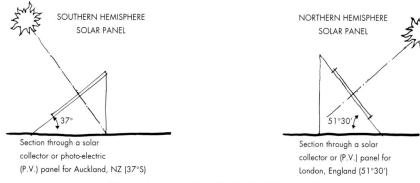

SOUTHERN HEMISPHERE
SOLAR PANEL

NORTHERN HEMISPHERE
SOLAR PANEL

37°

51°30'

Section through a solar
collector or photo-electric
(P.V.) panel for Auckland, NZ (37°S)

Section through a solar
collector or (P.V.) panel for
London, England (51°30')

Solar panels may be positioned (in plan) from 15° east to 15° west
of the sun's direction at noon

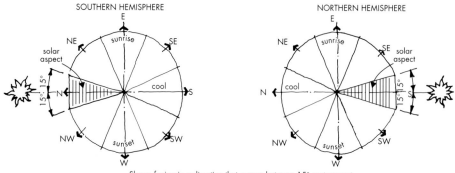

Slopes facing in a direction that ranges between 15° east or west
of the sun's direction at noon are satisfactory for the principal
facade of an energy efficient building designed on passive–solar design principles

Figure 2.6: Slope and aspect analysis showing the basis of optimal siting of photovoltaic cell solar collectors

should be within the range of the orientation of solar collectors. In other words, solar collectors can be faced in all directions that lie between 15 degrees west and 15 degrees east of solar north. To find solar north, place a short stick in the ground so it casts a shadow. Note that the shadow's direction, which is solar (true) north is different from magnetic north, for every place on Earth.

WIND ROSE ANALYSIS

Meteorological data on the prevailing winds for an area may be very generalised. Once the design process has reached a stage that warrants a greater investment of time, local winds should be recorded on a continuous basis and a wind rose diagram drawn for the site. Visit the site night and day to discover how breezes affect it and enquire from neighbours whether unpleasant winds cause problems during summer and winter. Although you have already considered the proximity of major highways or industrial areas to ensure that prevailing winds will not carry polluted air to your site, visit the site early on a windless midsummer morning and again at night during the week, when traffic pollution is at a maximum. Ideally, check whether the pollution control authorities have any records, comparative maps or advice concerning pollution levels in the area.

RAINFALL AND EVAPORATION RECORDS

From the meteorological bureau obtain rainfall and evaporation data collected from the earliest possible date to the present. If records are unavailable, local knowledge on flooding heights is invaluable.

SUN PATH AND SHADOW ANGLE ANALYSIS
(SOLAR ACCESS)

Using one of the standard methods of plotting the altitude and direction of the sun at the various seasons of the year, record the sun's position in relation to the site on an overlay diagram. Existing trees and neighbouring buildings should then be drawn, along with the shadows they cast. This is necessary to ensure that there is enough space on-site to allow sunlight to enter the house and gardens in winter and to plan for excluding sunlight in summer. Your architect will draw these shadow tests for you, or a reference such as Phillips (1992) can be used.

VEGETATION SURVEY

It is just as essential to keep your house naturally cool in summer to save energy costs as it is to keep it warm in winter. Some sunlight is essential in every room, so the idea is not to block out all of the summer sun, but to properly control it. This can be achieved with roof overhangs, shading devices and landscaping. Survey all trees and shrubs and plot them on another transparent overlay to the base plan. Record trunk diameter, canopy diameter, estimated height and whether evergreen or deciduous. Note if any of the trees are twisted, infected with borer or other insects, stunted, or leaning over, as these could be signs of nutritional deficiencies, GMF anomalies or potential land-slip. Figure 2.7 shows how to estimate the height of a tree if a clinometer or similar instrument is not available.

Once the heights of trees (or nearby buildings) are known, it is possible to plot the shadows they will cast. While this is the task of an architect or landscape architect, there is one important test you can conduct that graphically determines the angles of the sun (above a level plane) for the site in question at midday in midsummer and midwinter. In an atlas, find (to the nearest degree) the latitude of the site in question. For example the latitude of a site in London is 51° 30'N (51½°) and of a site in Auckland, New Zealand, is 37°S. To determine the angle of the midsummer sun at midday, subtract the latitude from 113½°. To determine the angle of the midwinter sun at midday, subtract the latitude from 66½°. For London the midsummer angle would be 113½°–51½° = 62° and the midwinter angle 66½°–51½° = 15°. For Auckland, the angle in midsummer would be 113½°–37°, that is, 76½° and in midwinter 66½°–37° = 29½°.

Remember that these angles refer to due solar north or south only. Later or earlier in the day and at intermediate times of the year the various angles change. These angles give a good idea of how far the building needs to be set back on the north (or south) to avoid or take advantage of the altitude of the sun. Should you wish to understand sun angles in greater detail than this, consult Appendix B. There you will find how to plot the position of the sun in the sky at any time of the day for midsummer and midwinter, the maximum and minimum for the year. To calculate sun angles for other times of the year, it is advisable that you consult a specialist in the field.

INSOLATION RECORDS

The number of hours of sunshine a country receives at any location is usually mapped by a relevant government authority. Otherwise the information on the number of hours of sunshine you can expect each season is obtainable from the meteorological department for your region or state.

GROUND FROSTS

Information about the incidence of ground frosts is beneficial for the planning of your garden. Records of ground frosts are best obtained from local nurserymen or farmers, otherwise residents in the locality of the site may be able to help you. Low-lying land often allows cold air pockets to form. Cold night air flows like treacle and fills depressions, encouraging frost to form.

GEOMAGNETIC SURVEY

A geomagnetic survey should be undertaken to determine the gradients in the Earth's magnetic field

Figure 2.7: Estimating the height of a tree

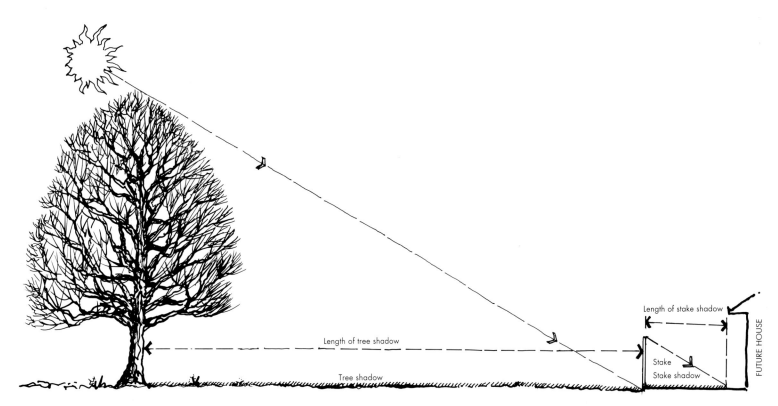

TO FIND HEIGHT OF A TREE (on any sunny day of the year)
1. Find a straight stick and drive it into the ground; measure its height above ground.
2. Measure length of the tree's shadow.
3. Measure length of the stake's shadow.
4. Then height of tree = height of stake multiplied by length of tree shadow and the result is divided by length of stake shadow
TO CALCULATE THE MAXIMUM AND MINIMUM LENGTH OF THE TREE'S SHADOW (at noon)
For midwinter angle: 66½°minus latitude of your site, eg for Auckland, NZ (latitude 37°), the angle is 66½°– 37° = 29½°
For midsummer angle: 113½° minus latitude of your site, eg for Auckland, NZ (latitude 37°), the angle is 113½°– 37° = 76½°

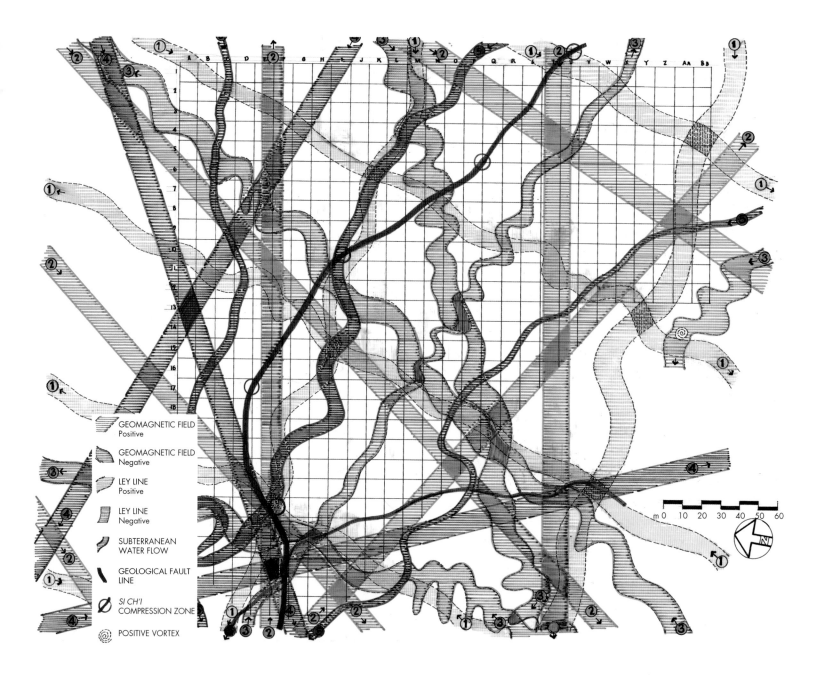

Legend:

- GEOMAGNETIC FIELD Positive
- GEOMAGNETIC FIELD Negative
- LEY LINE Positive
- LEY LINE Negative
- SUBTERRANEAN WATER FLOW
- GEOLOGICAL FAULT LINE
- SI CH'I COMPRESSION ZONE
- POSITIVE VORTEX

Figure 2.8: A full geomantic survey of the Lokasi Hotel site, Djakarta, Indonesia (Courtesy: J. Schmidt, *feng shui* consultant and geomancer)

for the site. This will reveal any anomalies which can affect the health of the occupants of the house. Distorted or twisted trees should be noted on the geomagnetic survey as potential locations of geomagnetic anomalies that should be measured with instruments.

It is claimed that a child will retreat to the corner of a cot away from earth radiation and will sleep with its feet towards the radiation. Dogs, pigs and other animals are said to avoid areas where subterranean water veins intersect. Trees will branch down towards radiation and ants will nest above radiation lines. Bees are said to produce more honey when their nests are built over such zones. Wasps tend towards zones of radiation and cats prefer to rest over them (Tietze 1988).

A magnetometer, preferably a proton magnetometer, can be hired in most capital cities or by inter-city delivery (see Resources List). You will need some professional advice on its use from the hirer.

The results of this survey are best plotted as an overlay contour plan to the base plan. Geomagnetic highs and lows are to be noted as anomalies indicating potential areas of radioactivity. Care must be taken that the interpretation of the results are given by an expert as, for example, subterranean steel or iron can produce false readings as can the proximity of moving vehicles and other factors.

Areas where the GMF is measured at higher than 500 gamma, alternatively known as 500 nanoTeslas or 5 milliGauss, should be avoided when siting your house or relaxation areas in your garden.

RADON SURVEY

The amount of radon$_{222}$ in the soil, air and water of a site can be determined by the use of small detectors located in canisters placed in the soil, the toilet cistern, water tanks and in a protected position in the outside air, for example, under the eaves. The water tests could be conducted in a neighbour's cistern, but this may be impractical as all detectors have to be in place for a few seasons, even a full year. (See Resources List for radon detectors.)

Another option is to use a portable nuclear radiation monitor to detect the levels of alpha radiation at ground level and 1.5 metres (5 feet) above ground. The ground level readings record the emission of radon (as gamma and alpha radiation) direct from the ground while the readings above ground show how much alpha radiation is dispersed by the movements of air. By taking these measurements it is possible to isolate sites where long-term detectors need to be installed to gather detailed data. See the Resources List for suppliers of radon detectors.

DOWSING AND *FENG SHUI* SURVEY

The practice of dowsing, classifiable as parascience, was first recorded in Europe in 1240, though it probably dates back to the neolithic period, and certainly to the ancient Egyptians. In their attempts to find underground anomalies, such as water, mineral ores or 'ley lines', dowsers use a Y- or L-shaped divining rod, a bowed twig, a L-shaped length of metal or a pendulum. Professor H.D. Betz of the Physics Department at Munich University undertook a 10-year comparison of dowsing and conventional water detection techniques. A dowser worked on 691 sites and isolated the areas where water could be found. When drilling was performed, water was found in 96 per cent of the locations. The dowser's predictions regarding the yield and purity of the water were accurate 80–90 per cent of the time. (Technological methods for such predictions are not yet available.)

Ley lines are paths of ionising radiation. Their effect can be positive or negative, so it is advisable to locate your house away from them.

It may be difficult to find a reliable, reputable dowser; if that is the case, you can collect much of the necessary data using a proton magnetometer. If you are successful in finding a dowser, ask them to locate underground water veins and geopathogenic stress zones, ley line field distribution and the Hartmann and Curry Net grid lines. Plotting these on an overlay will help you avoid unhealthy zones when siting your house, planning the layout of rooms, and placing furniture. Figure 2.8 shows a geomantic survey which was developed by a *feng shui* practitioner and dowser.

A related geomantic survey can be undertaken by a *feng shui* consultant, but they are also difficult to find. A *feng shui* survey should correlate with the dowser's survey in regard to ley lines, geomagnetic field distribution and underground water concentrations. It should also map the movement of *ch'i* over the site.

ANALYSING YOUR OVERLAYS

By plotting all of the previous information on transparent overlays, then referring to them laid over the original base plan of the site, it will be possible to locate the most desirable place to build your house. This is even easier if your survey information is on computer. (The above procedures need to be conducted for each site if you wish to compare various options.) If all this is too complicated, it can be undertaken for you by an architect or landscape architect skilled in the use of instruments to measure geomagnetic fields.

Remember that your family's health will, to a large extent, depend on whether you make wise decisions at this early stage. Such decisions cannot be made without having all the information available to you. Allocate adequate funds for research early on and you will benefit later.

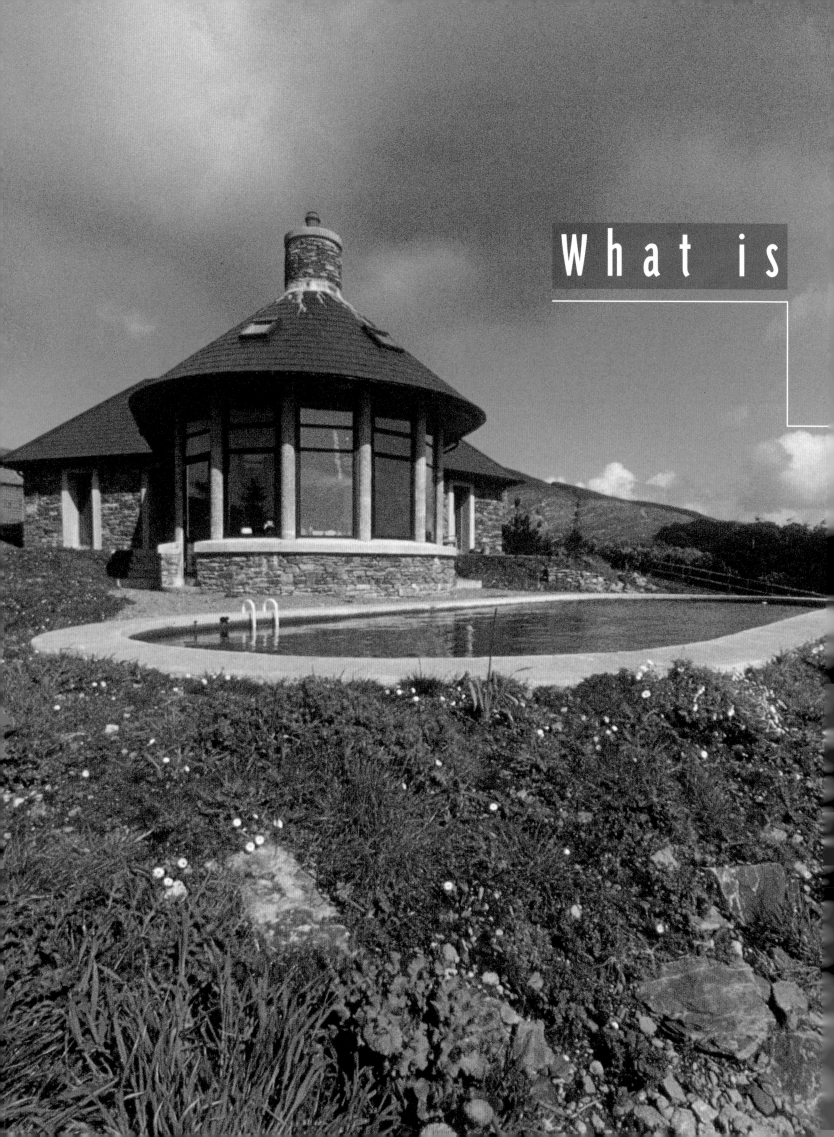

What is

a healthy house?

to create a healthy living environment, we need to banish fantasies of the 'intelligent' house of the future, in which electronic gadgetry fulfils every need and our trust can be placed in the latest developments in synthetic building products, paints and furnishings. Such a house is far from intelligent — it exemplifies an unhealthy environment, dominated by harmful electromagnetic and electrostatic fields and indoor chemical pollution. Instead, think of your house as an organic structure which is going to 'grow' around and with you. A holistically designed building conserves natural energy in all its forms. Unobtrusive in the natural environment, it utilises the mechanisms of nature rather than the electronic gadgetry of humanity. It puts health and ecology first and egocentric architectural style last. It creates an environment conducive to spirituality, personal growth and beauty; it does not implement technological fixes to attain environmentally short-sighted goals or in the name of architectural fashion.

The housing of the future should be organic in planning, like the cross-section of a living organism. It is not enough to simply borrow forms from the animal, vegetable or mineral world. A building suitable for human beings now has to express empathy and continuity with nature. As British architect Christopher Day has stated, it is necessary to: 'listen to the place, listen to the idea and find ways in which they are compatible' (Sweet 1994). To which we would add: 'and listen to Gaia and her

Think of your house as an organism which, like you, must breathe. Choose only materials that allow for the transfer of air and moisture. Utilise the mechanisms of nature rather than electronic gadgetry.

needs'. The house of the future should be simple in layout and appear to belong to the Earth itself, reflecting the building's relationship to nature: part of, rather than distinct from, the natural environment.

The degree of difficulty associated with 'making over' an existing house to create a healthy environment is daunting, and often the best solution is to begin again by constructing your own home according to healthy building principles.

The healthy building has a sound structural system (or building 'envelope') with adequate services and correctly fitting components. Indoor pollutants are minimised to avoid threatening the health and wellbeing of the occupants.

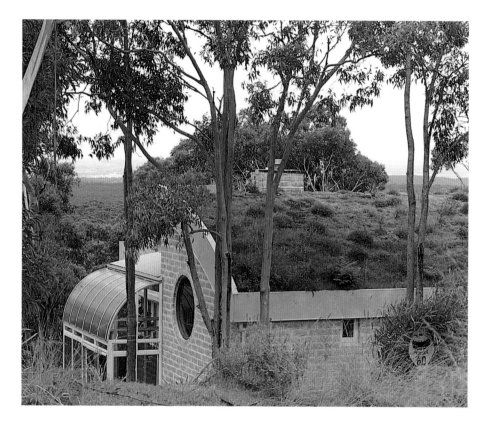

A turf roof healthy house with earth-brick walls and wood-framed floors and roof in the Blue Mountains, NSW, Australia (Design architects: S. and D. Baggs)

Ideally, a healthy house uses sun, wind and water for as much of its energy requirements as possible and incorporates methods of passively storing and reusing energy. It is sited to optimise winter sun and summer shade, the cooling effects of breezes and the temperature-modifying effects of the soil. The healthy house emits minimal amounts of pollution into the surrounding air, water and soil. It incorporates a composting system, utilises waste water and relies on the latest pest control procedures that avoid chemical pesticides. A healthy house is supplied with filtered water, or rainwater where possible. It is sealed against

ingress of radon from the soil. It optimises negatively ionised air in bedrooms and balances the ratio of positive to negative ions in work and living rooms. It utilises natural, not mechanically-forced, ventilation. Fragrant herbs and shrubs in the garden bathe window and door openings with pleasant aromas.

A healthy indoor climate is created by incorporating natural materials that do not give off polluting chemicals or induce electrostatic field effects, and by design features and permeable building materials that control air temperature, humidity and flow. A healthy house is not sited near harmful electromagnetic fields, such as power lines (and avoids the build up of electromagnetic and electrostatic fields from electrical equipment), or geological faults or ground water flows that distort the Earth's electrical and magnetic fields and produce zones detrimental to health. If it is not possible to avoid locating a building over such zones, protective strategies should be incorporated to modify the effects on health. Also, bed and sitting room furniture should be placed in their respective rooms so that effects of these harmful fields are diminished. *Feng shui*, the Chinese method of siting a building in relation to the topography and earth-energy of a location, can be applied in the design process.

A quiet atmosphere is created in a healthy house by insulating it from exterior noise and orienting it to the sounds of nature. Well-lit interior spaces are provided that do not need artificial light in the daytime; fluorescent lighting is avoided completely. The healthy house is integrated with its ecosystem, utilising native trees, shrubs and flowers to attract wildlife, and exotic plants to achieve specific design requirements.

In the construction of the healthy house, non-toxic, non-polluting, renewable, biodegradable materials and products produced with low environmental and social costs have been used. If materials are not biodegradable, they should be modular or demountable so that they can eventually be recycled when the useful life of the building is over.

We need homes that support rather than hinder us, and we need new aims and priorities for living. Our homes should be designed for the health of the body and to provide a peaceful, healing environment. It would then be up to those who occupy such a house to adapt their habits and lifestyles to their new environment.

A Question of Structural Type

Having decided on a suitable site, the next consideration is what type of house to build. There is no absolute solution. Each house type has its own benefits and deficiencies which need to be evaluated before coming to a final decision.

◎ The pole house ◎

Termite attack can cause disastrous structural damage to a pole house, so you need to have a totally infallible system of termite control set in place and undertake regular inspections. A pole house also creates the perfect conditions for a fire to start in the face of an advancing bush or forest fire. However, it has a wonderful aesthetic and creates a sense of living in the treetops. It can also leave the soil and natural ground water and run-off patterns beneath it relatively untouched, and hence fertile and productive for plants suited to shaded environments. Finally, it is ideal for steeply sloping sites.

◎ The wooden-floor house ◎

The use of pervious building materials is vital for a healthy house. While a wooden floor is very pervious, it has a low thermal mass, hence lacks the capacity to store solar heat in winter or act as a cold sink in summer. It is also vulnerable to termite attack, however termiticides are not necessary if the floor is well lit, well ventilated and high enough from the ground to allow inspection access. If termite attack does occur, the damage is rarely life-threatening, unlike the pole house. While clear access to sub-floor areas and good ventilation are essential, it is recommended that sub-floor areas be sealed with masonry fender walls to prevent bush or forest fire damage. Sub-floor ventilators should be covered with insect mesh (non-plastic) to prevent the admission of sparks. When a wooden-floor house is sited into the ground, particular care must be taken to intercept the natural flow of ground water to prevent the sub-floor space from becoming wet and harbouring mould (and termites if they are prevalent). Figure 3.2 indicates how ground water is diverted around the house.

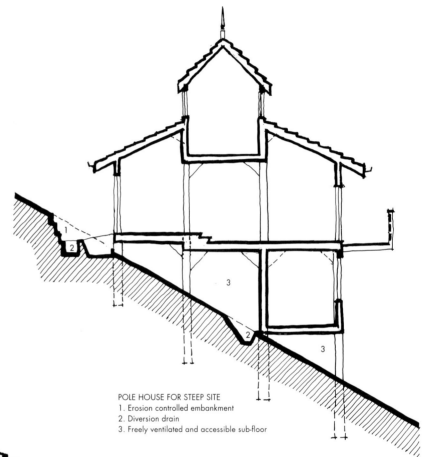

POLE HOUSE FOR STEEP SITE
1. Erosion controlled embankment
2. Diversion drain
3. Freely ventilated and accessible sub-floor

WOODEN-FLOOR HOUSE EXCAVATED INTO SITE
1. Erosion controlled embankment
2. Drain to divert surface run off (uphill from building) around it
3. Generous sub-floor ventilation

Figure 3.1: Pole house for steep site

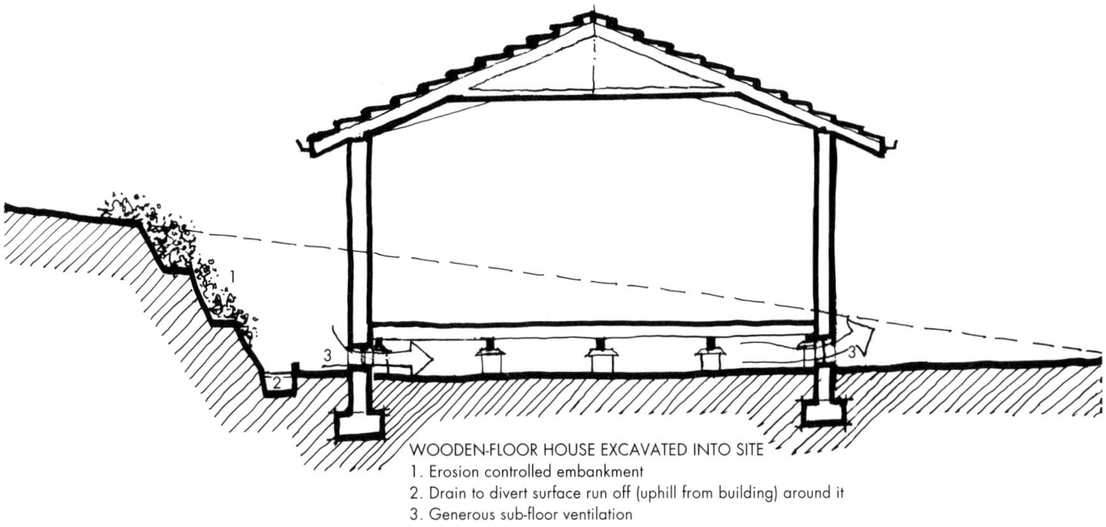

Figure 3.2: Wooden-floor house excavated into site

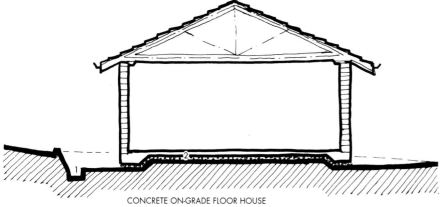

CONCRETE ON-GRADE FLOOR HOUSE
1. Diversion drain
2. Atmospheric pressure is balanced (and hydrostatic pressure from ground water released) by either cellular drainage panels or coarse aggregate non-capillary drainage bed

Figure 3.3: House with concrete on-grade floor with hydrostatic pressure-release layer

Figure 3.4: Earth-sheltered, concrete-floor house, the ultimate in energy-efficiency strategies. It can be a challenge to make such a building 'breathe', but ventilating when exterior air temperature and humidity is appropriate will help to alleviate the problem, as will the use of diffusive materials

@ The concrete-floor house @

Concrete floors are used to control the upward push of hydrostatic pressure (water pressure) and to store solar or excess heat from the building. A layer of hardcore brick, crushed brick, or stone filling is placed beneath the concrete slab to entrap air, which relieves the hydrostatic pressure. The water then drains away.

Concrete floors contain steel reinforcement which, by disrupting the GMF, can cause health problems for the building's inhabitants, so it is not a preferable floor type for the healthy house. However, sometimes this system of flooring is acceptable, for example when a house requires the energy-efficient thermal storage properties of concrete in order to cope with climatic extremes. If the house is correctly sited to avoid geomagnetic anomalies, the pathogenic conditions associated with such zones will not be distributed throughout the building if the reinforcing steel is non-continuous and earthed (grounded) using correct electrical earthing procedures. See Chapter 9 for further details.

@ The earth-sheltered, concrete-floor house @

The earth-sheltered, concrete-floor house represents a highly efficient thermal energy conservation strategy, provided an efficient, natural air-exchange system is included in the design. The advice of an experienced architect is required to ensure infallible waterproofing of the reinforced concrete walls, roofs and floors. It is the most energy-efficient design strategy available, but the same health considerations surround this type of housing as the concrete-floor house discussed above.

A LOW-ALLERGY HEALTHY HOUSE

Chemicals, electrical stimuli, and air and water pollution can result in a vast range of symptoms in people who are allergic to them. Designing a building that does not foster allergy or ill health is a major task. A low-allergy healthy house should minimise as much of the unhealthy emissions from the outside environment and the interior of the building as is practicable within the project budget.

@ Radon emissions from the ground @

Raised well above the ground, the pole house is an ideal house type for avoiding radon emissions. Radon gas and its radioactive daughter products emitted at ground level are diffused by wind currents before they have a chance to enter the building. This means that the building will only be exposed to the general level of environmental radon in its local geographical area.

The earth-sheltered, concrete-floor house must be totally waterproofed in order to keep out radon. A sub-floor waterproof membrane which is continuous with the wall and roof membranes will ensure that all

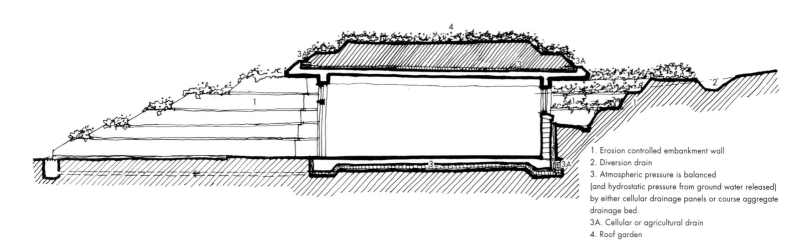

1. Erosion controlled embankment wall
2. Diversion drain
3. Atmospheric pressure is balanced (and hydrostatic pressure from ground water released) by either cellular drainage panels or course aggregate drainage bed.
3A. Cellular or agricultural drain
4. Roof garden

House type	Radon penetration without controls	Cost to control radon	Unchecked pollution intrusion to interior	Cost to exclude exterior pollution	Total score (0 = best case; 40 = worst case)	Comments
Pole house	2	0	10	10	22	Vulnerable to exterior air pollution
Timber-floor house on ground	10	10	8	10	38	Vulnerable to exterior air pollution
Concrete-floor house	5	5	6	5	21	Sub-floor waterproof membrane may cause outgassing. Radon seals will solve this problem
Earth-sheltered, concrete-floor house on ground	1	5	1	1	8	Continuous waterproof membrane may cause outgassing. Radon seals will solve this problem

Adapted from: A Consumers' Guide to Safe Pest Control; 10 = highly significant; 0 = insignificant

gaps at slab and wall penetrations are sealed. The homogeneity of this waterproofing system will provide an automatic barrier to radon penetration.

◎ Air exchange between interior and exterior ◎

As cells of high and low air pressure move through a geographic area, air moves into and out of the building through all the openings, cracks and gaps connecting the interior to the exterior. The rate of exchange depends on the gross area of all apertures, hence an old building with many cracks and vent openings will exchange air with its outside environment more quickly than one that is sealed.

Earth-sheltered, energy-efficient houses are totally sealed and have minimal air exchange with the outside environment, so while they are resistant to external pollution, they are susceptible to high levels of interior pollution and require total air-flushing every few days.

The pole house is particularly vulnerable to external pollution and it is inadvisable to construct one near a major highway, airport or in the air-drainage pattern of a major city. The ground level

Table 3.1: Relative degree of freedom from exterior and interior pollution of four house types. This is an approximate guide to selecting a house type for an area where the ground has a high radon content and high air pollution levels from industry, airports, traffic, etc

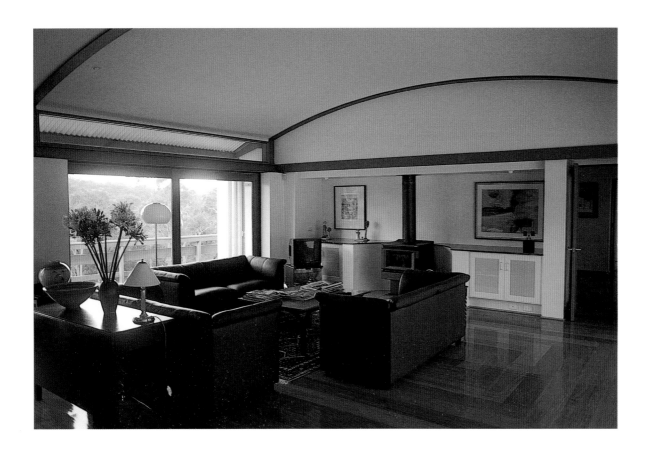

The living room of 'Bidri Park' in the Southern Highlands of NSW, Aust. (Architect: C. Pattinson, Arcoessence; Photograph: C. Pattinson)

house with a wooden floor is less problematic, but needs to be moderately altered to inhibit the intrusion of too much outdoor air.

Outdoor air pollution should be monitored and the stale air flushed out of the house when pollution levels are low and temperature, wind and moisture readings are favourable. It is desirable to utilise a 'stack-effect' ventilating chimney with the appropriate sensors (see Chapter 8).

Low-allergy retrofit to an existing house

While it is ideal that you construct your own house using holistic principles, it is possible to make alterations to an existing house or apartment to improve its health-promoting qualities. Such a retrofit will always be a compromise, yet much can be achieved if you follow the advice given in Chapters 9 and 10 regarding vents under the house, radon control strategies, painting, floors and floor coverings, and furniture.

If you are about to buy a house, it is far better to buy an old house needing renovation rather than one renovated prior to sale, as such renovations are usually undertaken with little consideration for healthy procedures. Do not tackle everything at once, but work in stages.

Pest control

When buying a house, try to locate the pest control firm that supplied the vendor with the pest control certificate. Ask for documentation of the application rate, the type of chemicals, and the degree of dilution of each chemical used on the property prior to sale. Find out whether the pest control firm had to treat the property for infestation, what type of infestation, the chemicals used, and how recently. This information may not be available because, in some countries, there is no requirement that the poisons used to eradicate pests must be registered. Organochlorines remain active for 20 to 30 years, and it may be possible that the house has been

The kitchen of a low-allergy, wooden-framed, earth-sheltered house with concrete floor: the 'Pit House' in Sante Fe, New Mexico, USA (Architect: J. McGowan; Photograph: K. Prescott)

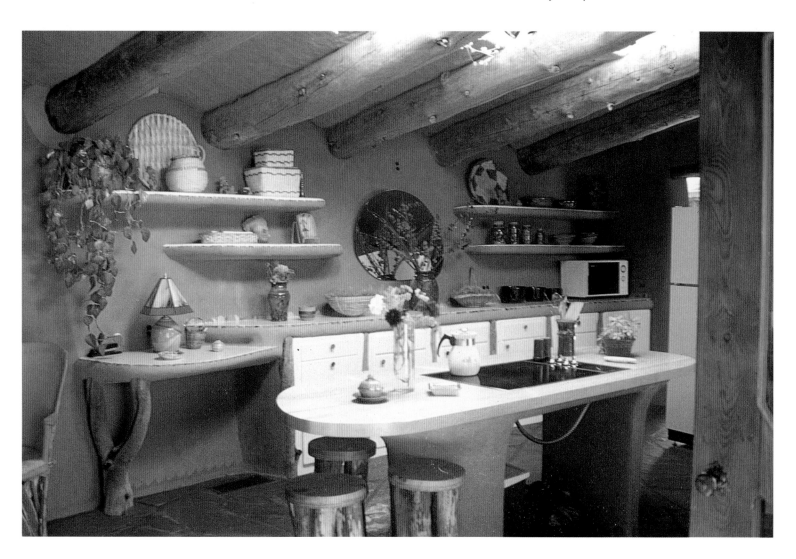

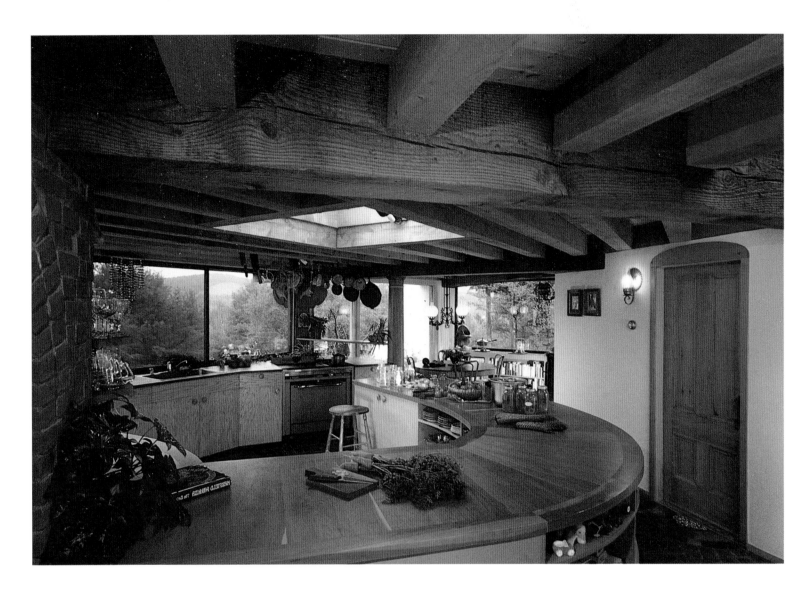

treated with them, or other toxic chemicals, within that time.

Organochlorines have now been banned from use in pest control in many countries, including Australia. The long-term health effects of substitute organophosphates are still not understood, but they too are poisonous.

Faced with the choice between using potentially dangerous chemicals to control termites and increasing the risk of houses falling down, Australian regulatory bodies have opted to protect our homes [rather than us] (Higgins 1989).

Have the site inspected by a holistic pest control company which will be able to guide you on alternatives to synthetic chemicals. If termites are found, they can be eliminated using environmentally sensitive procedures. It is now possible to make a new building termite-resistant, but for an existing building, an integrated termite management program should be implemented by someone qualified in both entomology and building construction. If you live in a house that has been sprayed for termites in the past with toxic chemicals, make sure that you keep the house well ventilated and try to use natural, non-toxic materials in the interior of your home.

This issue may dictate whether you buy an existing house or build a new house, because there is no way to undo the toxic impact of a chemical treatment for termites or other insects, other than to wait for perhaps 30 years for the chemicals to become so weak that outgassing stops.

Low-allergy, earth-sheltered house, California, USA (Architect: D. Metz)

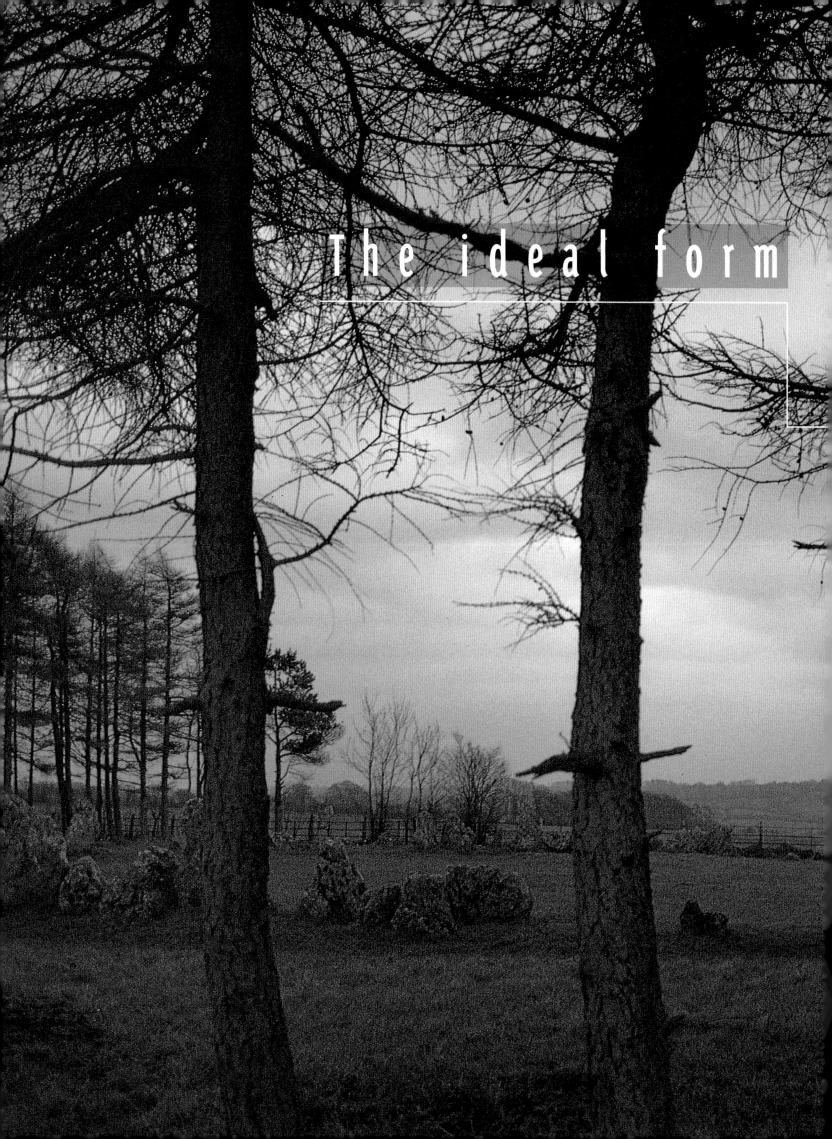

The ideal form

for the healthy house

a healthy house must be worthy of human beings, a benign and health-supporting shelter within which the family can grow and develop in physical, emotional, mental and spiritual health. These factors are affected by the shape, symbolism and pattern of the structures around us.

Symbols created by human beings possess an innate capacity to influence their surroundings. They resonate with the qualities and ideas inherent in their design. This resonance conveys those qualities and ideas to the living things around them. The standing stones of an ancient stone circle at Tsbyty Cynfyn in Wales, the United Kingdom, (overleaf) have become part of the enclosing garden wall of a church. This temporal continuity is an example of symbolic resonance. Inherent to both the old and new geometry of the site is the special purpose of the construction.

Do the shapes surrounding us in our daily lives affect our health and wellbeing? Is it possible to adopt a holistic approach to design so that the shapes of our houses positively influence our health and enhance our quality of life?

MORPHIC RESONANCE

In the 3rd century BC, Plato put forward the idea that the form of physical objects was governed by eternal archetypes, and Aristotle posited that each thing had a spirit or soul from which its form arose. In the 5th century BC, Democritus and Leucippus introduced the concept that the smallest component of all forms was the atom. This idea was the seed from which developed materialism, a system of thought which

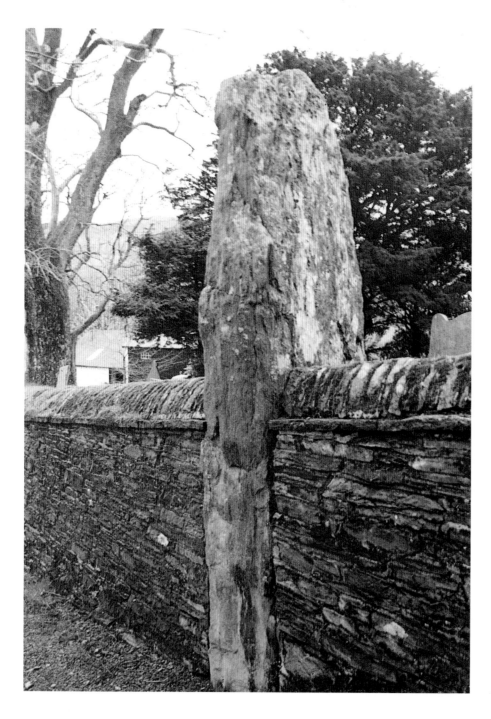

Ancient standing stone as part of the enclosing wall of a Christian church, Ysbyty Cynfyn, Wales, UK

Page 52: The Rollright Stone Circle, Oxfordshire, UK. These stones were investigated by Robins (1985) and Brooker (1988) who found that the GMF formed a spiral pattern diminishing in strength towards the centre

past which has been conserved and still operates to influence the present and the future of the organism; in it is contained all that the organism is and does in the present; and finally, in it is contained all that the organism vaguely points to in its own future development and that of its offspring. The whole is there carrying all its time with it. (Smuts 1926)

Sheldrake, in his controversial books *New Science of Life* (1987) and *The Presence of the Past* (1989), suggests a similar concept to Smuts. He considers that the DNA in our genes plays an important role in determining how proteins are made, but that such things as our form, appearance and instinctive behaviour can be attributed to morphic fields: fields of 'influence extending in space and continuing in time'. The morphic field contains all that ever was of every form or pattern, a memory of all habits, laws of nature and crystals that make up objects. The longer such forms and concepts have existed, the more powerful the morphic field. He holds that each type of cell, tissue, organ and organism has its own kind of field which operates over great distances and across time. The new seed or fertilised egg 'tunes in' to its field; the cell of a potential feather takes on the characteristic of 'featherness' from its morphic field.

It is anticipated that tests planned by Swedish physicists working in the area of low temperature superconductors will provide more conclusive results than presently exist regarding Sheldrake's hypothesis. The scientists will monitor the development and performance of new superconductive materials the first few times that these materials are made. Being new materials, there are no pre-existing atomic relationships. If Sheldrake's hypothesis is correct, the 'memory' of the atomic relationships will improve over time and the materials' development period will shorten.

When Sheldrake, in his attempts to use this hypothesis of causative formation to counteract materialism in the biological sciences, likens it to a contemporary version of Aristotle's 'soul', he is trying to reanimate nature. If correct, his hypothesis will universalise the idea that there is 'life in every atom' and hence in everything. It would mean that the life in you is in every creature and every object, whether organic or inorganic.

insists that all questions can be settled by observation but not by intuition. Today's dominant scientific attitude developed from the basis of materialism, even though many of the great empirical scientists reject systematic materialism. Modern molecular biology tells us that the secret of how organisms are formed can be decoded from the 'language' of chromosomes. But one scientist, Rupert Sheldrake, is working to counteract materialism in the life sciences, making the ideas of past thinkers such as Aristotle relevant once more.

The organism and its field is one continuous structure, and in this continuum is contained all of the

The Pattern Effect

Doctor Andrew Stanway, in his book *Alternative Medicine, A Guide to Natural Therapies* (1979), argues that the ancient Egyptians and Greeks realised the power of pattern and shape to affect the body's health and wellbeing. This effect may originate at the subatomic level where every particle in the physical world corresponds to a specific pattern. Smith and Best (1989) have described how allergies can be triggered by nearby microwave installations and metallic structures like railings, because of their pattern. Schizophrenic patients are said to improve in a trapezoidal-shaped ward, wounds of mice heal faster in spherical cages and beer deteriorates in taste if stored in square cans rather than cylindrical barrels.

The Pyramid as the Form for a Healthy House

As architects, we have experimented with various building forms, particularly curved forms because of the subtleties of light such buildings create. Curved forms are most suited to earth-sheltered houses. Above-ground buildings, on the other hand, are more likely to use materials with planar surfaces, so curved forms are less of an option. The most interesting possibilities in terms of the shape of above-ground houses are provided by the pyramid.

◎ Squaring the circle: the *true* pyramid ◎

It is often assumed that the Great Pyramid of Egypt, the archetype for pyramid investigations, is based on the equilateral 60 degree triangle, but it is not. Over the years, many tried to accurately calculate the angle of the sides of the pyramid, coming up with a range of results between 40 degrees and 60 degrees. The angle is 51°50'34", but this figure proved elusive because those who tried to measure it were unaware that the Egyptian priests knew how to 'square the circle'. If the vertical height of the pyramid is used as the radius of a circle, the circumference of that circle will be equal to the length of the perimeter of the square base of the pyramid. Another general way to express this is that the perimeter of the base is to the height as the circumference of a circle is to its radius (2Π). From this it can be calculated that the angle is 51°50'34".

To understand the significance of squaring the circle to the ancient Egyptians it is necessary to look into the esoteric meaning of the symbols involved. Obviously the Egyptians placed great significance on these symbols because they had the knowledge to use the far simpler geometry of the 60 degree pyramid, yet chose not to use it.

◎ Symbolism of the pyramid form ◎

According to the famous 19th century esotericist H.P. Blavatsky, the pyramid represented a tree; at its apex the link was made between heaven and earth. The original Great Pyramid was thought to be capped with gold over the limestone casing to symbolise the importance of this mystic connection with heaven.

In the 'Mysteries of Egypt ... the measurements of the great pyramid were studied as emblematical of the proportions of the Universe' (Leadbeater 1926). The Mystery teachings concerning the pyramid (and hence the inverted, universal-tree symbol) were taken up by the Hindus as *Aswartha* (Blavatsky 1960) as well as by the Qabbalists, and the Tree of the Sephiroth resulted (Figure 4.1).

The symbolic value of the circle in original Sanskrit sources was that it circumscribed the extent of creation. Figure 4.2 shows symbolically the various

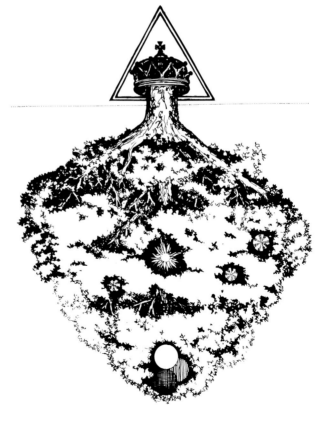

Figure 4.1: The Tree of the Sephiroth (redrawn from Hall 1962). The branches reach down into the earth and thence 'to the four cardinal points of the universe of matter' (Leadbeater 1926)

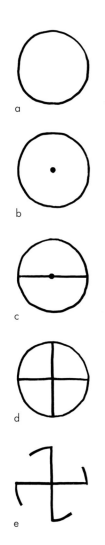

Figure 4.2: Aspects of the creative forces (a) the universe is circumscribed; (b) the seed; (c) the dual aspects of the universe; (d) the bipolar 'egg' of the universe is rotated 90 degrees; (e) matter is energised and the physical world is forming, symbolised by the rotating cross (Besant 1954)

Figure 4.3: (a) The Cross of Matter upon which is constructed Square of Matter within the Circle of Creation (b) the Pyramid is its third-dimensional expression

stages in creation from the first ordering of chaos to the creation of matter. The symbolism of the Hindu *Vedas* was adopted by the early Egyptians and resulted in the symbolic 'squaring of the circle' in pyramid design (Blavatsky 1960). It allowed the circumscribing circle of creation (see Figure 4.3) to be transformed into the circumscribed circle of the square pyramid base. The square base of the pyramid, a symbol for physical matter, is contained within the circumscribed universe (the circle).

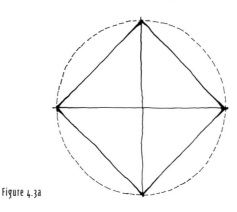

Figure 4.3a

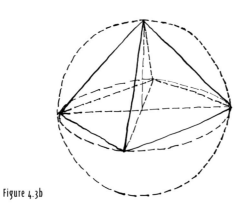

Figure 4.3b

The symbol had become the plan of a pyramid, but the symbol of creation did not contact the apex of the pyramid. This is where the ancient Egyptians appear to have taken a step beyond the Hindu *Vedic* symbols. They reduced the circumscribing circle (sphere) until it touched the apex of the pyramid. As the apex was the 'primordial point' of the first aspect of the Creative Force, it had to be in contact with the circumscribing circle. To relate the qualities of creation to those of the created world, the summation of the four sides of the square (symbol for physical creation) was made equal to the circumference of the inscribed circle (symbol for the whole field of creative activity). The circle had been squared while maintaining the integrity of all symbols.

Pyramids and healing

In the 1930s, the Frenchman Antoine Bovis found inside the Great Pyramid several small, dead, dehydrated animals. The animals' skin, bone and hair were intact, though in normal circumstances they would have decomposed. Fascinated, he returned to his laboratory and built a lightweight, scaled-down replica of the Great Pyramid. He found that in the climate of France, he could reproduce the results he had observed in the Great Pyramid in Egypt. The variables of the high thermal mass of the Great Pyramid and the low humidity of Egypt were seen to be irrelevant to the result. He went on to preserve fruit and vegetables in the same way. He, and later researchers in the 1940s, Verne L. Cameron and Ralph Bergstresser, were ridiculed because of their work, probably because the results could not be explained in terms known to empirical science.

In the late 1940s, Karl Drbal, a Czechoslovakian radio technician, discovered that he could resharpen blunt razor blades by placing them beneath a cardboard pyramid. He patented his discovery, but it took metallurgists a further 10 years to agree on how it worked. Minute air pockets in the steel trapped moisture, and it was found that entrapped moisture could reduce the strength of steel by some 22 per cent. When the pyramid and the blade were aligned north-south, the water dried out and restored the strength, and hence sharpness, of the steel (Stanway 1979).

Researchers Kerrill and Coggin (1975) found that they could alter the taste of food — make coffee taste less bitter, improve wine, lower the acidity of fruit juices — by utilising pyramids. Their experiments on enhancing plant growth with pyramidal canopies are said to have been successfully replicated.

In one experiment conducted by Kerrill and Coggin, blindfolded subjects had a pyramidal canopy lowered over them without their knowledge. After 30 to 45 seconds, their electroencephalograph readings showed that the alpha and theta components of their brain wave activity had doubled. Alpha rhythms indicate a state of relaxed composure, as in contemplation, and theta rhythms occur during deep sleep or meditation. Subjects reported a sense of weightlessness, warmth and tingling, accompanied by feelings of tranquillity and relaxation, and even time distortion, visions and dreams. Some reported clairvoyant and clairaudient (mental perception of sounds beyond the range of human hearing) experiences (Stanway 1979).

In other experiments by Kerrill and Coggin (1975), children who knew nothing about the experiments were placed in pyramid-shaped tents. Five of the 18 tested noticed no change, but 13 said that they felt warmth, tingling and other bodily sensations. One hyperactive child became happier and more contented and read his school books for a longer time than was previously possible. Women sleeping beneath pyramids for 4 to 16 weeks noticed altered and less painful menstrual cycles (Stanway 1979).

Stanway has hypothesised how the pyramidal form may work, by suggesting that:

> … certain electromagnetic waves are concentrated and condensed by the particular configuration of the pyramid. Conventional magnetism may be involved … because a Gauss meter [magnetometer] placed at the centre of even a non-magnetisable pyramid … shows a positive reading which increases in strength as the pyramid is brought into north-south alignment.

The effect is heightened with a steel pyramid, suggesting an association with the GMF, as such a steel casing would normally shield the interior from stray magnetic fields in its vicinity.

⊚ The pyramid's place in healthy house design ⊚

Though research into the effect of pyramids is continuing, for our purposes the case is strong enough to warrant consideration of the mathematically correct 51°50'34" pyramid form for the design of the healthy building. The remaining critical angles and dimensions are shown in Figure 4.4. Such a strong roof form may not appeal to everyone, though it is an ideal shape for generating a relaxing atmosphere conducive to alpha and theta brain rhythms.

A certain level of exposure to the pyramid form has beneficial effects on our health, but too much exposure may have the opposite effect. It is not advisable to follow the 'broad-brush' application of pyramidology practised by certain people, for example the American architect, Robert Bruce Cousins (Toth and Nielsen 1985). So how can the design of a healthy building safely utilise the principles of

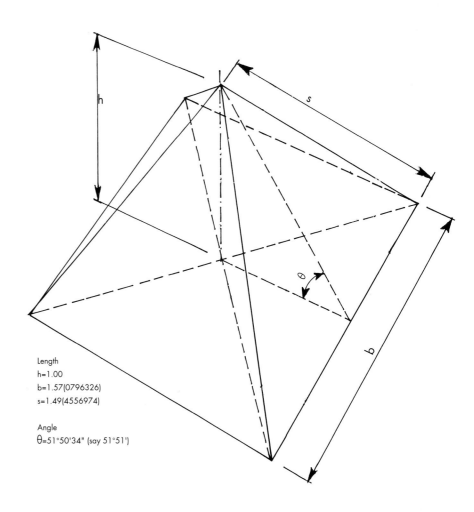

Length
h=1.00
b=1.57(0796326)
s=1.49(4556974)

Angle
θ=51°50'34" (say 51°51')

pyramidology without overexposing occupants to what Toth and Nielsen (1985) call 'anoxia', a condition caused by the body tissues not receiving enough oxygen? By using the pyramid (in its pure geometrical form) only over a courtyard and not over the remainder of the residence, it is possible to limit the exposure of occupants to the effects of the form.

Organic, rather than metallic, materials are generally preferable for permanent roofing, however, aluminium may be acceptable as it is unlikely to create its own magnetic field. Such a structure is better erected away from the main building where it can be used for meditation rather than continuous occupation.

One approach to handling the bioenergy enhanced by the pyramid form is to construct a frame pyramid over a central atrium or rainforest garden. The function of such a structure is to stimulate the growth of plants, not to stimulate the frequencies in the human brain related to spiritual thought and feeling. Such a frame is best constructed of an organic material such as solid or laminated wood.

Figure 4.4: The mathematically correct pyramidal form which can be used in the design process of a healthy building

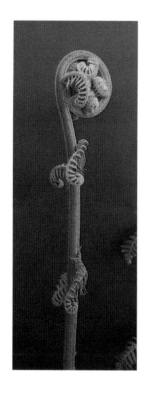

The spiral form occurs everywhere in nature: *Cyathea australis*, tree fern

Figure 4.5: Development of the golden spiral from the Golden Section rectangle

Hardy (1994) reports that all of the pyramid houses he knows of have been vacated after 6 months of occupation. His explanation is that the pyramid form caused the occupants to accumulate psychic tension and anxiety which could not be discharged. However, according to Schul and Pettit (1986), many pyramid house dwellers use buildings that are far from pure in form and are still living happily in them. The occupants claim to have become more 'healthy and spiritual' and that the growth rate of their children has been enhanced. There is a good case for long-term post-occupancy surveys to ascertain the real effect of dwelling within the pyramid form. Until such surveys are done, it may be wise to use the pyramid form mostly for the benefit of plant growth.

The ideas put forward by pyramid experts Hardy and Killick (1987) fit well into the Gaian philosophy. They emphasise the need to rehabilitate the planet after millennia of abuse of its resources, and the need for purity of intention without egotism. We believe the pyramid form can be incorporated into a lifestyle that respects Gaia, if it is used only in certain areas of the house: meditation spaces or atriums which stimulate the growth of plants. It is not a suitable form for a permanent dwelling, as it seems to energise the physical at the expense of unbalancing or overstimulating other aspects of the person, in particular the emotions and mind.

Were the builders of the Great Pyramid conscious of stimulated electromagnetic forces at times of sunspot activity? If so, the geomagnetic activity of the Earth must have been significant to the functioning of the structure. Schul and Pettit (1986) point out that many pyramids lie on agonic lines, lines which link parts of the Earth's surface that have zero magnetic declination. It seems reasonable to suggest then that pyramid builders were aware of magnetic declination and that zero declination must have had some importance in the building of the pyramids.

BIOHARMONICS

Having seen the effect that the patterns of our surroundings can have on our health and wellbeing, we now turn our attention to the question of how the dimensions and proportions of the house (including its furniture, fixtures, and fitments) can be integrated with the patterns of life and growth expressed in natural forms. This process is referred to as 'Bioharmonics' by Reinhard Kanuka-Fuchs (1993), director of the Building Biology and Ecology Institute of New Zealand.

⊚ Patterns of life and growth ⊚

The graceful appearance of a tree is the result of ease, economy of force, and effort. Although the beauty of a tree is not due to its precise observance of any archetypal mathematical formula of growth, but to its subtle differences from such a formula, the growth of plants in general can be described by certain geometrical formulae. The study of the geometrical patterns underlying plant growth is termed phyllotaxis.

In the 3rd century BC, the Greek mathematician Euclid defined a formula known variously as the 'Golden Rectangle', 'Golden Section' or 'Golden Mean', which architects such as Le Corbusier subsequently adopted in an attempt to develop proportional rules for controlling the overall design of a building and creating integrated architectural details.

The Golden Section rectangle (see Figure 4.5) is formed by drawing a square with four points: A, B, C and D, halving one side DC at H, then with a centre on the half-point H and a radius to the corner B of the square, an arc is dropped down to the base of the square, extended to F. The rectangle AEFD forms the

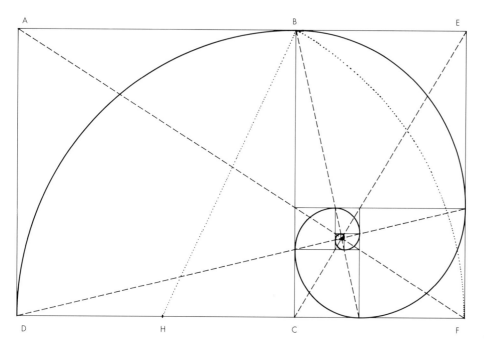

Golden Section, the sides of which form the ratio 1:1.618. The leftover rectangle BEFC has the same proportions as the Golden Section. If the new rectangle has a square marked off from it, the residual rectangle, again, is a Golden Section, and so on.

The 20th century architect, Le Corbusier, used the Golden Section because he thought that human life was 'comforted' by mathematics. This innate feeling for an integration of mathematics with art and architecture was also experienced by Leonardo da Vinci.

The proportions of the Golden Section are 1:1.618, or $(1+\sqrt{5})/2$, known as *phi* (a letter of the Greek alphabet). Try this yourself. First take three ordinary postcards (postcards are about the same proportion as the Golden Section) and cut a slot in each as in Figure 4.6(a).

Now interlock the cards and notice how their corners link up and describe the points and edges of a regular icosahedron, one of the Platonic solids.

◉ The Fibonacci series ◉

In 1202, the Italian mathematician Leonardo da Pisa (Fibonacci) described a mathematical problem, known as the Fibonacci series, which he illustrated with the example of the breeding of rabbits. A pair of rabbits produce another pair of rabbits. That pair, and all successive offspring, after they have reached 8 weeks of age, produce one pair of rabbits per month. In the first month, there is only one pair of rabbits. In the second month, there is still only one pair. But by the third month, the offspring have begun to breed, so there are two pairs. In the fourth month there are three pairs, in the fifth month there are five pairs, and so on. This process produces the numerical series: 1, 1, 2, 3, 5, 8, 13, 21, 34, 55 ... Each number in the series is always an addition of the previous two numbers. As the numbers in the series increase in magnitude, when a number is divided by the one before it, the resulting number approaches the value of 1.6180 or *phi*, the Golden Section, as follows: 1, 2, 1.5, 1.6, 1.6, 1.625, 1.6154, 1.6190, 1.6176, 1.6182.

Any series with this *phi* relationship between one number and the number before it is termed a 'Fibonacci series'. Scientists have since discovered the same pattern in nature, in the spirals of sunflower heads and snail shells, the coiled fern frond, the arrangement of leaves on stems, the spiral rotation of leaves growing one above the other on the same

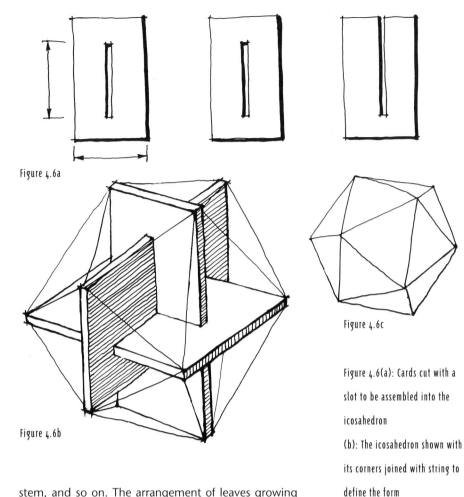

Figure 4.6a

Figure 4.6b

Figure 4.6c

Figure 4.6(a): Cards cut with a slot to be assembled into the icosahedron

(b): The icosahedron shown with its corners joined with string to define the form

(c) The icosahedron as a solid

stem, and so on. The arrangement of leaves growing alternately, that is, one leaf on one side of the twig, the next on the other such as in the maple or fig, is called 'half phyllotaxis'. In beech and hazel, one-third of a turn separates leaves, hence, 'one-third phyllotaxis'; in oak and apricot there is two-thirds of a turn; in poplar and pear five-thirteenths, and so on. Here is one of the 'mysteries' of pattern, the innate Golden Section and *phi* ratio in nature.

◉ Platonic solids ◉

Plato stated that any three-dimensional space can be filled, with no space left over, using any one of the five shapes known as the Platonic solids (see Chapter 1). The dodecahedron, which is made up of three Golden Section rectangles, is one of the solids. If these five solids exclusively fill all three-dimensional space, it is easy to see how they could also interact to produce the archetypal patterns of the crystal formation of matter.

The Platonic solids are one of many symbolic patterns which have been shared by vastly different cultures throughout history: the Tau cross (or Tau Key, see Figure 4.7), Celtic cross, ankh, swastika, the Platonic solids and the spiral.

Table 4.1: Comparison of the characteristics of the Platonic solids and their link to the Tau key

Platonic Solid	Number of Apexes	Number of Surfaces	Number of Triple Tau Keys	Number of Right Angles in all Surfaces of Solid	Symbol of 5 'Planes' of Nature in. Platonic and Eleusinian Mysteries
Tetrahedron	4	4 triangles	1	8	Fire (Atma)
Octahedron	6	8 triangles	2	16 (8 surfaces x 2 right angles)	Air (Mental)
Hexahedron (cube)	8	6 squares	3	24 (6 surfaces, each a square x 4 right angles each)	Earth (Physical)
Icosahedron	12	20 triangles	5	40 (20 triangular surfaces)	Water (Astral)
Dodecahedron	20	12 pentagons	9	12 (12 x 6 right angles to each pentagon)	Buddhi

* Note: A geometrical 'rule' says that the interior angles of any regular solid are equal to twice as many right angles as the figure has sides plus four right angles

Links have been found between symbolic forms used by prehistoric builders and the pattern of the GMF at sites on which they constructed mounds and megaliths. For example, at the ancient Rollright Stone Circle in Oxfordshire in the United Kingdom, it was found that the GMF was weakest at the centre and spiralled outwards in seven rings, increasing in intensity until it reached ambient field strength at the eastern portal of the circle.

The spiral has been a very important symbol throughout human history, first appearing on megalithic structures, dolmens and menhirs (ancient stone structures). Related to the spiral was the labyrinthine symbol which was incorporated into the megaliths in all continents and into the narthex of many cathedrals. The labyrinth was the path to be trodden by the penitent or the initiate, and probably permitted the human body to adjust gradually to the different intensity of GMFs prevailing at the centre of the path. At the centre the initiate suffered a symbolic death and a three day entombment followed by a 'resurrection' into the world of spiritual life. The spiral, the Tau cross and the Platonic solids are powerful symbols, an integral part of what Jung calls the racial unconscious.

Figure 4.7(a): The Tau key (b): The Triple Tau made of three Tau crosses, mnemonic for the hexahedron Platonic solid. Angle θ = 90°; 8 x θ = 720°

☺ Life fields ☺

Why does the practice of *feng shui* advise us to use octagonal or curved spaces around our bodies, or to change rectangular spaces by using screens in corners? Why do the shapes of food containers influence the quality of yoghurt and beer? Can the shapes that surround humans affect their health and wellbeing?

It is probable that, at the subatomic, atomic and molecular levels, the geometrical structures of our physical world influence our biological electromagnetic fields. It may be that resonance is at work, or that 'highly coherent electromagnetic energy is very probably what is involved in many varied, popular descriptions of the unknown and intangible, such as "vital energy", "life forces", "earth forces" and so forth' (Smith and Best 1989). In 1981 Rupert Sheldrake wrote: 'according to the organismic theory, systems of "organisms" are hierarchically organised at all levels of complexity … referred to as morphic units'.

Here is the 'archetypal pattern' or field of Pythagoras, the archetypes of the unconscious of Jung, the holistic field of Smuts and the morphic field of Sheldrake, the 'growth pattern' we have been considering. Perhaps this explains the mystery of single, human, embryo cells that beat to the rhythm of a heart, when no heart is yet present.

In the 1950s and 1960s Professor H.S. Burr (1972), neuroanatomist at Yale School of Medicine, demonstrated that physical forms and structures are organised and controlled by electrodynamic fields. He described life-fields, 'L-fields', which surrounded young salamanders. The salamander's L-field was

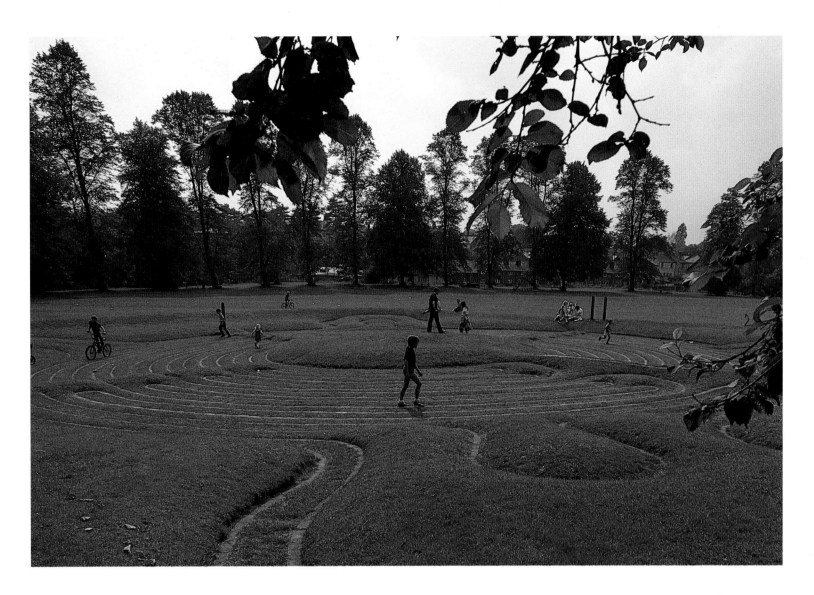

approximately the shape and size of an adult salamander, and its electrical axis originated in the egg before fertilisation. With bean seeds, the field approximated the adult plant. From these studies he concluded that an organism develops following a predetermined growth pattern. Along with Northrup, his colleague from Yale, Burr gathered conclusive proof that the human body's electrical potential correlates with an electrical pattern that organises the morphogenic nature, form, growth pattern and evolutionary direction of the organism.

Consider the cell division that takes place when a lizard loses its tail and grows a new one. Why a tail and not a leg? The lizard's growth pattern is affected by the 'tailness' morphogenic field. Sheldrake (1981) states that changes within a system can lead to variations and distortions of the morphogenic field. Consider how the electromagnetic pollution from a computer terminal could potentially modify the morphogenic field of the foetus of a pregnant computer operator. Sheldrake's theory may also explain the environmental changes that produce diversity in growing children, plants and animals. Polluted environments should be avoided, and current sources of pollution removed. Exposure may cause allergic reactions and disease in adults, but more importantly, could specifically affect the growth of the young.

It is time that science re-examined the ancient ideas of a universal, transforming energy or spirit which guides nature. The concept of an ordering field or archetypal pattern should be reviewed so that a more human and holistic vision of the energies currently referred to as electricity and magnetism can be developed. These energies define and sustain nature's patterns of growth. Once these patterns are better understood, the spaces in which we live can be designed scientifically so that they resonate with the healthy human body. Such holistic designs will create conditions that enhance the quality of life; the form of the pyramid has already shown that this is possible.

An ancient spiral maze, 115 m (75 ft) in diameter and 1500 m (4921 ft) long at Saffron Walden, UK

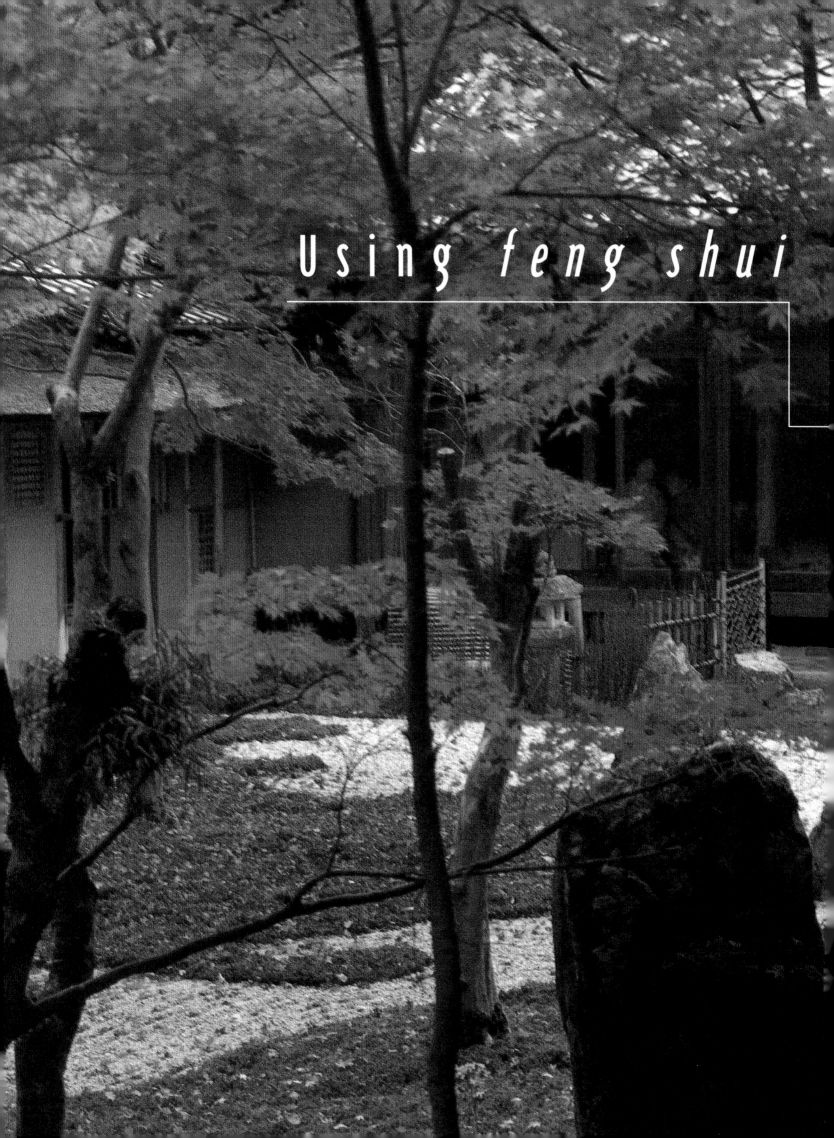

Using feng shui

in the healthy house

a blend of geomancy and astrology, the Chinese practice of *feng shui* is based on the principle that location in the universe affects our destiny. When buildings are harmoniously positioned in accordance with *feng shui* practice, life patterns are in balance and harmony with nature and the universe. Prosperity, health and equanimity follow for the inhabitants.

Ch'i is an energy that creates and breathes life into all organisms on the planet. It is important to understand its qualities and behaviour as its movement through a house affects health, prosperity and happiness.

EASTERN ASTROLOGY

Eastern astrology is an integral part of *feng shui*. Practitioners utilise astrology to gain an insight into the people who will be living in the house, then use that information to create a building which best suits their needs. For this reason, we need to have a basic understanding of eastern astrology. The Chinese zodiac animals are familiar to most of us. Each year is controlled by one of the zodiacs, for example 1995 was the Year of the Pig and 1996 the Year of the Rat. These zodiacs do not relate to constellations of stars, as we are accustomed to in western astrology.

The planet Jupiter takes 12 years to complete its circuit around the sun. The Chinese call this the 'Great Year', each 'month' of which is an ordinary year. Every year was termed an Earthly Branch in the ancient Chinese texts and the Twelve Earthly Branches defined a Jupiter planet–cycle.

About 1000 years ago these Earthly Branches were given animal names (See page 83).

Purple Crepe Myrtle method

The Purple Crepe Myrtle method traces the fate of the individual through the influences of the principal stars of the Great Bear constellations and its neighbouring stars. Purple is the symbolic colour of the Central Palace of the Heavens (including the Great Bear constellation referred to in China as the Northern Ladle) and the Crepe Myrtle is a revered Chinese landscape tree. Purple Crepe Myrtle astrology deals with the fixed stars, not planets (which are called the 'wandering stars').

THE TWENTY EIGHT LUNAR MANSIONS

There is a fundamental difference between Chinese and western astronomy and hence their respective systems of astrology. To people in ancient times, the sky appeared to rotate around a fixed point in the sky. For the northern hemisphere, in the present day, this point is the Pole Star in the constellation of the Great Bear. Thousands of years ago, this star did not coincide with the rotation point, but over time, a gradual shift has occurred. To ancient observers, the direction of that rotation point in relation to a person standing on the ground was always the same. The moon and the planets ('wandering stars') appeared to move along approximately the same path in the sky as the sun (called the ecliptic in western terms), but at varying speeds.

The sky was thought to rotate as a giant bowl with its axis joining the observer to the Celestial Pole. The axis was slanted up to the sky, as was the equator. This celestial equator was called the Red Path. The path travelled by the sun, moon and planets was called the Yellow Path. Certain stars along the Red Path were identified as signposts. The four seasonal stars were called the Green Dragon, the Red Bird, the White Tiger and the Black Tortoise. Ultimately, each quarter of the Red Path was divided into seven, making 28 divisions, known as *hsiu*. These 28 divisions can be imagined as uneven segments of an orange, and in this sense they are similar to the western zodiac principle, except that they are divisions of the sky and not the path of the sun, moon and planets.

Basically, the 28 *hsiu* or Lunar Mansions rule each day and determine an individual's destiny in two ways. As in western astrology, the first influence is from the presence of the Celestial Messengers, that is, the planets. The second is the direction in which each mansion lies.

THE PALACES

The sky is divided into five 'palaces'. There are two extra palaces (the first and last in the list below) that are not 'visited' by sun, moon or planets. Each of the palaces is associated with a direction in relation to magnetic north.

The palaces are:
- The Purple Palace of the Crepe Myrtle (*Tzu Wei*): celestial north
- The Green Palace of the Dragon: east
- The Black Palace of the Tortoise: north
- The Yellow Palace of the Emperor: centre
- The White Palace of the Tiger: west
- The Red Palace of the Bird: south
- The Jade Green Palace: south

PLANET	ELEMENT	CHINESE ASTROLOGY	WESTERN ASTROLOGY
Jupiter	Wood	The planet of *yin*, the feminine; rules over creation, birth, motherhood, creativity, physical appearance, virtuous love, happiness; Negative aspects: coldness of heart, slovenly appearance, uncaring, conceit	Creativity; Negative aspect: conceit
Mars	Fire	Symbolises government and administration; military leadership; courtesy	Top executives; military leadership
Saturn	Earth	Happiness and long life, safety, prosperity; Negative aspects: danger, disasters of the land	Conscientiousness
Venus	Metal	Associated with masculinity, *yang*, honesty; when visible in the daytime, indicates prosperity and change; Negative aspects: dishonesty, secrecy	Kindness
Mercury	Water	Symbolises knowledge; influences effects of other planets; Negative aspects: lack of commonsense	Influences the effects of other planets

Table 5.1: Comparison of Chinese and western planetary influences

FENG SHUI AS A DESIGN TOOL

As the 20th century comes to a close, interest in geomancy, or divination based upon observation of certain aspects of the Earth's behaviour and appearance, continues to grow. The popularisation of the Gaia hypothesis, the increased profile of dowsing societies, the revival of Earth-mother philosophies, and a re-evaluation of the feminine role in society have all contributed to this growth. Throughout the world, more and more people are beginning to embrace the concept that the Earth is a living entity. Ancient cultures treated certain sites where they believed Earth-energies were focused, as sacred. The rites associated with such places gradually led to forms of geomancy. These magico-religious rites and ceremonies were used to integrate human settlement with Earth-energies. From the Ohio and Pueblo Indians of North America to the prehistoric cultures of England and Europe, the relationship of Earth-energies to human life may be seen in the symbols and designs of the earth-mounds and megalithic structures which they built.

Arguably the oldest and most philosophically formalised of the ancient systems of integrating human settlements with Earth-energies is the practice of *feng shui* (pronounced 'fung shway'), a tradition which began in China, spread throughout Asia, and is now influencing building design in the West. The roots of *feng shui* can be found in the ancient book the *I-Ching* (pronounced 'yee jing'), or *Book of Changes* which was written during the *Chou* dynasty (1123–221 BC). The use of oracle bones, ancestor worship and worship of the spirits of nature date back even further, to the *Shang* Dynasty (c 1751–1111 BC). When *feng shui* is implemented, a vast resource of wisdom is tapped — wisdom that reaches back more than two millennia.

Taken literally, the term *feng shui* means 'wind and water', but in essence, it refers to the blending of spirit and matter. It is 'a thing like wind which you cannot comprehend and like water which you cannot grasp' (Michel 1975). It is based on an animistic belief that everything in the universe, whether organic or inorganic, has life.

Feng shui is used to divine the forces at work in the heavens and on Earth so that we can live in balance with them. Once we understand the forces at work in the cosmos and in the Earth's systems, we can harmoniously integrate our buildings with them, to optimise the health and good fortune of all occupants. According to the principles of *feng shui*, each living thing has its own niche to which it is best suited. *Feng shui* practitioners endeavour to refine the link between people and their niches, and to balance any prevailing disharmonies, thus creating harmony with the natural as well as the built environment.

Feng shui is neither a superstition nor a religion and, as science progresses, some of its causes and effects will be measurable in the future.

Yin and yang

Integral to ancient Chinese thought, including *feng shui*, is the concept of *yin* and *yang*. They are two polar energies that, through their fluctuation and interaction, cause the universe to exist. From the interaction of *yin* and *yang*, the Five Elements arose (Wood, Fire, Earth, Metal and Water), and from these the natural world was created. All things in the universe are governed by the duality of *yin* and *yang*, with *yin* characterised as the feminine, passive, dark principle and *yang* as the active, male, light principle. All inorganic and organic things, and natural phenomena, arise from the interaction between *yin* and *yang*.

According to the ancient Chinese, the first human was born from an egg which was dropped down from heaven to Earth, into the waters. Consider how this myth coincides with the scientific hypothesis that the first life on this planet resulted from the impact of a meteor.

Chinese texts describe how a continuous line of *yang* curved like the circumference of a circle to circumscribe the boundaries of creation, into which *T'ien*, the primal cause, breathed the primary creative energy, symbolised by the centre of the circle. This point moved outwards, to the limits of creation (the circumference), dividing the circle in two. *Yang*, as the first causative principle, and *yin*, are the dual aspects of creation, and the first and second lines respectively. The double line symbolises the two axes (the x and y axes of mathematics) that can generate two dimensional forms between them. This 'cross of matter', as it was termed by Blavatsky (1956) has its expression in the next dimension as the x, y and z axes, capable of generating three-dimensional forms when positive and negative poles generate a field between them. This field, in symbolic terms, is the polarised web upon which matter is created. On the line separating *yin* and *yang* a third

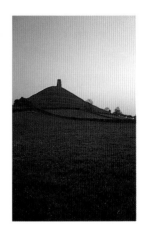

High prominences once used as foci for Earth energies in old astronomical religions became the sacred sites of historic times as in the St Michael Mount or Glastonbury Tor (with St Michael's tower at the summit) Somerset, UK

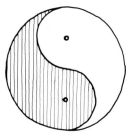

Figure 5.1: The symbol of *yin* and *yang* in creative rotational activity

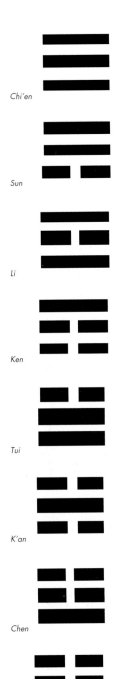

Chi'en

Sun

Li

Ken

Tui

K'an

Chen

K'un

Figure 5.2: The eight Trigrams

rotational force occurred, a stirring of all creation. This was the active aspect of Creation and is symbolised by the divisional line rotated through 90 degrees to form the 'cross of matter'. The trailing flames of the whirling cross become the swastika, ancient symbol of creative activity for eastern cultures. *Yin* and *yang* are manifestations of the Creative First Cause, *Tao* (pronounced 'dow'), or 'the way'. *Yin* manifests itself as the Earth and *yang* as heaven. The rotation required to create matter may be seen in the *yin-yang* symbol.

◎ The Trigrams ◎

The Trigrams are a series of eight symbols which were developed during the *Chou* Dynasty (1123–221 BC). *Yang* is symbolised by a solid line, and *yin* by a broken line of two dashes. All possible combinations of *yin* and *yang* are summarised symbolically by the eight Trigrams, each consisting of a different arrangement of three lines (either solid or dashed).

Each Trigram is read from the bottom line upwards. Those with a *yang* line at the bottom are more stable than those with *yin* on the bottom line. Remembering that the solid lines are *yang* and the broken lines are *yin*, you can see the gradation from total *yang* in the form of *ch'ien*, through to the development of *yin* in *Li*. Then follows *K'an* in which *yin* becomes greater until *K'un*, the completely female aspect, is reached. As the sun is in the south in the northern hemisphere, warmth and *yang* are also in that direction while *yin*, representing cold, is in the south.

◎ Ch'i ◎

Fundamental to the practice of *feng shui* is an understanding of *ch'i* (pronounced 'chee'), the energy that creates and breathes life into all organisms on the planet. It is important to understand the qualities and behaviour of *ch'i* because its movement through a house affects health, prosperity and happiness.

WHAT IS CH'I?

Ch'i is very difficult to define, and opinions vary on how to describe it. It flows like cold viscous treacle, or like cold air. For instance, the flow of *ch'i* can be controlled with doors. It can accumulate, becoming stagnant and exhausted, just as air can in a stuffy, crowded space. It can also be deflected and blocked in its path by the use of mirrors, just as light can. Yet it is neither light nor radiant energy.

Water can absorb certain kinds of *ch'i* in the same way that it can absorb gamma radiation, and *ch'i* has been found to carry radiation from a radioactive isotope. However, it cannot penetrate matter as gamma rays do, so it cannot be gamma radiation.

Ch'i is stimulating to the activity of the mind, so it may have something in common with the beta rhythm of the brain; focused thought can deflect *ch'i*. It may also be linked with the beneficial effect of an abundance of negions in the air. Like negions, a greater abundance of *ch'i* occurs on cliffs and hillsides, and it is said to be conducive to stimulated brain activity (as are negions), but not to relaxation or sleep. This activity is reminiscent of alpha brain rhythms and ELF electromagnetic field effects. However, it is not an ELF effect, as it does not carry electric charges and interact with electromagnetic fields.

To have all of these characteristics yet not really *be* any one of them, *ch'i* is certainly unusual. What the *feng shui* practitioner can be certain of, however, is that *ch'i* is active at every level. On an individual level we can observe *ch'i* as the energy flowing in the body's acupuncture meridians. In agriculture, it is what brings fertility to crops and vegetation. In our climate, it is the energy in the wind and water. To the Taoist, *ch'i* is also related to sexual energy, making sexual intercourse an act charged with cosmic energy.

Ch'i interpenetrates both heaven and Earth. There are three main types of *ch'i*: Earth *ch'i*, living in the 'dragon veins' of the Earth; heaven *ch'i*, which can overrule Earth *ch'i*; and weather or climate *ch'i* which mediates between heaven and Earth. Climate *ch'i* is made up of rain, fine weather or sunshine, heat, cold and wind *ch'i*. The wind (*feng*) carries and disperses *ch'i* while water (*shui*) contains it. Thus an optimum site for a house is one where the wind has been controlled to a gentle breeze and the house is contained by the curved shape of a watercourse or ponds.

The flow of *ch'i* varies throughout the day. *Yang ch'i* (vital *ch'i*) flows most readily from midnight to noon. Torpid *ch'i* (*yin ch'i*) flows as the sun declines, from noon to midnight. As the sun moves from east to west, the directions from which both *yin* and *yang ch'i* emanate alternate like the ebb and flow of the tide. These cycles are diurnal and seasonal, within the framework of the 60 year cycle upon which the Chinese calendar is based.

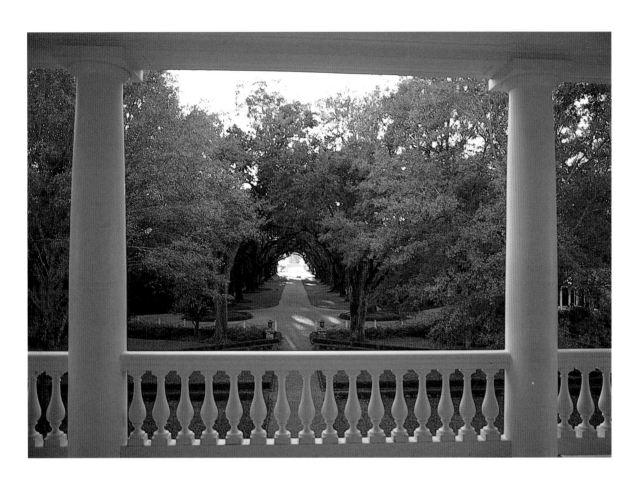

THE THREE ASPECTS OF *CH'I*

Sheng ch'i, the dragon's trail, is a meandering flow of vitality that has the potential to either improve or weaken the energy flow of a site.

Si ch'i is the name given to a curving path of ch'i which has been disturbed by the presence of a large structure, or even a large tree in the wrong place. *Si ch'i* eddies instead of flowing, and a stagnant condition results, deleterious to the health of the people in the building.

Sha ch'i is a carrier of unfavourable currents and if present, it must be deflected away from a site. *Sha ch'i* travels in straight lines and is focused by a line of power poles or transmission lines, a road, or a line of buildings angling toward a site. It is also present where geological faulting occurs, hence its link to geopathogenic zones. A long, central passage in a building causes *ch'i* to dissipate rapidly, hence such a corridor is considered a carrier of *sha ch'i*. *Sha ch'i* can also be channelled by valleys, gullies, tunnels, paths, roads, and corners of buildings, through a room by entering in one window and out the other or by being contained by opposite enclosing walls, by stairs located opposite entrance doors and by tall, vertical elements, whether natural or artificial.

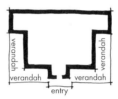

Fortuitous
1. This shape is often found on large rural properties in Australia

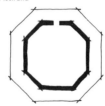

Fortuitous
3. This shape is good for finances, scholarships and marriage, hence, it an ideal family house shape

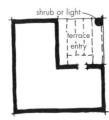

Unfortuitous
6. 'L' shape plan

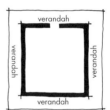

Fortuitous
2. Regular shapes are ideal for good *feng shui*

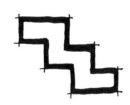

Fortuitous
4. This strong shape (resembling a lightning bolt) is often used in contemporary design as a series of linked pavilions giving good solar access and individual privacy to each section. The form of the roof should emphasise strength

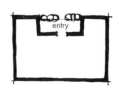

Unfortuitous
7. 'U' shape plan

Figure 5.3: Outline house plans showing various *feng shui* principles. These shapes have been chosen for their suitability to contemporary as well as traditional architecture

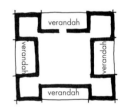

Fortuitous
5. This shape particularly enhances the accumulation of wealth, if this is required

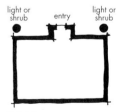

Unfortuitous
8. 'T' shape plan

Most unfortunate shapes can be corrected by locating bushes or exterior lights where dots are shown, or by squaring the shape with a verandah or pergola. This principle can be applied to other irregular plan shapes. In general, regular compact shapes are best. Complicated, irregular shapes need considerably more effort to reverse unfortuitous aspects.

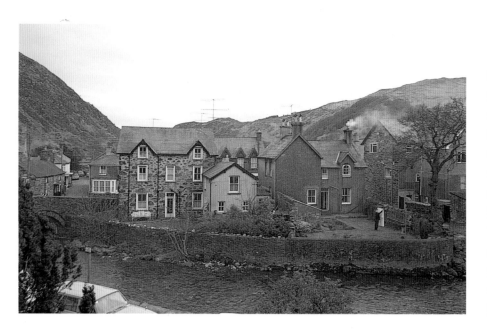

The maximum generation of *ch'i* occurs where the Dragon mountain of the west conjoins the Tiger mountain of the east. Beddgelert, Wales U.K.

CH'I AND ACUPUNCTURE

Said to have been practised in China for 5000 or so years, acupuncture deals with the movement of *ch'i* as it flows along what are known as meridians in the human body. The meridians are the pathways which connect 365 acupuncture points on the skin with specific organs of the body. While meridians do not exist in the same physiological sense as veins and nerves do, there is a perceptible decrease in the skin's electrical resistivity for a few millimetres (approximately $\frac{1}{10}$ inch) around the acupuncture points. *Ch'i* circulates around the body, through these meridians, 50 times a day.

In an experiment conducted by two French doctors, Darras and Devernejoul (Darras 1986), a solution containing a radioactive isotope (technetium) was injected into an acupuncture point and the movement of the radioactivity was traced using a gamma-ray camera. The velocity at which the radioactive material moved through the body was 3–5 centimetres (1–2 inches) per minute, which correlates with the rate of *ch'i* circulation through the body predicted by acupuncturists. The radioactive material moved along the paths recognised by acupuncture as the *ch'i*-carrying meridians of the body. It did not enter the blood or lymphatic systems, actually passed through a tourniquet, and diffused in the direction of a target organ. The rate of diffusion increased when the relevant acupuncture point was stimulated with a needle. The 'dragon path' of *ch'i* had been identified. It leads one to question whether it may be possible in the future to detect a similar meridian network in the body of the Earth. Only time will tell.

⊚ Does *feng shui* apply to all places on the globe? ⊚

Solar graphs used to find the angles of the sun in the sky and thereby determine how much sun will enter a site are designed around the sun being in the south of the sky (for the nothern hemisphere) and in the north of the sky (for the southern hemisphere). One is just an inversion of the other. Based on this, some have argued that the *feng shui* principles should be similarly inverted when used in the southern hemisphere. There is disagreement amongst many practitioners, some of whom believe that all the rules of *feng shui* apply in both the northern and southern hemispheres, while others claim that only certain rules apply to both, depending on the site itself.

When we set out to write this chapter we originally tried to follow the precept that all references to the sun in *feng shui* should be inverted for the southern hemisphere. This produced some strange, even ridiculous, results. Arguments made by Derek Walters, who has spent many years researching, writing and lecturing on the topic, were found by us to be convincing and reasonable. We concluded that the northern and southern hemispheres have no bearing on the way that *feng shui* should be applied to a given site, as evidence shows that the Chinese were well aware of the existence of the southern hemisphere, their astronomical pantheon even including *Lao Nan Chi*, the Old Man of the South Pole. The principles of *feng shui* relate to the position of the Earth in space, in a three-dimensional setting, thus the orientation of the stars significant for *feng shui* divination always remains the same, regardless of whether the site is in the northern or southern hemisphere.

Early Chinese settlers to Australia saw no need to alter *feng shui* practices for the southern hemisphere, as evidenced by several of their buildings which are still standing in Victoria. *Feng shui* was banned on the Chinese mainland with the advent of Communism in 1949, but as these buildings were constructed during the gold rushes of the 1850s, they exemplify the ancient traditions of *feng shui*. The buildings, located in Bendigo and South Melbourne, were built using northern hemisphere siting principles, such as facing the entrance to the southeast and making sure that no doors or windows pointed to the unfortuitous northwest.

Though the conflicts between solar access and correct *feng shui* practice place certain demands on building designers in the southern hemisphere because of the conflicting requirements of solar orientation and traditional *feng shui* principles, it is clear that those principles should be followed without alteration. We should ignore the exhortations of those who argue that inversion is necessary in order for the building to have adequate solar access. Thoughtful design can overcome such problems.

The practice of *feng shui*

Those in powerful positions [in Asia] do not take chances where feng shui *is involved … Hard-working businessmen [use]* feng shui *as an added tool to clinch deals, enhance corporate clout, or expand their businesses.* (Lip 1990a)

If we accept the Gaian hypothesis that the Earth is a sentient and self-sustaining entity, and the ancient Chinese belief that *ch'i* flows along the Earth's meridians, we are close to the model upon which *feng shui* is based. The *ch'i* flowing along the Earth's meridians can become sluggish under certain circumstances, creating zones that harbour pathogenic conditions. The *ch'i* can be stimulated by certain actions on the part of a *feng shui* practitioner, thus improving the health of the people living on the site.

For many thousands of years, southeast Asian and Japanese planners and architects have employed *feng shui* consultants when planning houses, villages, towns and cities. Although some modern Asian people, having lost touch with the tradition, treat *feng shui* like a superstition, many others, particularly in Hong Kong, Taiwan and other parts of Asia, including Japan, consider that no building should be designed without consulting a practitioner. The Singapore Hyatt Hotel's business is reputed to have improved greatly when the entrance doors and landscaping at the front of the hotel were redesigned following the advice of a reputable *feng shui* consultant. Not only do large corporations like the Chase Manhattan Bank, Citibank and Morgan Guarantee Trust employ *feng shui*, but also home owners, decorators and restaurateurs. Even grave sites are chosen using *feng shui*. It is accepted as an art, and reputable practitioners are often highly paid.

Feng shui practitioners use the balancing forces of *yin* and *yang* to harmonise people with nature by integrating the functions of a room, building or city with the *ch'i*, or 'dragon energy', of a site. *Feng shui* can be classified as geomancy, that is, divination utilising portents shown by the Earth. It complements and overlaps astrology. Its principles are carefully followed by a variety of communities, whether Buddhist, Muslim or secular. *Feng shui* can be successfully integrated into the western lifestyle, especially as it has some factors in common with modern landscape and architectural design.

Though they may not understand how acupuncture works, some medical practitioners use it empirically because its efficacy is well established. Similarly, though the exact workings of *feng shui* may also not be understood, benefits can be obtained by putting its principles into practice. Both acupuncture and *feng shui* are based upon the flow of *ch'i*, however, while the results of acupuncture can easily be observed (for instance, in the relief of pain), it may be a considerable period before the results of *feng shui* are detectable. With thousands of years of practice behind it, *feng shui* is worth including in our design process, even if some of the concepts involved challenge accepted notions.

The two schools of *feng shui* thought

There are two schools of *feng shui* thought, the Form and the Compass Schools. The Form School (or the *Kiangsi* Method) was the first to be formally established. Its patriarch has been generally acknowledged as Yang Yun-sung (sometimes known as Shuh Mei), who lived from AD 840 to 888. Yang Yun-sung's text, which used examples from the scenic formations of the beautiful Guilin district in which he lived, became the standard text for the Form School.

The school follows sets of rules about the placement of a building, its rooms and furnishings. Adherents to the Form School seek to interpret the surrounding landscape and environment, concentrating on the shapes of mountains, the directions of watercourses and the influence of the Dragon.

The Compass School (or *Tsung miao chih fa*) does not follow prescribed rules, but uses the *feng shui* compass to link aspects of a site with the personal astrology and familial status of the people who will occupy the building. Similarly, it can link the status of a company with the astrology of its founder (or date

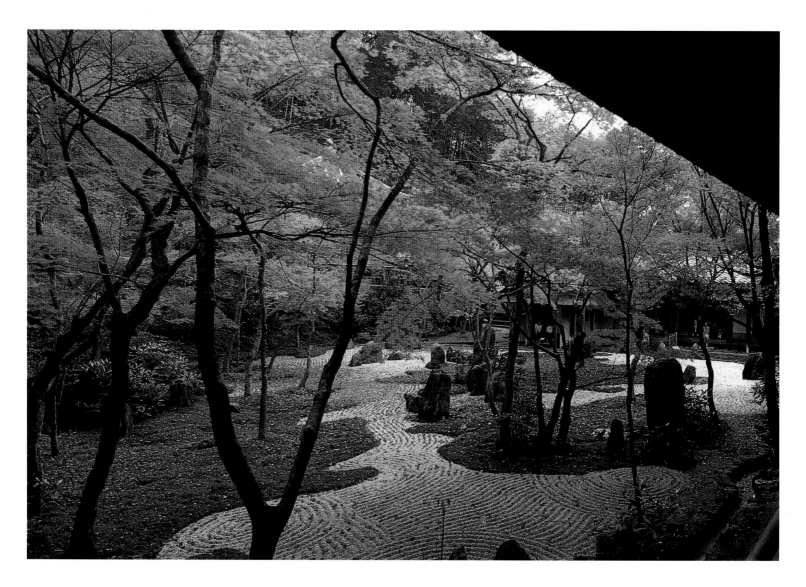

Vertical rock forms in the symbolic landscape of a Japanese *feng shui* garden: Konyogii Temple, Kyoto

of founding), to determine the location of a suitable site. The Compass School was formalised around AD 860 as a system which combines every influence that heaven can exert on Earth and on human affairs. It pays minimal attention to the configurations of the landscape and emphasises instead the planets and the Trigrams.

Planning for the circulation of *ch'i*

Many years ago we took note of some advice given by a Professor of Historical Geography: 'you should search for the symbolic form or pattern of architecture for the coming century'. After becoming involved in the design of earth-sheltered buildings (geotecture), it gradually dawned on us that the creation of curved voids (for example the 'dugouts' of Coober Pedy in South Australia and White Cliffs in New South Wales, Australia), seemed to reflect the general shift in collective consciousness towards a *yin* type of space

which was an expression of the feminine aspect linked to the feminist movement, the rediscovery of the 'earth-mother' archetype (as in the Gaia hypothesis), and the search for a female aspect of the Godhead in various religions. Our response to the professor's words is that the *gestalten* of contemporary building design seems to be the ovoid (*yin*) shape — the shape of containment — as exemplified by the cave. It is expressed in curved, hexagonal and octagonal forms, rather than rectangular ones. If rectangular forms are used, the structure should allow for the corners of rooms to be rounded or splayed.

Architecture based upon curvilinear shapes, such as geotecture, avoids sharp corners which create stagnant *ch'i*. Symmetrical rather than irregular plan shapes should be favoured. In the past, many have believed that conventional furniture will not fit into a curved-wall house, but you can avoid any such problems by making sure that the radius of the curve is greater than 3.5 metres (11.5 feet).

Ch'i follows a curvilinear course, thus if the front door is opposite the back door, *ch'i* will pass straight through and the beneficial effects of its meandering will be lost. To avoid this in an already existing house, use deflecting screens to elongate the flow path, remembering that *ch'i* behaves like cold, viscous air. The ideal condition is that the *ch'i* is able to enter through the front door, meander around the house without escaping, and eventually pass out the front door (or near the front door) again. In this way, the occupants will have maximum exposure to its beneficial effects. *Ch'i* can escape from open windows, but furniture can be used to deflect it.

◉ *Feng shui* terms ◉

THE SITE

The site is the specific place being analysed, whether an allotment of ground, a building or a room. *Ch'i* should be encouraged to enter the site and meander through it before leaving from the side opposite to where it entered. If a room is for working and concentrating, *ch'i* can be trapped for a while by reflecting it with mirrors. All rooms should have one opening door or window for *ch'i* to enter and one by which it can leave. Rooms that have one opening are only fit for use as storerooms.

THE LOCATION

The location contains the site and is usually limited to the surroundings visible from the site. It may be in bush or forest, desert, town or city. In all cases the panoramas from a site at any location are limited by some elements of the natural or built environment, such as tall trees, a spire or electrical supply poles.

THE ENVIRONMENT

The environment refers to the qualities of a location. It must be determined whether the environmental qualities of a location are detrimental or beneficial to the *feng shui* of a site. Detrimental features are to be counteracted and beneficial ones enhanced. This assessment requires the development of an eye for features in the environment, with the philosophical assumption that natural features are preferable to built ones. To try and develop the skill of isolating features in the environment, go to a window in the building where you are at present and observe both the natural and built features in the environment outside. Then find a window through which you can see as many features as possible, with a minimum of 20 or so.

Some features to observe are:
- In built-up areas: roof shapes against the skyline, blind walls, the closeness of adjoining structures, walls or any elements angled to form an arrow pointing towards you, parapet or roof ornamentations on nearby buildings, paths, drives and roads directed towards you, stairs, plumbing and electrical piping, natural features such as trees, grass, vegetated areas;
- In industrial areas: chimneys, tanks for storage of gas, water, chemicals, etc, cooling towers;
- Residential structures: houses, apartment buildings, terrace housing, large, isolated houses;
- Public buildings: schools, hospitals, churches, monuments and decorative 'follies' camouflaging sewer ventilation shafts, theatres and places of entertainment, obelisks, ornamental gates, civic monuments and arches, open civic spaces, market places, public incinerators;
- Public utilities: power poles and wires, high-voltage power lines and towers, street light poles, drains and culverts, water supply pipelines;
- Artificial features: ponds, reservoirs and dams, hedges, canals, sluices and conduits, public and private fountains, roads, bridges, railways, quarries, garbage dumps, tunnels, mine shaft openings, cuttings for road and rail;
- Natural features: mountains, hills and prominences, unusual rock forms, unusual skyline silhouettes or even small indentations in a distant skyline, large isolated trees, particularly pines, groups of trees, fields, lakes, lagoons, ponds and seashore, rivers, streams, creeks and rivulets, waterfalls, valleys and gullies, strata in rock faces.

In assessing such features, their magnitude and importance need to be kept in mind. Magnitude refers to the physical size or scale of the features. Importance refers to their impact on the individual, or on society in general.

ORIENTATION

Orientation refers to the compass direction that a site faces. A normal magnetic compass, or a Chinese compass (*Lo P'an* compass) can be used. The *Lo P'an* compass consists of a saucer-shaped dial rotating inside a square base plate. The base plate is fitted with two threads which are taut against the circular dial,

Figure 5.4: The Productive Sequence of elements:

Wood→ Fire→ Earth→ Metal → Water

Figure 5.5: The Destructive Sequence of elements:

Wood→ Earth→ Water→ Fire → Metal

Figure 5.6: The Mutual Control sequence of elements

Figure 5.7: The presence of Earth ameliorates the threat of Fire to Metal

Table 5.2: Relationships between the elements, planets, seasons, colours and cardinal directions*

and are aligned with the sides of the square base. In *yin-yang* symbolism, the Earth is the square (the base plate of the compass) and heaven is the circle (the rotating dial of the compass).

Derek Walters has expertly adapted the *Lo P'an* for use by westerners. On page 82 you will find a simplified version of his adaptation which principally reverses the north and south poles. (The standard western compass has its needle pointing to north, at the top of the compass, while the *Lo P'an* has the needle pointing to the south pole, at the top of the compass.) The compass housing (a small dial in the centre of the dial plate) is referred to as the 'Heaven Pool' after a constellation of Chinese astronomy close to the Pole Star. Moving outwards from the Heaven Pool, the first ring is inscribed with the Trigram symbols for the cardinal points, or 'Eight Directions'.

An exception to the normal use of the *Lo P'an* compass must be made when an existing house is being analysed. Should the front door not face the direction best suited to the principal occupant (discussed on page 81), then it is to be assumed that South on the *Lo P'an* compass is in the direction faced by the outside of the front door. The *Lo P'an* is then used without reference to its central magnetic needle.

◉ *Feng shui* and the five elements ◉

Fundamental to Chinese philosophy is an understanding of the five elements: Wood, Fire, Earth, Metal and Water. The elements are believed to form the link between all things in the universe. They correlate with five planets of great importance to Chinese astrology: Mercury (Water Star), Mars (Fire Star), Venus (Metal Star), Jupiter (Wood Star) and Saturn (Earth Star). The five elements are also related to the five cardinal points of the compass (Earth symbolising the centre of the compass), and to the seasons and colours: see Table 5.2.

Depending on the sequence in which the five elements are used, their relationships to each other can be either productive or destructive.

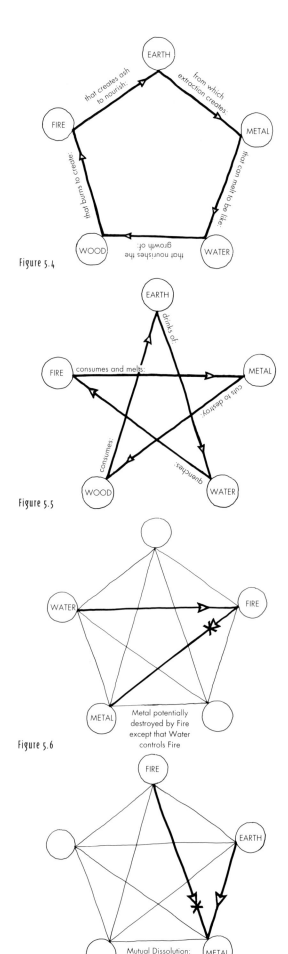

Figure 5.4

Figure 5.5

Figure 5.6

Metal potentially destroyed by Fire except that Water controls Fire

Figure 5.7

Mutual Dissolution: Fire threatens Metal and is ameliorated by Earth

ELEMENT	PLANET	SEASON	COLOUR	DIRECTION
Wood	Jupiter	Spring	Blue/green	East
Fire	Mars	Summer	Red	South
Earth	Saturn	Late Summer	Yellow	Centre
Metal	Venus	Autumn	White	West
Water	Mercury	Winter	Black	North

*Adapted from Skinner (1982)

THE PRODUCTIVE SEQUENCE

Follows the seasons of the year, as seen in Figure 5.4:

> Wood (fuel for Fire)
> Fire (produces ash which nourishes the Earth)
> Earth (from which Metal can be extracted)
> Metal (which can melt to become like Water)
> Water (which nourishes Wood).

THE DESTRUCTIVE SEQUENCE

When used in the destructive sequence, each element overpowers the next as in Figure 5.5.

THE MUTUAL CONTROL SEQUENCE

In the mutual control sequence (see Figure 5.6), one element will not be destroyed by the second because the third element can destroy the second. The destructive element is controlled by another element produced by the element under threat. For instance, metal would be destroyed by fire if it were not for the fact that water controls fire.

MUTUAL DISSOLUTION SEQUENCE

When one element is badly aspected by another, the presence of an intermediary element ameliorates the adverse influences of the threatening element. If Metal is threatened by Fire, the presence of Earth between them neutralises the situation, as in Figure 5.7.

INFLUENCE OF AN ELEMENT BY ITS ABSENCE

If all the elements except one are present, the missing element is the most noticeable because its negative aspect becomes dominant.

The *Po Hu T'ung* is a text which records the discussions of a council of classical scholars in AD 79. According to the *Po Hu T'ung*, Water is positioned in the northern quarter, where it nourishes all creation. As a *yin*-fluid it is always level, nourishing all things equally. In this sense, it is suggestive of the function of the universal ether of the ancient Greeks, as discussed in Chapter 1. It is also represented as the universal essence, or *monoke*, which, according to the Japanese religion, Shinto, interpenetrates all physical matter.

Wood is positioned in the eastern quarter, where the *yang*-fluid originates and the creation of things begins. Fire is located in the southern quarter, where the *yang* essence is superior and all created things burgeon and change. Metal is in the western quarter, where the *yin* begins to rise and created things cease to develop. Water is in the northern quarter, where *yin* is at its optimum level. Earth is located in the centre, the point from which all created things are brought forth. Each element has an associated landform and building shape.

With an understanding of the five elements basic to *feng shui*, it is now possible to consider what type of building is appropriate for a particular location with certain environmental features. The form and character of the building can be determined, as well as the appropriate plan shape and ideal arrangement of rooms. The elemental qualities of a building are determined principally by the building's form, not by the materials used in its construction.

Table 5.3: The five elements as metaphors for natural and built environment forms

ELEMENT	DIRECTION	COLOUR	SEASON	LANDSCAPE	BUILDING FORM	MATERIALS	APPROPRIATE FUNCTIONS
Earth	Centre	Yellow	Late Summer	Mesa or flat plain	Flat-roof buildings	Brick, earth-brick, earth, concrete	Storage, stock areas, occasionally-used areas, eg, lounge, parlour, garages
Metal	West	White/silver	Autumn	Rounded hills	Domed or vaulted buildings	Earth and metal combined, ferro-cement, rein-forced concrete	Functions incorporating metal equipment, tools, instruments, furniture, etc. Functions in which financial success is important, eg, banking, commerce, industrial production
Water	North	Black	Winter	River or lake, undulating irregular hills	Irregularly curved roofs	Major areas of glass (wood or metal framed); irregular curved roofs	Communications, public libraries, media and advertising offices, music rooms, brewing and distilling processes, computing and word-processing offices, places where electrical energy is a major use, eg, theatres, laundries
Wood	East	Green	Spring	Columnar mountains	Skyscrapers, vertical monuments or buildings constructed of wood	Timber	Functions involving: creation and growth, eg, studios, workshops, plant nurseries, kindergartens (play and rest); nourishment, eg, restaurant, kitchen; or residential buildings, eg, dining rooms, bedrooms, conservatory
Fire	South	Red	Summer	Triangular mountains	Steep pitch-roofed buildings, spires, churches	Metal	Intellectual functions, eg, university and school libraries; educational facilities; stove location in a residential kitchen

Feng shui's emphasis on form and shape is reminiscent of contemporary theories of pattern therapy and bioharmonic design, theories which state that the patterns and shapes around us have a critical effect on our lives and can be instrumental in helping cure disease.

CONTROLLING ADVERSE ELEMENTS

Consider a site that presents a potentially adverse environment, such as an Earth type of environment in which a Water type of house has been built. The juxtaposition of Earth and Water is a destructive sequence because Earth threatens to pollute Water. There are two means of controlling the situation. The first would be to introduce a third element to destroy the threat of Earth, such as Wood. Metal could also be used as a buffer, as Earth generates Metal and Metal contains Water. A design element symbolising either Metal or Wood should be introduced as part of the design. (See Table 5.5.)

It is important to note that the symbol of the element is dominant over the actual material used. In the case of Metal, for example, the symbol is the dome or arch. Any dome or arch, even if it is made from brick, will be a Metal symbol.

Another approach is to introduce a major material of an element which strikes a balance. This can be achieved by using materials that are of the Water element, such as glass, and metals like steel or iron. The Fire element is present in most materials that are manufactured by a process involving heat, such as fired bricks and metal products, however in metal products, the element Metal dominates over Fire as the principal element. With its combination of metal and concrete, reinforced concrete represents both Metal and Earth.

APPLYING THE FIVE ELEMENTS TO ROOM DESIGN

Consider the example of a room containing a window with a view of a power pole. The pole is vertical in shape, therefore is of the Wood element. A fish bowl with red goldfish is introduced into the room. The red of the goldfish is Fire, and the bowl is Water. As Water, Wood and Fire follow one another in the productive sequence of elements, harmony prevails and the threat of the power pole is neutralised. These principles can be extended to threats from any other element in the room by following Figures 5.4 and 5.5.

Table 5.4: Elements used to control threats*

ELEMENT OF THE SITE	THREATENED BY	TO CONTROL SITUATION USE EITHER
Wood	Metal	Fire or Water
Fire	Water	Earth or Wood
Earth	Wood	Metal or Fire
Metal	Fire	Water or Earth
Water	Earth	Wood or Metal

*Compiled from Walters (1991)

Table 5.5: Elemental features of an environment that can threaten a site (following Form School principles)

THREATENING ELEMENTS	THREATENING FEATURES	STRATEGIES TO CONTROL THREAT
Wood threatens Earth	Power poles, columns, pillars, trees outside a south window	A traditional three-element strategy is the goldfish bowl. Although the Water generates Wood, apparently increasing the threat, the red goldfish, Fire, is generated by Wood, thus balancing the Three Elements. Alternately, use metal railings or sculpture. Painting walls white (symbol of Metal) may also be appropriate
Fire threatens Wood	Pointed roof gables, hips and dormers; spires and pointed towers	Introduce a fountain, drinks dispenser or a tap. A compound solution is Wood (generates Fire) and Earth (generated by Fire) — a potted plant supplies both. (In general, consider a fire-control system in such cases.)
Earth threatens Water	Flat roof blocking out half a window; church with a tower (as 'demons' dispelled by a church occupy a nearby building); *sha* horizontal lines of threat	Wood is the controlling Element here, also the colour green and plant life. Perhaps a wooden carving, green decoration or the use of tall evergreen trees behind the building (never in front) could be used
Metal threatens Wood	Curved roof of a gas tank, statues with metal swords, spherical or curved water tanks	The symbol of Fire controls Metal, so consider candlesticks, incense holders or a hearth fire. For a compound solution use Earth and Water such as a water garden with stones
Water threatens Fire	Inauspicious shapes of water bodies in view; electrical installations	Single element remedy is Earth, represented by a large rock or ceramic ornaments. The compound solution involving Metal and Wood can be derived from a dried-flower arrangement in a metal pot. Metal and wooden chimes or sculpture would also suffice

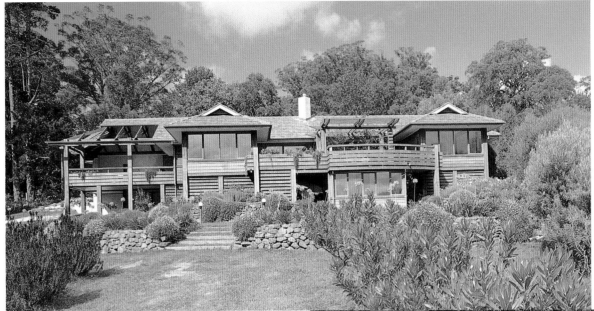

Left: Trees substitute for a hill at the back of this rammed-earth healthy house, NSW, Aust. (Architect: C. Pattinson, Arcoessence; Photograph: C. Pattinson)

◎ Building orientations ◎

When orienting a building on your site using *feng shui*, the following landscape features should all be taken into consideration:

• A building is ideally backed by a hill or mountain. Trees or high buildings can be substituted if it is not possible to locate your building near hills or mountains, because beneficial *ch'i* flows into the building while detrimental *ch'i* is deflected away.

• Conversely, the building should not face a mountain, high trees or buildings, as *ch'i* is restricted or prevented from entering a building by such blockages.

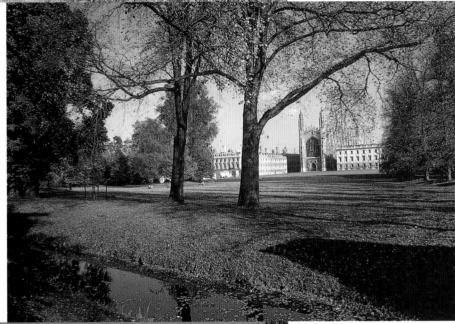

Above: The front entrance of King's College Chapel, Cambridge, UK, faces the river

Left: An adobe residence fortuitiously sited with hill behind, Sante Fe, New Mexico, USA (Architect/builder: J. McGowan)

The Healthy House

An arrow of *sha* (negative) *ch'i* is often created inadvertently, as in this restaurant in Sydney, NSW Aust.

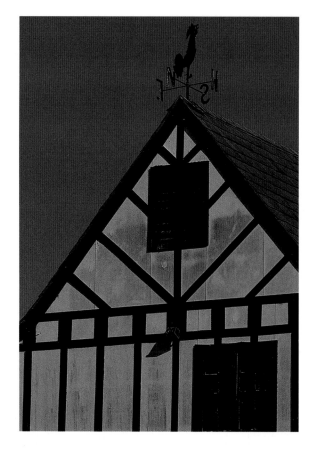

◉ The celestial animals ◉

Amongst the celestial animals of Chinese astrology are the Dragon, Bird, Tiger and Tortoise. These animals are significant to *feng shui*, and are represented by points of the compass, as shown in Table 5.6.

They also correspond to certain spaces within a given site. The Bird is the front door. The Dragon is at the right-hand side of the site to a person standing at the front entry. The Tiger is the left-hand side of the site, and the Tortoise is at the rear of the site.

The Dragon and Tiger are mutually coexistent. The Dragon and Tiger may not appear to be present in the landscape of a given site, but as they are omnipresent forces of the Earth, they are assumed to be present. The ideal site is one where each of these symbols is distinguishable in the form of the natural scenery. This sometimes requires the imagination of a child who sees fantastic shapes in the clouds. The more symbols that are visible the better, but at least the Dragon should be present. If symbols are not visible, statues of rock-shapes suggestive of the Dragon, Tiger, Bird and Tortoise can be used.

◉ The Water Dragon ◉

The Water Dragon Classic, written by the great philosopher Chiang Ping-chieh around AD 600, sets out the ideas of the Water Pattern School, a division of the Form School of *feng shui*. The Water Pattern School was developed by practitioners working in areas dominated by flat plains with few mountains. Without the presence of mountainous elements, practitioners in those areas needed to concentrate on another landscape element, such as water.

- The best situation is when the land and buildings on the left side of the front door are higher than on the right-hand side, as the flow of beneficial *ch'i* from the Dragon direction is deflected into the front door.

- The front entrance should not face a T-intersection of roads.

- When rivers, water bodies or waterways are nearby, the front entrance should face the water.

- When building near bridges or road and rail flyovers that seem to curve in onto the building site, the entrance should face away from these curved elements so they do not appear to re-curve back onto the building.

- Avoid all 'arrows', such as the forms of building corners pointing towards the house. Cover battens on gabled buildings can also produce problems. Such arrow shapes mean that *sha ch'i* will flow into the site.

WATER AND THE LANDSCAPE

- The ideal house has a flat, open stretch of land in front of the building, free from unfavourable arrows of *sha ch'i*. This clear area in front of the house should contain a semicircular pond, known as a *Ming T'ang*. This can be substituted with a wide courtyard.

- It is better to have water flowing towards a site rather than away from it. Water should approach the house in a sinuous line, rather than a straight one. If it flows in a straight line it becomes a carrier of *sha ch'i*.

- Water flowing away from a site should not be visible from the house or building. This can be

Table 5.6: Animals and associated season, direction and colour in *feng shui*

Animal	Season	Direction	Colour	Spatial relationship
Dragon	Spring	East	Green	To right hand of front door
Bird	Summer	South	Red	Front door
Tiger	Autumn	West	White	To left hand of front door
Tortoise	Winter	North	Black	Opposite to front door

achieved by ensuring that there is a curve in the river or stream so that the river bank hides the water. It is also possible to use a pipe inlet to divert the water underground, or a bridge to physically obscure the view of its exit downstream.

• Water flowing towards a site and then around it is beneficial to the occupants.

• Water flowing towards a site turning away is not beneficial to the occupants. Benefits are carried towards the site but never arrive.

• The use of water flowing along the Tiger (western) side and from the Tortoise (northern) direction (symbolising the Water element) is considered to be propitious. Ideally it should slow down and move through a *Ming T'ang* curved pool to the south (or entry side) of a building and out again. Beneficial *ch'i* will accumulate without becoming stagnant because it is eventually released at the outlet and flows away.

• A site at the junction of two streams has the added benefit of two flows of *ch'i* coming towards it.

• A site situated just downstream from the junction of two streams is ideal, as the full flow of *ch'i* from both streams passes each side of the site.

• Building sites are best located within branches of a watercourse where inner *ch'i* (the minor flow) is carried. Outer *ch'i* (the major flow) is carried in the main body of the river.

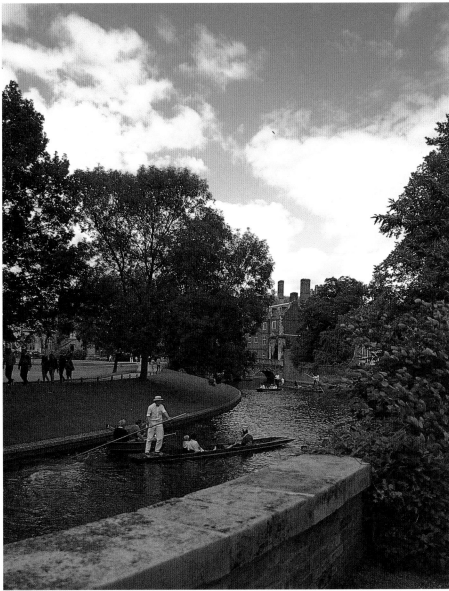

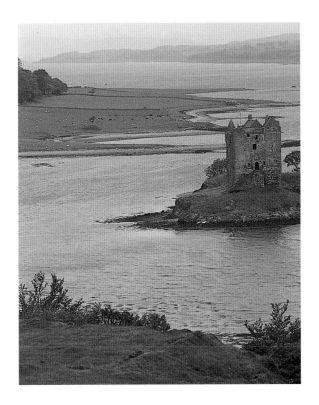

• The animals of the cardinal compass points, the Bird of the South, Dragon of the East, Tortoise of the North and Tiger of the West are not only linked with the seasons but also with the courses of rivers and streams: 'All dwellings are very honourable which have on the left [east] flowing water which is the Azure Dragon, on the right [west] a long path which is the White Tiger in the front a pool, which is the Red Bird, and behind hills, which are the Sombre Warrior [another name for the tortoise]' (Feuchtwang 1974).

⊙ *Feng shui* and interior design ⊙

The interior design and arrangement of rooms and furnishings is just as important to *feng shui* as the choice of a location and orientation of the house to the surrounding landscape. Following are some points to remember when designing the rooms of the house.

Above: Bridge obscuring the exit of water, River Cam, Cambridge, UK

Left: A medieval castle in Scotland where water flows towards and then around the site

THE BEDROOMS

We commence with the bedrooms, possibly the most important rooms in the house, given that at least one-third of a person's life is spent there, often in a passive state, receptive to all environmental influences.

General guidelines when designing the bedroom:

• Do not locate a bedroom over a garage or storage room, as stagnant *ch'i* is associated with such spaces.

• Except in tourist facilities, spectacular views should be avoided, as they provide too much energy for a bedroom.

• It is preferable that the bedroom have only one entrance. If the bedroom adjoins another room, that room should be one with slow-moving *ch'i*, such as a dressing room, another bedroom, or a sitting room.

• Avoid direct access to a bathroom. If an *en suite* is desired, buffer it from the bedroom with a dressing room or corridor.

• The bed should not face the door or be close to a window, as this will cause energy to drain away. If the bed must be near a window it should be separated from it by a table or chair. The door should open so that the head of the bed is not immediately in the line of sight. Ideally the door should be located diagonally to the bed.

• In an attic room, the bed should be situated so that the person in the bed lies parallel with the slope of the roof. There must not be any exposed roof beams over the area of the bed.

• The bedrooms should be the last rooms visited by *ch'i* as it meanders through the house.

• Because a state of quietude is desirable in the bedroom, mirrors are best avoided as they energise *ch'i*. If a mirror is necessary, it should be located so as to avoid giving a view of the door from the bed, or giving a view of the bed itself. Elsewhere in the house, mirrors may be used to deflect *ch'i* and move it around a room.

• The master bedroom should be sited away from the main entrance door to the house. A minor bedsitting room can be used as a buffer. Peacefulness is said to be improved by locating the bedroom away from the front door.

• The bed head should not be located behind the bedroom door (leaving only the foot of the bed visible from the door), as it is said to cause restlessness.

• If you were born in the autumn or winter, your bed head should face south, if in the spring or summer it should face north.

• Do not locate the dressing table opposite a door.

• Light colours are preferable in the bedroom. Strong colours should be used sparingly, for example as trims on a light background.

• Provided it does not actually reach the bed, light from the rising sun is beneficial in the bedroom, though it may be too strong for elderly people. Glare is adverse for all, so use sun-control devices such as blinds and shades. (O'Brien and Ho 1991)

THE DINING ROOM

Ideally, the dining room should be east of the kitchen; the second preference is south. It is best to have two entrances into the dining room, for example, from the kitchen and the sitting room. The dining room should not be closed off to the rest of the house, as this reduces the family's opportunities for becoming prosperous. In many Asian homes, the dining room is an extension of the living room.

Octagonal dining room tables are preferable, with each side facing one of the eight Trigram directions. Circular tables are also good as they symbolise heaven, and are said to improve the flow of *ch'i* between family members. A square table is considered acceptable if it is of the correct *feng shui* dimensions (this concept is discussed later). It is best that the table have four legs, but a single columnar base is acceptable. A rectangular table is less acceptable because it exaggerates the hierarchical relationship of the people seated. The effects of a rectangular table can be reduced by making sure it is not too long and is of the correct *feng shui* dimensions.

THE KITCHEN

In the kitchen, Fire and Water are in constant conflict, separated by the element Metal in the form of kitchen utensils. The kitchen should be located at the centre of the house, the centre representing Earth. If this isn't possible, it should at least be away from the entrance hall, which is the south or Fire side of the house, as this would conflict with the Water element of the kitchen. You should also avoid the north side of the house (the Water side), because Water threatens the Fire of cooking, but if you cannot avoid having the kitchen on the north side of the house, make sure it at least has west-facing windows, correctly controlled for heat and glare. The west (Metal) side of the house is a good compromise location for the kitchen.

The kitchen should be located away from the bathroom. If this is impractical, separate them with a passage or wall of storage space. A bathroom must never be located above the kitchen in a two-storey construction.

The stove should be located on the south (Fire) side of the room, separated from the sink by bench space. Metal utensils should be stored on the left-hand side of the stove. Should it be necessary to eat in the kitchen for informal meals, the space for that function should be separated from the space used for cooking and food preparation, and should be to the east or south of the cooking area.

THE STUDY/WORKROOM

A room for quiet study or work is best located on the north (Water) side of the house because of this element's connection with communication. In the northern hemisphere this provides ideal non-glare lighting conditions. In the southern hemisphere, it allows warm, winter sun to penetrate, but good solar control is required to eliminate glare, considered a source of bad *ch'i*. Working and writing tables need to be at an angle to the line of a window to reduce glare.

BATHROOMS AND LAUNDRIES

Bathrooms and laundries use a lot of water and hence they belong on the north (Water) side of a dwelling or of the rooms that they service. All toilets should have direct openings to the outside air, which is easily achieved by the use of ventilating skylights. Unless light is plentiful, plants should not be used in bathrooms, as they inhibit the flow of *ch'i*.

LIVING ROOMS

Winter warmth from the sun can be maximised in the living room by having north-facing windows in the southern hemisphere, or south-facing ones in the northern hemisphere, with a separate greenhouse to warm the overall space. This important room is compromised somewhat if it faces east or west, with solar control becoming more difficult. If you cannot avoid having the living room facing east or west, plant deciduous trees outside.

No chairs should directly face doors or windows, nor should they have their backs to them. Placement of furniture should be such that meandering *ch'i* can wander throughout the room. Guests should always be seated in the master position, facing south. Chairs should not be too close to coffee tables or positioned under ceiling beams, or facing the corners of projecting columns or wall junctions.

It is best to arrange the furniture in a regular pattern, especially an octagonal pattern, like the eight-sided mirror known as the *Pa Kua*, sometimes used by *feng shui* practitioners to protect a building from bad *ch'i*. Avoid L-shaped arrangements.

STAIRCASES

A hall with stairs facing a door destroys the flow of *ch'i* in a building. To counteract this effect, the staircase should be at right angles to the door, or out of sight of it. The staircase should not be in the middle of a building, but if this cannot be avoided, the lowest tread should be turned at an angle to the front door. Otherwise, a screen should be used in front of the stairs, or a mirror placed on the intermediate landing.

WALLS, DOORS AND WINDOWS

There should be at least one wall in a room which does not have doors or windows. That wall may contain a fireplace, but the best location for a fireplace is on the wall which contains the entry door, as this allows *ch'i* to fully circulate around the room then flow on.

Windows and doors should not face each other. If corner windows must be used, a free-standing screen can be employed in the corner to focus the outlooks of both directions. Windows should preferably open outwards. The use of air-circulating fans will also help move *ch'i* around the room.

If there is no view from a window, draw attention away from that fact by creating other attractive features in the room, for example, a permanent flower arrangement, a statue, indoor plants, or a wall hanging, and use curtains or blinds on the window, particularly if an arrow of *sha* is focused into the room, threatening the occupants.

COLOURS

Green, blue and turquoise tones are good for promoting growth and harmony in east-facing rooms. They also convey a sense of coolness in warm

ELEMENT	COLOUR	COMMENT
Wood	blue-green	blue of sky, green of plants
Fire	red	good fortune
Earth	yellow	yellow river silt, also means 'royal'
Metal	white	metallic and silver (silvery grey)
Water	black	brings good luck

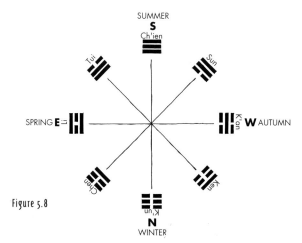

Figure 5.8

climates. Red tints and pinks are best used in south-facing rooms and are ideally suited to the southern hemisphere where warmth is needed because those rooms receive limited sunlight. Autumn tones and yellow pastels are good for rooms facing west, but in a hot climate, they may not be suitable, given the need for cool colours on the hot side of the house. If it is necessary to make a compromise, design the room using autumn tones.

In the north-facing rooms, pale colours are recommended, with the occasional black trim. In the southern hemisphere, such a colour scheme may be quite glary and need curtains or even shutters for hot summer days. If any of the colours conflict with taste or practicality, the *feng shui* practitioner would probably recommend a token use of the colour on small features in the room.

MIRRORS AND FISH TANKS

Mirrors can be used to stimulate the flow of *ch'i* around a room. Carved tracery screens are often used to deflect *ch'i*. They can be placed in difficult corners of a room to avoid an arrow of *sha* or the stagnation of *ch'i*. Fish tanks and pools of water can be used to collect *ch'i*, and as fish are thought to stimulate *ch'i* by their movement, the vortices they create make the body of water a resource of *ch'i*.

◉ Simplified Compass School method ◉

The Compass School of *feng shui* classifies a site or building according to its Trigram. Trigrams represent the essence of change, governing all choices and changes in life. Each Trigram has a cardinal direction and represents the type of use for which a space, room or location is appropriate. Before the Trigrams can be used to assess a site, it is necessary to know which Trigrams govern which directions of the compass and what their symbolism means.

FORMER HEAVEN SEQUENCE: This sequence is seen on the inner ring of the base plate of the *Lo P'an* compass and on talismans used by Chinese geomancers. Tradition holds that the Former Heaven Sequence was formulated by the Emperor Fu Hsia who was revered as one of China's first wise men and was the inventor of the Chinese calendar. In this sequence, the eight Trigrams are connected to the seasons. The absolute *yang* begins to wane in midsummer (*Ch'ien*), *yin* gradually interpenetrates at late summer (*Sun*), moving on to the balance of autumn (*K'an*), then midwinter (*K'un*). *Yin* begins to lessen as *yang* interpenetrates in *Chen*, moving towards the balance of Spring (*Li*) and on to early summer (*Tui*) and back to midsummer (*Ch'ien*).

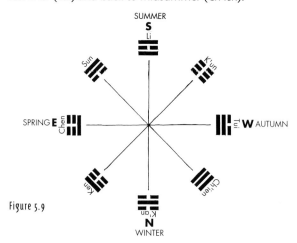

Figure 5.9

LATER HEAVEN SEQUENCE: In the *I-Ching* another sequence of these Trigrams is nominated, known as the Later Heaven Sequence. Its development is attributed to King Wen (1160 BC), who assigned cryptic interpretations to the Trigrams. This sequence appears on the base plate of the *Lo P'an* compass. The order of the Trigrams represents the balance of *yin* and *yang* at particular locations on the ground. A reading from the Earth (and site) is compared with a reading from the Former Heaven Sequence, thereby balancing the cosmic and localised *yin* and *yang*.

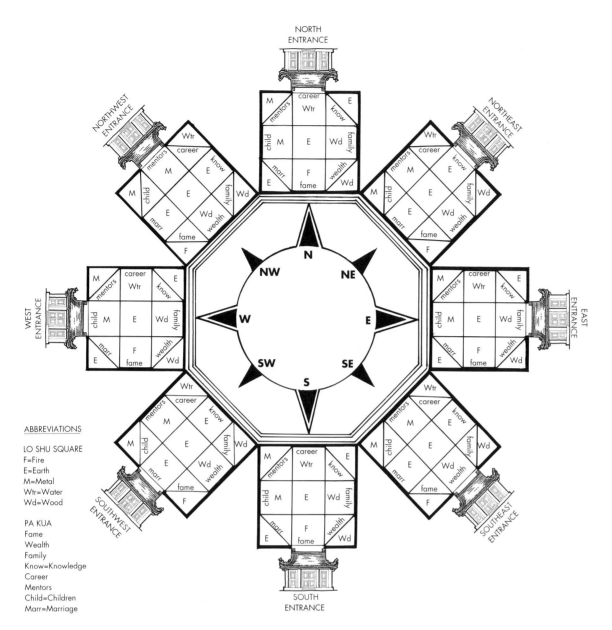

Figure 5.10: The Eight
Orientations and variations in
the Nine Portent Zones of each
(after Walters 1993 and Too 1993)

ABBREVIATIONS

LO SHU SQUARE
F=Fire
E=Earth
M=Metal
Wtr=Water
Wd=Wood

PA KUA
Fame
Wealth
Family
Know=Knowledge
Career
Mentors
Child=Children
Marr=Marriage

The Trigram relevant to a building is governed by the direction the front door faces, so our first step is to work out the orientation of the building. The Chinese classic, *Book of Rites*, prescribed the placement of rooms for the south-facing palace of the emperor. These precepts were subsequently adapted to suit the homes of people of lower rank, whose buildings did not face the warm south. These ideas became a formalised system for the correct placement of functions within a building to create harmony. Placement is determined by an interaction of the Former and Later Heaven Sequence of Trigrams.

Following is a simplified step-by-step version of a Compass School method for planning the layout of a house. A *feng shui* consultant would use a more complex, and hence more accurate, method but this one will be a good start towards planning your home.

STEP ONE: You will first need to collect the astrological details of the people who will be living in the house. You need to know each person's Chinese zodiac sign and the element that has the most favourable effect upon them, that is, the one that comes before theirs in the productive sequence of elements (discussed on page 72).

This information can be found by consulting Table 5.8 on page 83. Simply look up the year in which the person was born. (Please note that the years listed in the table commence on the first day of the Chinese New Year, which differs from year to year.) The person's zodiac sign can be found in the left hand column. Listed directly under their year of birth is their element. The element next to this in brackets is their favourable element. For example, a person born in January 1965 is a Wood Dragon and their favourable element is the one listed in brackets: Water.

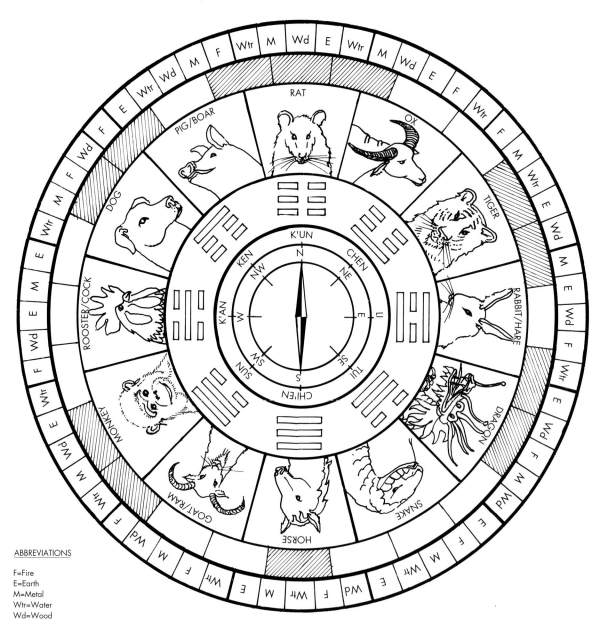

ABBREVIATIONS

F=Fire
E=Earth
M=Metal
Wtr=Water
Wd=Wood

Figure 5.11: Modified Western version of *Lo P'an* compass

(abbreviated from Walters 1989)

ANIMAL	NEW YEAR DATE/ELEMENT (FAVOURABLE ELEMENT) FOR THAT YEAR								
Rat	31 Jan 1900 Metal (Earth)	18 Feb 1912 Water (Metal)	5 Feb 1924 Wood (Water)	24 Jan 1936 Fire (Wood)	28 Jan 1948 Earth (Fire)	28 Jan 1960 Metal (Earth)	16 Feb 1972 Water (Metal)	2 Feb 1984 Wood (Water)	19 Feb 1996 Fire (Wood)
Ox	19 Feb 1901 Metal (Earth)	6 Feb 1913 Water (Metal)	25 Jan 1925 Wood (Water)	11 Feb 1937 Fire (Wood)	29 Jan 1949 Earth (Fire)	15 Feb 1961 Metal (Earth)	3 Feb 1973 Water (Metal)	20 Feb 1985 Wood (Water)	7 Feb 1997 Fire (Wood)
Tiger	8 Feb 1902 Water (Metal)	26 Jan 1914 Wood (Water)	13 Feb 1926 Fire (Wood)	3 Jan 1938 Earth (Fire)	17 Feb 1950 Metal (Earth)	5 Feb 1962 Water (Metal)	3 Jan 1974 Wood (Water)	9 Feb 1986 Fire (Wood)	28 Jan 1998 Earth (Fire)
Cat	29 Jan 1903 Water (Metal)	14 Feb 1915 Wood (Water)	2 Feb 1927 Fire (Wood)	19 Feb 1939 Earth (Fire)	6 Feb 1951 Metal (Earth)	25 Jan 1963 Water (Metal)	11 Feb 1975 Wood (Water)	29 Jan 1987 Fire (Wood)	16 Feb 1999 Earth (Fire)
Dragon	16 Feb 1904 Wood (Water)	3 Feb 1916 Fire (Wood)	23 Jan 1928 Earth (Fire)	8 Feb 1940 Metal (Earth)	27 Jan 1952 Water (Metal)	13 Feb 1964 Wood (Water)	31 Jan 1976 Fire (Wood)	17 Feb 1988 Earth (Fire)	5 Feb 2000 Metal (Earth)
Snake	4 Feb 1905 Wood (Water)	23 Jan 1917 Fire (Wood)	10 Feb 1929 Earth (Fire)	27 Jan 1941 Metal (Earth)	14 Feb 1953 Water (Metal)	2 Feb 1965 Wood (Water)	18 Feb 1977 Fire (Wood)	6 Feb 1989 Earth (Fire)	24 Jan 2001 Metal (Earth)
Horse	25 Jan 1906 Fire (Wood)	11 Feb 1918 Earth (Fire)	30 Jan 1930 Metal (Earth)	15 Feb 1942 Water (Metal)	3 Feb 1954 Wood (Water)	21 Jan 1966 Fire (Wood)	7 Feb 1978 Earth (Fire)	27 Jan 1990 Metal (Earth)	12 Feb 2002 Water (Metal)
Goat	13 Feb 1907 Fire (Wood)	1 Feb 1919 Earth (Fire)	17 Feb 1931 Metal (Earth)	5 Feb 1943 Water (Metal)	24 Jan 1955 Wood (Water)	9 Feb 1967 Fire (Wood)	28 Jan 1979 Earth (Fire)	15 Feb 1991 Metal (Earth)	1 Feb 2003 Water (Metal)
Monkey	2 Feb 1908 Earth (Fire)	20 Feb 1920 Metal (Earth)	6 Feb 1932 Water (Metal)	25 Jan 1944 Wood (Water)	12 Feb 1956 Fire (Wood)	30 Jan 1968 Earth (Fire)	16 Feb 1980 Metal (Earth)	4 Feb 1992 Water (Metal)	22 Jan 2004 Wood (Water)
Rooster	22 Jan 1909 Earth (Fire)	8 Feb 1921 Metal (Earth)	26 Jan 1933 Water (Metal)	13 Feb 1945 Wood (Water)	31 Jan 1957 Fire (Wood)	17 Feb 1969 Earth (Fire)	5 Feb 1981 Metal (Earth)	23 Jan 1993 Water (Metal)	9 Feb 2005 Wood (Water)
Dog	10 Feb 1910 Metal (Earth)	28 Jan 1922 Water (Metal)	14 Feb 1934 Wood (Water)	2 Feb 1946 Fire (Wood)	18 Feb 1958 Earth (Fire)	6 Feb 1970 Metal (Earth)	25 Jan 1982 Water (Metal)	10 Feb 1994 Wood (Water)	29 Jan 2006 Fire (Wood)
Pig	30 Jan 1911 Metal (Earth)	16 Feb 1923 Water (Metal)	4 Feb 1935 Wood (Water)	22 Jan 1947 Fire (Wood)	8 Feb 1959 Earth (Fire)	27 Jan 1971 Metal (Earth)	13 Feb 1983 Water (Metal)	31 Jan 1995 Wood (Water)	18 Feb 2007 Fire (Wood)

* from the *Chinese Ten Thousand Years (Perpetual) Lunar Calendar*. (The first day of the lunar New Year varies from year to year, and falls either in January or February.)

On a piece of paper, list all the members of the household, principal householder first. The major income earner is generally considered to be the principal householder. Write down the principal householder's zodiac sign and favourable element. Then list the favourable elements of the other householders.

STEP TWO: From a *feng shui* point of view, the most fundamental decision you need to make is which direction the house will face. In *feng shui* practice this means the direction the front door faces, that is, the direction you face if you stand at the front door and look out.

Now refer to Figure 5.11 (opposite page), which is the *Lo P'an* compass modified for western usage. (Unlike the Chinese *Lo P'an*, which has south at the top, our compass has north at the top, to conform to western convention.) Locate the animal sign of the principal householder on the *Lo P'an*. Moving outwards from the animal sign, look at the next ring, which is

Table 5.8: Eastern Astrological Chart 1900–2007*

Figure 5.12: Southern elevation of the case study family's house, incorporating a pyramidal structure over a central atrium

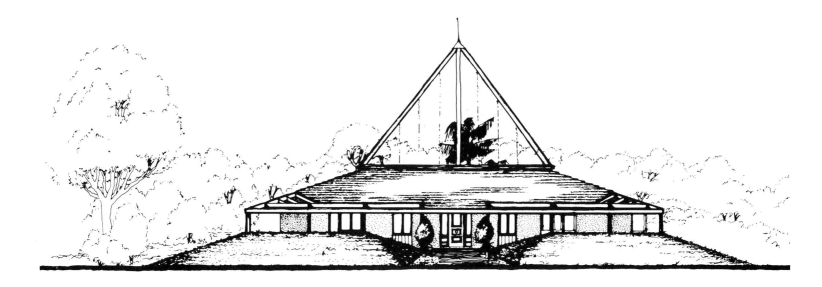

DIVISION	NAME	POSITION ON FENG SHUI SCALE (MM)	POSITION ON FENG SHUI SCALE (IN)	PORTENDING
I**	Ts'ai	0.00 to 53.88	0.00 to 2.12	Wealth
II	Ping	53.88 to 107.76	2.12 to 4.24	Sickness
III	Li	107.76 to 161.64	4.24 to 6.36	Separation
IV**	I	161.64 to 215.53	6.36 to 8.49	Righteousness
V**	Kuan	215.53 to 269.41	8.49 to 10.61	Promotion
VI	Chieh	269.41 to 323.29	10.61 to 12.73	Robbery
VII	Hai	323.29 to 377.17	12.73 to 14.85	Accident
VIII**	Pen	377.17 to 431.05	14.85 to 16.97	Source
		** Dimensions to be used for resonance with good fortune		

Table 5.9: Divisions of the *feng shui* foot and their portents (Walters 1988)

made up of a series of shaded and unshaded segments. If there is a shaded segment next to the principal householder's animal sign, look to the inner circle of the *Lo P'an* to see which direction the segment lines up with. This is the direction the front door of the house should face. If the ring includes two or three shaded segments, then the front door can face any direction within the range of those segments. To establish the direction with greater accuracy in such a circumstance, or if the zodiac sign has only blank segments next to it, move to the outside ring and find the principal householder's favourable element. The direction that it lines up with in the innermost ring is the most favourable direction for the front door to face.

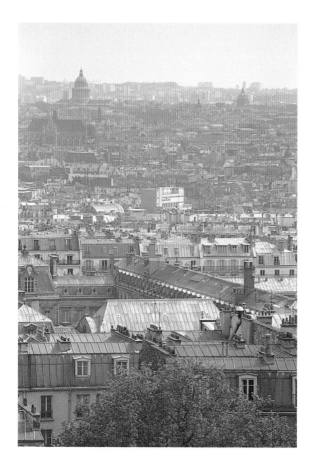

A line of *sha ch'i* is formed by the long roof in the foreground of this view of Paris. The arrow of *sha* points directly at the mansard-roofed tenements in the middle ground

STEP THREE: Now that you have chosen the direction of your front door, and hence the overall orientation of your house, you can calculate which zones of that building will be most suited as bedrooms for the people who will be living in the house. Go to Figure 5.10 on page 81 and find the house that has its front door facing the same intended direction as yours. Note that the house has been divided into nine zones, each of which is governed by a particular element. Compare each individual's favourable element with the elements of the zones of the house. An individual will be suited to a zone if it is the same as their favourable element. (If the zone is the same as the individual's actual element, the effect will be neutral.)

Note that the outermost zones of the house are marked with the words: wealth, family, knowledge, marriage, fame, children, mentors, wealth and family. These are known as the Eight Life Situations. A certain part of your life will be enhanced by the Life Situation of your favourable zone. For instance, if your building is south-facing and your favourable element is Water, the Life Situation corresponding to your most favourable zone is 'career', so your career will be enhanced by using that zone as your bedroom.

STEP FOUR: Lastly, you will need to decide the best location for rooms where a number of people will interact, such as the dining room and living room. Keeping in mind the general principles of room location (see pages 78 and 79), try to choose a zone that is of the same favourable element as that shared by the majority of people who will use the room.

⊛ Incorporating *feng shui* analysis ⊛
The information you gather through *feng shui* analysis can be summarised to show the relationships between the spaces allocated to various functions and the elements of the occupants. We have designed a house based on the birth details of all the members of a hypothetical family: a retired couple who have their children and grandchildren to stay for long periods. We will track the design process of the house in following chapters. It was decided that the most appropriate building form for the *feng shui* of the family's woodland site was the pyramid (see Table 5.11 on page 86). We incorporated the family's Chinese horoscopes into a house design which included the pyramid shape as a major design element.

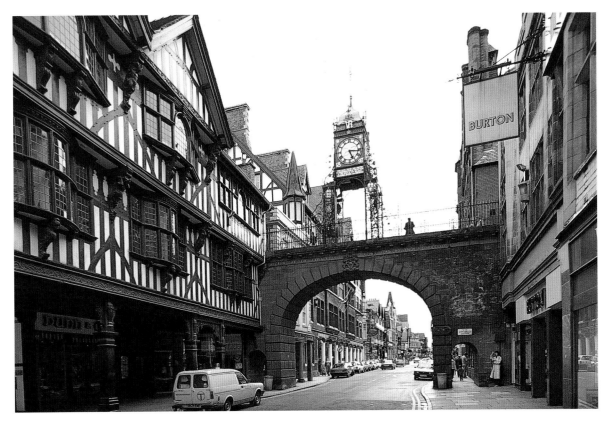

You may have entirely different needs, and will have your own unique data on which to base your design. Your information needs to be integrated with the design process to produce a final plan which reflects the needs of the people who will live in the house.

Buying a home using *feng shui*

There are several important things to keep in mind when buying someone else's property rather than building your own:

• The fortunes and the business successes and failures of the vendor and the vendor's family members are indicators of the potential fortunes of the purchaser of the house.

• Setting aside hereditary factors, the health of the house's occupants may be related to *feng shui*, or to other adverse environmental factors on the site, like pollution.

• You should not be influenced by how the previous occupants used the rooms of the house. Be creative, apply *feng shui* principles, and rethink how the rooms of the house can been used. It may be appropriate to change the functions of certain rooms, or even the orientation of the front entrance of the house.

• The entrance door is always assumed to face south for *Lo P'an* analysis, regardless of the direction it actually faces.

Choosing an appropriate street number

Generally speaking, from the *feng shui* viewpoint, multiple rather than single house numbers are preferable. Even numbers are *yin* and uneven are *yang*. The Chinese language operates on a tonal system where different inflections give different meanings to a particular word. Thus, when the Chinese numerals are spoken out loud, they make sounds which could be considered similar to other words. Numbers are thought of as fortuitous when their combined sounds are reminiscent of fortuitous Chinese words — others are considered unlucky because of the unlucky words they mimic. For some numbers, this also applies to the shape of the characters used.

FORTUITOUS		UNFORTUITOUS	
NUMBER	SOUNDS LIKE	NUMBER	SOUNDS LIKE
28	'Easy growth'	24	'easy death'**
48	'Lot of growth'	58	'no growth'
64 (=8x8)	The number of diagrams in *I-Ching*	174	'all dying together'
81 (=9x9)	Number of chapters in the Taoist: *The Way of Virtue*		
92	'Easy growth and expansion'		

* Walters, 1988; Too, 1993
** Walters considers this fortuitous as there are 24 divisions in the Chinese calendar year

Table 5.10

Figure 5.13: The *Ting Lan* Scale Rule of *feng shui* feet and inches. Unpropitious divisions are shown in half-tone. (Please note this ruler is not true to scale.)

Table 5.11: Choosing an appropriate building shape to suit the environment

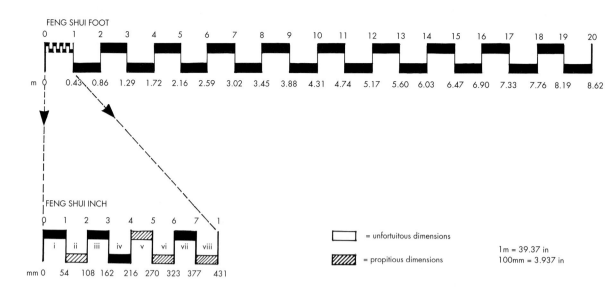

FENG SHUI FOOT

| 0 | 1 | 2 | 3 | 4 | 5 | 6 | 7 | 8 | 9 | 10 | 11 | 12 | 13 | 14 | 15 | 16 | 17 | 18 | 19 | 20 |

m 0   0.43 0.86 1.29 1.72 2.16 2.59 3.02 3.45 3.88 4.31 4.74 5.17 5.60 6.03 6.47 6.90 7.33 7.76 8.19 8.62

FENG SHUI INCH

| 0 | 1 | 2 | 3 | 4 | 5 | 6 | 7 | 1 |
| i | ii | iii | iv | v | vi | vii | viii |

mm 0   54   108 162 216 270 323 377 431

☐ = unfortuitous dimensions
▨ = propitious dimensions

1m = 39.37 in
100mm = 3.937 in

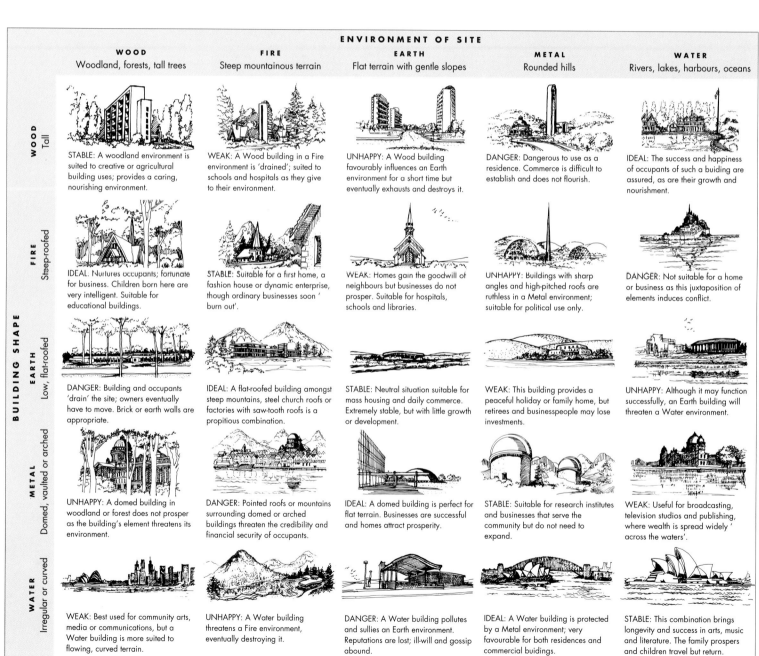

ENVIRONMENT OF SITE

	WOOD Woodland, forests, tall trees	**FIRE** Steep mountainous terrain	**EARTH** Flat terrain with gentle slopes	**METAL** Rounded hills	**WATER** Rivers, lakes, harbours, oceans
WOOD Tall	STABLE: A woodland environment is suited to creative or agricultural building uses; provides a caring, nourishing environment.	WEAK: A Wood building in a Fire environment is 'drained'; suited to schools and hospitals as they give to their environment.	UNHAPPY: A Wood building favourably influences an Earth environment for a short time but eventually exhausts and destroys it.	DANGER: Dangerous to use as a residence. Commerce is difficult to establish and does not flourish.	IDEAL: The success and happiness of occupants of such a building are assured, as are their growth and nourishment.
FIRE Steep-roofed	IDEAL: Nurtures occupants; fortunate for business. Children born here are very intelligent. Suitable for educational buildings.	STABLE: Suitable for a first home, a fashion house or dynamic enterprise, though ordinary businesses soon ' burn out'.	WEAK: Homes gain the goodwill of neighbours but businesses do not prosper. Suitable for hospitals, schools and libraries.	UNHAPPY: Buildings with sharp angles and high-pitched roofs are ruthless in a Metal environment; suitable for political use only.	DANGER: Not suitable for a home or business as this juxtaposition of elements induces conflict.
EARTH Low, flat-roofed	DANGER: Building and occupants 'drain' the site; owners eventually have to move. Brick or earth walls are appropriate.	IDEAL: A flat-roofed building amongst steep mountains, steel church roofs or factories with saw-tooth roofs is a propitious combination.	STABLE: Neutral situation suitable for mass housing and daily commerce. Extremely stable, but with little growth or development.	WEAK: This building provides a peaceful holiday or family home, but retirees and businesspeople may lose investments.	UNHAPPY: Although it may function successfully, an Earth building will threaten a Water environment.
METAL Domed, vaulted or arched	UNHAPPY: A domed building in woodland or forest does not prosper as the building's element threatens its environment.	DANGER: Pointed roofs or mountains surrounding domed or arched buildings threaten the credibility and financial security of occupants.	IDEAL: A domed building is perfect for flat terrain. Businesses are successful and homes attract prosperity.	STABLE: Suitable for research institutes and businesses that serve the community but do not need to expand.	WEAK: Useful for broadcasting, television studios and publishing, where wealth is spread widely ' across the waters'.
WATER Irregular or curved	WEAK: Best used for community arts, media or communications, but a Water building is more suited to flowing, curved terrain.	UNHAPPY: A Water building threatens a Fire environment, eventually destroying it.	DANGER: A Water building pollutes and sullies an Earth environment. Reputations are lost; ill-will and gossip abound.	IDEAL: A Water building is protected by a Metal environment; very favourable for both residences and commercial buildings.	STABLE: This combination brings longevity and success in arts, music and literature. The family prospers and children travel but return.

(left side label: BUILDING SHAPE)

The following gives a brief idea of meanings associated with the numbers 1 to 9:

1 One Chinese Dictionary has 67 meanings for the character for number 1. Another takes 923 pages to discuss it, but basically 'one' is the Undivided, the Perfect Entity

2 'Easy'

3 'New beginnings'

4 'Death' (However, 44 is thought by some practitioners to be acceptable as the number adds up to 8, an auspicious number)

5 'The Five Elements'

6 'Bringing wealth'

7 Although a *yang* number, seven is considered as *yin* because the rhythm of female development appears to be based on a seven year cycle.

8 'Becoming rich'. This is the second-best number (after nine). Though it is an even number, and hence *yin*, eight is linked to the male.

9 'Longevity'; the fullness of heaven and Earth. All numbers containing only the numeral nine can eventually be reduced to the number nine by adding the digits (for example, by adding the digits of 9999 you arrive at 36, and 3+6 = 9), hence the numeral has mystical connotations, as well as being associated with longevity.

If you are unsure of the connotations of a multiple house number, add the numerals again and again until you reach a single numeral. For example, if the number of the house is 374, 3+7+4=14 and 1+4=5, so the relevant numeral is 5.

MEASUREMENTS IN *FENG SHUI*

In *feng shui*, a special unit of measurement is used for room sizes, ceiling heights, mounting heights for power and light switches and fittings, doors, furniture, furnishings and so on. The *feng shui* foot corresponds to 43 centimetres (1 foot 5 inches). Measured using the *Ting Lan* scale-rule, a *feng shui* foot has eight divisions (inches), each corresponding to one of the eight Trigrams. A *feng shui* inch is 5.39 centimetres (approximately 2 inches).

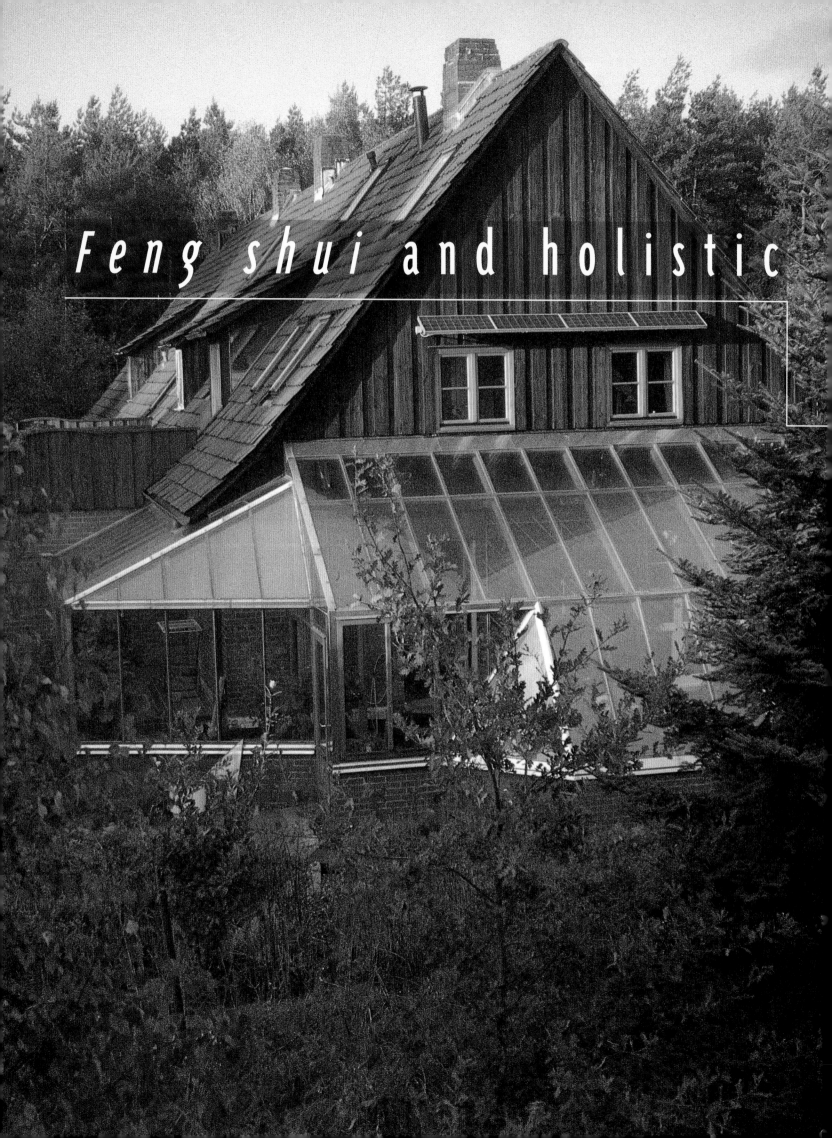

Feng shui and holistic

design principles

the term holism (GK: *holos* meaning 'whole' or 'entire') is frequently used in ecology, the health sciences and quantum physics. When health professionals use the term, they mean that a person's body, feelings, thoughts and even psyche (soul) should be considered as a whole when treating the health of the person. The whole person is greater than the sum of all their separate parts.

The notion of underlying unity is shared by most mystical traditions: '. . . while multiplicity and separateness are characteristic of manifest reality, the deep order is one of mutual enfoldment and oneness' (Combs 1992).

Similarly, the city has an existence that is greater than the sum of its people, buildings, open spaces, roads and communication networks — but holism does not stop at the level of the city. In its broadest sense, it embraces the total environment, of which humanity is one part. The house and its occupants, the street, village, town, city and countryside are integral parts of a total living organism, the planet itself. The complex ecological web of the Earth's interrelated natural and human environments responds to change and modification either in a positive, beneficial way, or in a negative, detrimental way. Our actions, thoughts and feelings produce effects which modify our social, natural and built environments. They in turn modify us.

So what is holistic architecture? There are very few examples of holistically designed buildings to which we can refer. It is perhaps easier to define what holistic architecture is *not*.

Most buildings in our surroundings are non-holistic in their design. A non-holistic building generally has an unsound structural system and enclosing envelope. It has cracks, leaks and dampness, and probably inadequate water, electrical and gas supply services. Indoor pollutants can be found in heavy concentrations, threatening the health and wellbeing of the building's occupants. Energy conservation would not have been considered in the building's design. This places unnecessary demands upon the building users' finances and the community's power sources, and adds to pollution. The non-holistic building has not been designed to express the needs and desires of its occupants, and hence is made up of spaces that are the wrong size and have inappropriate relationships with each other. The soul and spirit of the building would not satisfactorily reflect those of its users. The feelings engendered by the building may be ambiguous, or even the antithesis of the building's purpose.

The exterior of a building should prepare a person entering it for what they will experience inside; there should be no psychological shocks awaiting them. This does not apply to certain types of buildings, such as theatres. These are designed to change the mental attitude of the visitor, preparing them for a temporary suspension of reality. This may be appropriate in a theatre, but do we need whole districts that are a chaotic mixture of 'stage-set' styles, appealing to the lowest common denominator of public taste? The decisions we make today affect the visual quality of our suburbs and cities, which must be endured for decades.

The non-holistic home fails to elevate the spirit of the resident. It does not stimulate activity when it should, nor does it sooth and refresh when necessary. It denies the occupant an opportunity to express their identity. Alienation at both personal and social levels follows.

You have no doubt seen in glossy magazines the wonder house of the future, virtually an electronically controlled plastic capsule. All its inventions and expensive gadgetry may seem to service the physical needs of the household, but the house fails to meet one very important criterion of holistic design: to serve the senses and thereby the occupants' emotional needs. In this 'wonder house' the abundance of electromagnetic fields and plastics covertly pollutes the building's interior environment.

The holistic house, on the other hand, is beneficial to our health and emotions, reflects our lifestyles, accommodates the priorities in our lives and expresses our personalities. As individuals, we need to be involved in the design of the house, giving full rein to our imaginations, experimenting with natural materials, lighting and fabrics — and enjoying every step of the process.

Ideally, holistic architecture satisfies the needs, aspirations and desires of the individuals who are to use a building, and of the society and culture to which they belong. The building's social significance and context must be considered, along with its aesthetic and physical presence in the landscape, streetscape and overall environment. It should be a valid expression of the needs, drives and the physical, emotional, mental and spiritual characteristics of the people it is to house. Such buildings should not only have minimal physical impact on the surrounding natural and built environments, they should become part of those environments. The design process should include procedures to minimise any temporary impact upon the environment during construction.

The holistic house should provide its occupants with opportunities for life-enhancement beyond those created by a shelter designed only to satisfy the most basic physical needs of its occupants. The holistic house becomes an organism or third skin (the second being clothing) into which people are integrated. Each individual home can contribute to improving the health of the planet itself.

HOLISTIC ARCHITECTURE

Holism is a relatively new idea in architecture, and the procedures for creating a holistic house are necessarily more complex than those for customary house design. Holistic design requires the skills of architects or designers who have the training, maturity and experience to embrace all aspects of a family's lifestyle. Such a task may seem daunting at first, but the process can be undertaken step by step and will provide a fascinating insight into your family. It is an ambitious undertaking for which architects and designers must be willing to invest more time than is normally allocated for the interview and design process. You must also be prepared to spend time undertaking the analytical and enquiry work yourself.

It is necessary to undertake an analysis of physical factors such as the slopes, soils, surface drainage and vegetation of the site and non-physical factors, such as views. You need to analyse outdoor pollution, the effect construction will have on the ecosystem, and the site's GMF and geopathogenic zones. It is also necessary to analyse the social and cultural environment (the neighbourhood) of the new home and the civic environment (residential and civic building design, parks and open spaces, other recreation facilities, proximity to schools, shops and educational facilities). The aesthetic environment of the new home must also be taken into consideration, for example, whether the site is in a suburban or bushland setting, what the streetscape is like and the type of buildings already existing in the area.

Holistic architects and designers must have a thorough knowledge of passive-solar design; what comprises an environmentally healthy house in the biological and ecological sense; and landscape architecture. They should also have background knowledge of psychology, philosophy and possibly even comparative religion. They should be able to design the landscaping of a site as well as the actual building, so they need to understand the soil, the surface and sub-surface flow of water on the site, and the site's flora, fauna, geology, GMF and ionised radiation levels.

Holistic architects and designers must understand that we need homes that support us, rather than hinder us. They should be aware of the larger issue of designing houses not only for harmony with the site, but harmony with the planet. Their task is to provide a healing environment — the rest is up to the people who occupy the house.

As well as understanding these issues, they should also be able to apply bioharmonic proportions to the building design, and have a knowledge of bioenergetics. An enquiring mind and a willingness to experiment across the sciences, into the area of the parascientific, is perhaps the greatest value of all for a holistic architect or designer.

All this may seem idealistic and unreal. It is not. It is the standard that should be required of any professional who claims to design holistic buildings. Public awareness continues to grow of how a healthy house should be designed, what triggers allergies, which building materials contain toxic, outgassing chemicals, how radon levels need to be controlled, and the electrical pollution caused by the incorrect

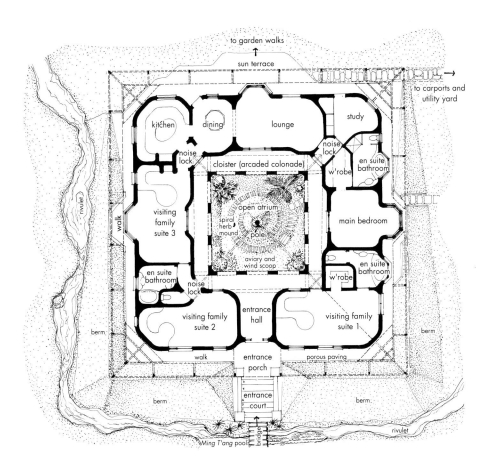

layout of wiring, or choice of electrical equipment. The time will possibly come when professionals who do not keep up to date with these matters may become answerable in law for what amounts to professional incompetence; such situations have already arisen in the United States and Germany (Kanuka-Fuchs 1994).

◎ Designing your own safe and healthy home ◎

In the previous chapter we introduced a hypothetical family, a retired couple whose children and grandchildren visit for prolonged periods. Figure 6.1 illustrates how we have combined the *feng shui* process with a western, holistic design approach to derive a house suitable for them. It is now up to you to design an environment that will reflect *your* outlook on life, *your* needs and desires.

PASSIVE-SOLAR CONSIDERATIONS

Early in the design process it is necessary to consider how your general building plan and form can best be combined with passive-solar design principles. The passive-solar system should be suited to the microclimate of your site and the floor plan you have

Figure 6.1: The final design plan for the case study family's house. It features an open, central atrium and accommodation for visitors

designed. The microclimate is the climatic conditions around your building, as opposed to the climate of the surrounding landscape (the topoclimate) or of the whole region (the macroclimate). Prior to this step, you would have considered solar access in choosing your site (see Chapter 2). The solar-collecting windows must be oriented to the sun, or within 15 degrees either side of north (in the southern hemisphere) or south (in the northern hemisphere).

The building's design should make maximum use of the cooling effects of winds. Natural vegetation can be used as a shading device in summer; in arid climates vegetation also increases the relative humidity within the building.

Conservatories can be used for direct solar gain, and when combined with a high thermal mass floor (one that absorbs and stores solar heat, in winter releasing it when the sun has set, and in summer, losing it to the air at night) can control heat gain and storage. In temperate and hot climates, a conservatory attached to the house must have shading devices to shield the glass from the sun's radiant heat, or the entire house will overheat. If the conservatory is designed to be sealed as a separate heating chamber, it can act as a resource of preheated air in winter. In summer, it is essential that heat can be released from an opening at a high level in the conservatory in order to balance the air temperature. In cold climates this is less of a problem and the conservatory functions most successfully.

All windows that are used for winter solar heat gain should be complemented by a floor pad just inside the window to absorb the heat from the winter sun. A floor pad is an area of material that has a high thermal mass, such as brick or compacted earth. High thermal mass materials in the floors and walls will provide radiant thermal solar energy heating during winter. Roof overhangs exclude sunlight in summer and permit its entry in winter. By referring to the chart in Appendix B you can calculate how large the roof overhang needs to be to provide shade in summer, yet allow sunlight to enter in winter. Similarly, you can calculate the amount of shadow cast by a tree or house (see Chapter 2).

In the southern hemisphere, the number of windows should be minimised on the south of the house, and on the north in the northern hemisphere. Cross ventilation should be provided and high-level louvres in walls used for heat distribution. Living rooms need to have summer and winter zones, and the heating source should have a flue that shares its winter warmth with other rooms in the house. It is best to avoid skylights in the roof, unless they are double-

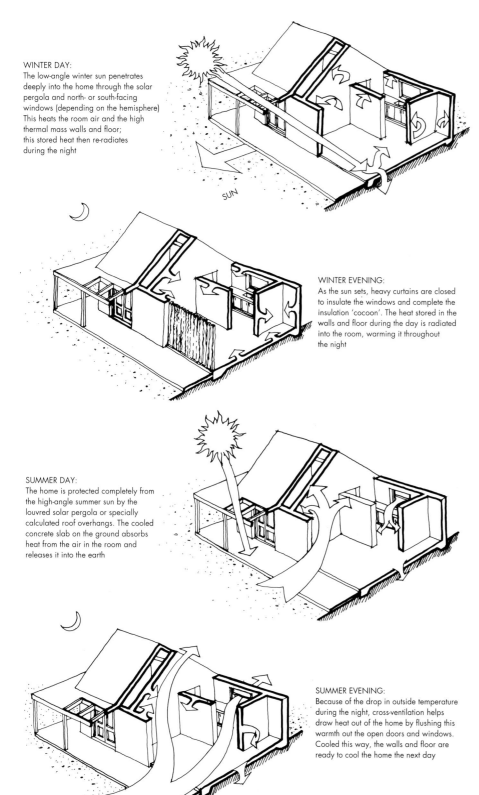

WINTER DAY:
The low-angle winter sun penetrates deeply into the home through the solar pergola and north- or south-facing windows (depending on the hemisphere). This heats the room air and the high thermal mass walls and floor; this stored heat then re-radiates during the night

SUN

WINTER EVENING:
As the sun sets, heavy curtains are closed to insulate the windows and complete the insulation 'cocoon'. The heat stored in the walls and floor during the day is radiated into the room, warming it throughout the night

SUMMER DAY:
The home is protected completely from the high-angle summer sun by the louvred solar pergola or specially calculated roof overhangs. The cooled concrete slab on the ground absorbs heat from the air in the room and releases it into the earth

SUMMER EVENING:
Because of the drop in outside temperature during the night, cross-ventilation helps draw heat out of the home by flushing this warmth out the open doors and windows. Cooled this way, the walls and floor are ready to cool the home the next day

glazed with assisted ventilation and sun-control louvres. When only one wall of a room contains windows, the width of the room, measured at a right angle to the windows, should be related to the amount of daylight entering, so that the wall opposite the windows receives a suitable level of light. To ensure this, the room should not be more than two and a half times deeper than the height of the glass in the windows. In rooms where there are windows on opposite sides of the room, the width of the room should be no more than five times the height of the windows. (If there are venetian blinds or a tree outside obstructing the light, the room depths should be reduced.)

A wet-back slow combustion stove with dual combustion is not only used for cooking but also provides hot water for general household use and heats the room air. In the United States, Australasia and other countries where they are available, they can be combined with a solar collector system as a back-up. In Europe, a Kachelofen (a tiled masonry oven) can be used instead of a wet-back stove.

⊚ Functional analysis ⊚

The next step is to establish each family member's personal needs, desires, goals and dreams. What positive aspects need to be encouraged or supported? What negative aspects need to be changed? Consider the special health needs, preferences and tastes of your family members, as well as their interests. The full range of their needs is more far-reaching than simple physiological ones, so consider their interactions with other family members, their sense of security, social life, creative interests, and so on.

In our case study family, the two parents permanently reside in the house, while the son and two daughters, and their children, stay during holidays. We have so far calculated where all the rooms of the house need to be located in terms of passive-solar requirements, *feng shui* principles and the magnetic field of the Earth.

The next step is to integrate the separate personal spaces in accordance with the needs of every member of the family. Each person should be asked about their eating and working or studying habits, their storage and privacy needs, their hobbies, and how much space they need to exercise, meditate and entertain in. Musical preferences also need to be considered, as problems often arise in households

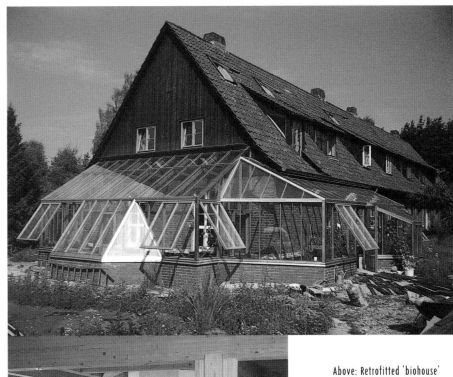

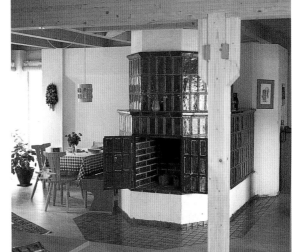

Above: Retrofitted 'biohouse' built in 1935 in Steyerberg, Germany (Architect: Prof. D. Kennedy; Photograph: Prof. D. Kennedy)

Left: A healthy house in Germany, designed by Baubiologie™ containing a Kachelofen (tiled oven) which can draw pre-heated or pre-cooled air into the room (Photograph: D. Pearson)

when family members play different types of music in close proximity to each other.

For the case study family, when the surveys of individual family members were completed and analysed, it became clear that individual privacy was a primary concern. A good choice of house would be a heavy, earth-wall construction that attenuates noise, and incorporates 'neutral-zones' such as bathrooms that will act as buffers to unwanted sound.

Room sizes must be firmed-up and budgetary constraints calculated to arrive at the affordable total building area. In the process, a plan was developed around a central court or atrium in which plants are used to stimulate oxygen and carbon dioxide exchange to enhance healthy air and ionisation. The building was designed around an atrium because it is harmonious with the *Pa Kua* (the eight-sided shape

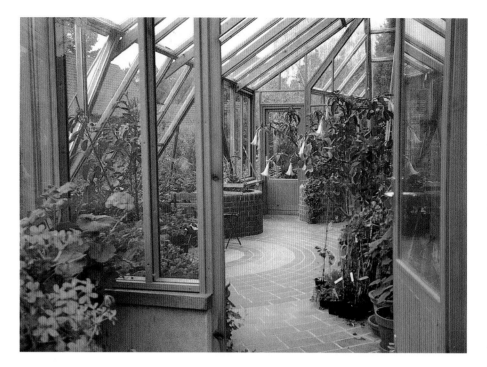

A cold climate conservatory forms part of the energy conservation strategy for this residence at Steyerberg, Germany (Architect: Prof. D. Kennedy; Photograph: Prof. D. Kennedy)

Figure 6.3: Heat and air flow strategies in the final house design

incorporating the eight Trigrams). The shape also represents the mouth, which is associated with the spleen, the 'characteristic quality of which [is] trustworthiness and reliability' (Eberhard 1989). It also symbolises 'posterity' (Lip 1993).

Figure 6.1 on page 91 and Figure 6.4 on the opposite page indicate the final design that satisfies the brief for our hypothetical family. It provides an open court in the centre for family gatherings. The *yin* form of the open court is complemented by the *feng shui* Fire element in the form of a pyramidal roof frame over the courtyard. The horizontality of the site and its surrounds presents an environment of the Earth element, symbolising stability. As fire burns, it produces the organic matter that forms earth, so the relationship between the elements is a productive one.

Thermal performance of the building

When you are satisfied with the design, calculations can be made of how the building will perform thermally, depending on which materials you choose for the windows, doors, roofing, walls and insulation. The walls and roof, their claddings and finishes should breathe enough to avoid interior condensation, and hence fungal moulds, while still keeping out the weather. Materials have to be selected to avoid outgassing while other materials such as interior linings and furnishings should be chosen to balance negative to positive ions in the building. (This means avoiding polishes, paints, fabrics and other surfaces that allow the accumulation of electrostatic fields.)

Your consulting architect will then determine the insulation R-value for each exterior material. (R-value is a measure of a material's resistance to the transfer of heat.) He or she will calculate the total area of the various materials that form the weather skin between the inside and outside of the house, and will determine the exterior and interior temperatures for the coldest months of the year.

The rate of heat loss through each exterior surface area will be calculated, room by room. Also to be considered is the sol-air effect, the amount of the solar radiation on, and air temperature at, the skin of the building which separates the interior environment from the outside weather. Included in the sol-air calculation are: the solar radiation on all building surfaces, the outside air temperature, orientation of the building, the thermal mass, conductivity, colour and texture of external materials, any movable insulation, the shade falling on external surfaces, and the positions and sizes of the windows.

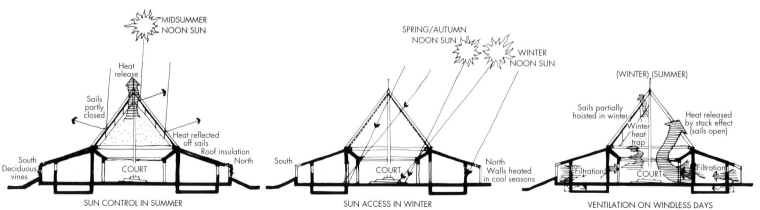

HEAT AND VENTILATION CONTROL STRATEGIES USING SCOOP-SAILS OVER CENTRAL COURT

The total heat loss will be calculated for the entire structure over a given period. For each room, the infiltration heat loss (through cracks in doors, windows or at junctions between wall and ceiling linings), and for the building as a whole, will be determined. The consultant will then add together overall, infiltration and slab-edge (heat lost through the edge of a slab exposed to air) heat losses, and balance those with the heat produced from the use of electrical equipment and human body heat. This will indicate how much winter heating will be necessary — in the best solar design no heating should be needed, except in extremely cold climates. If the total heat loss exceeds 50.5 watts per square metre (16 BTU per square foot) of floor area per hour, window areas will have to be reduced and infiltration heat losses checked.

He or she will then determine how much solar energy can be collected for use on a typical day each month, based on the total collection area, allowing for shading, cloudy days, and so on. The percentage of the total heat available in a normal season from solar collection will be calculated. This is related to the probable maximum duration of winter cloud cover between clear days, during which your building will have to perform on stored heat alone. This gives an indication of the period when solar heat storage will probably be needed.

The consultant will also calculate the volume and heat capacity of the thermal storage mass (the walls, concrete floor and so on). If the total storage capacity is less than the total heat loss, you may have to include storage units such as a mass of rocks or

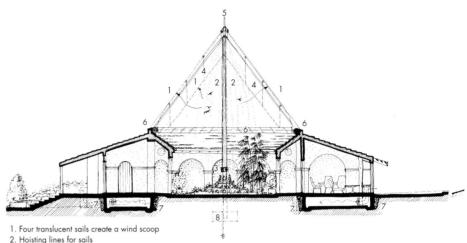

1. Four translucent sails create a wind scoop
2. Hoisting lines for sails
3. Auto winches for hoisting lines
4. Guy guides
5. Lightning arrestor system
6. Spring-loaded rollers for sails
7. Agricultural pipeline keeps sub-floor space dry
8. Footing to central pole and earthing for lightning arrestor

concrete, or water tanks as part of the overall design. Alternatively, you could include more thermal mass in the building plan, use auxiliary heating or seal infiltration zones better.

It is then necessary to check the possibility of using natural lighting, ventilation and air circulation. Strategically locate doors, windows and vents to allow for natural air circulation, daytime lighting and the removal of odours and excess heat.

The architect should then build a scale model of the house to give you an understanding of how the building will actually look in three dimensions, how it will relate to the site and express the plan shape you have chosen and how it will respond to the sun at different times of the year (by using a torch).

Figure 6.4: Cross-section of the case study family's house at a site in the subhumid zone

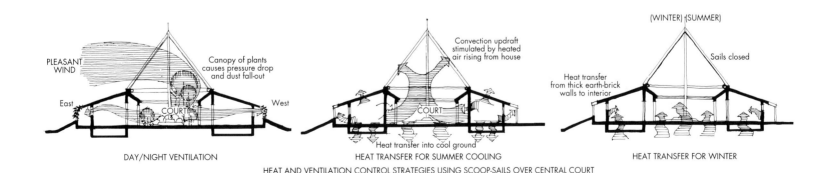

HEAT AND VENTILATION CONTROL STRATEGIES USING SCOOP-SAILS OVER CENTRAL COURT

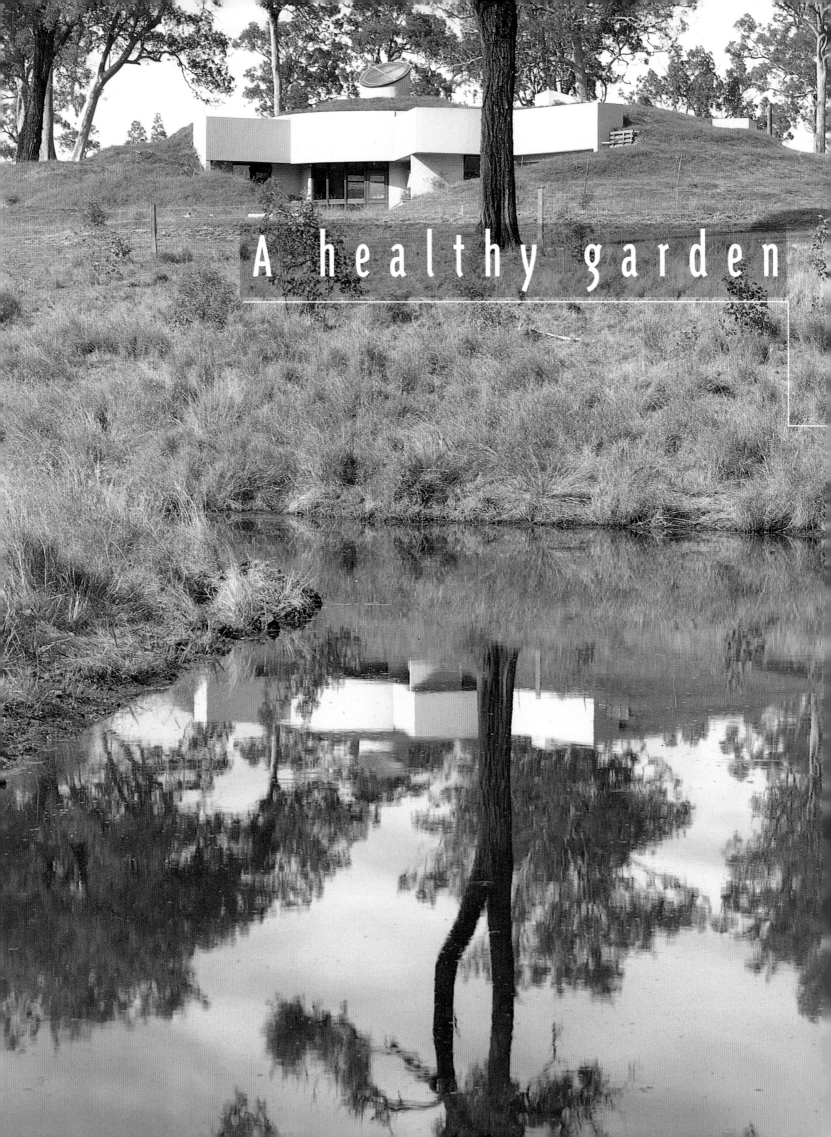

A healthy garden

for the healthy house

fifteen years ago, while doing research in the United States, we came across a meticulously fabricated and faithfully reproduced, full-size plastic tree — complete with plastic oranges — in a shopping centre north of Fresno, California. The popularity of such plastic trees has since grown, and they can now be found in buildings all over the world. The cleaner who was dusting the 'tree' explained that synthetic specimens were so much easier to maintain than live plants. This plastic tree made us feel uncomfortable, but why? Was it because we have a fundamental need for other living things in our environment?

All living things have an associated biological energy field. If sentient life is absent we probably sense this at some level not yet accessible to the rational mind. Nature should be part of our daily experience. We need to integrate with, and become part of, the natural environment.

The Old Testament instructed humanity to 'fill the earth and subdue it; and have dominion over the fish of the sea and over the birds of the air and over every living thing that moves upon the earth' (Genesis 1:28). From the Judaeo/Christian viewpoint, our task would be to subdue nature, our servant. A large proportion of the world's population has been raised with the Judaeo/Christian ethic that nature is there for human beings to use. Yet there is a growing ecological awareness that we are not dominant over nature, but that we are part of it. It is time to re-establish the role of

Contact with nature is a basic human need but 'for the moment it seems we have lost our touch . . . We must regain the old instincts, re-learn the old truths . . . we must rediscover Nature'.

(Simonds 1961)

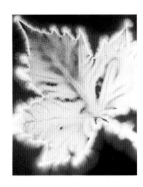

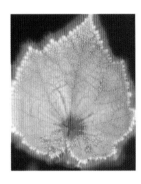

Kirlian photographs of a Japanese maple leaf (top) and a grape leaf, taken with an Auragraph camera (Photograph: Graydon H. Rixon)

Page 96: A prize-winning earth-sheltered home where the roof is used for agistment. The walls and roof are fire-proofed by deep soil cover. Hunter Valley, NSW Aust. (Architects: ECA Space Design Pty Ltd)

the sympathetic steward of nature, once encouraged by the Celtic Christians of Glastonbury, Eire and by pre-Christian cultures. It is time that we heeded the words, so often used to illustrate the message of Gaia, of Chief Seattle of the Suquamish Indians:

> *How can you buy or sell the sky, the warmth of the land? … You must teach your children that it is sacred … tell your children that the rivers are our brothers, and yours, and you must henceforth give the rivers the kindness you would give any brother. Teach your children what we have taught our children — that the earth is our mother. Whatever befalls the earth, befalls the sons of the earth. If men spit upon the earth, they spit upon themselves.*

Humans can be seen reaching out constantly for contact with nature, in daily life, recreation, and in business as well, as evidenced by the reintroduction of real, rather than artificial, plants into the workplace. This may be the expression of a basic need. Nature contact may be essential for our survival, health and wellbeing. H. F. Searles (1960) found that he could cure mentally ill patients by exposing them to natural environments. What was lacking for the patients was contact with the nonhuman, organic environment, that is, nature contact. It follows that withdrawal from nature can create ill health and disease.

Doctor Roger Ulrich (1983) found that patients in rooms with a view of trees spent less time in hospital than those with a view of a brick wall. Those with a view of trees only needed aspirin compounds and had fewer post-operative complications than the other group who had more complications and needed potent narcotics. Nature contact is conducive to mental and physical health and a lack of such contact is detrimental to our emotional, mental and physical equilibrium.

LIFE ESSENCE

Many religions and philosophies describe the essential energy of life by using terms such as life essence, vital essence, universal essence, *prana, ch'i, manas,* health aura, *monoke, mulaprakriti,* universal plastic medium, *vril,* serpent current, *anima mundi,* and light-etheric force. In the 1950s, Doctor Semyon Kirlian and his wife, Valentina, used an alternating current of high frequency to 'illuminate' their subjects, and claimed to have captured life essence on light-sensitive paper.

The Kirlian imagery suffices to show that some type of field effect prevails between living organisms. As two organisms draw closer to each other, this force bridges the gap. When a Kirlian image is made of a leaf, even if a portion of the leaf is missing, it appears as though it is still whole.

◉ Biological energy fields ◉

When a device, known as the Superconducting Quantum Interference Device (SQUID), is used to measure the extremely low electromagnetic forces within the human body, magnetic signals can be detected that are 50 million times weaker than the Earth's magnetic field. The body also has a strong electric field of some 10 million volts per metre, far greater than that experienced near high voltage power lines. The whole of a person's body is like an antenna; the larger the organism, the weaker the field it can detect.

Human beings have an 'all-or-nothing' threshold of sensitivity for electromagnetic fields. A person who is allergic to electromagnetic forces may feel perfectly well until, through overexposure to environmental toxins their immune system becomes weak, they reach their tolerance threshold and suddenly become ill when exposed to electromagnetic pollution.

In the same way that the eye has evolved to be very sensitive to movement and hue, the pineal gland in the brain has become sensitised to changes in the GMF of the Earth and to ELF fields. The pineal gland is light-sensitive and performs a time-keeping function for the body. When we come into contact with another living organism, an energy flux occurs between our field and the organism's. This is demonstrated in the movement of the dowser's pendulum or rod.

Perhaps the human organism senses the falseness of an artificial plant and reaches out to naturalness in environmental stimuli, in the same way that very young children, over an extended period of time, will seek out foods containing the nutrients their bodies require. Adults may eventually expose young children to foods that introduce distortions of taste, but until that happens, they have innate discrimination. Perhaps our taste for the natural in environments in preference to the fake is an uncultivated, innate preference for contact with energised rather than debilitated biological energy fields, or non-living objects which do not have such fields.

An inner conflict exists for many though, between their awareness of being part of nature and their feeling of 'being apart from all the rest of nonhuman nature' (Searles 1960). While subjected to the laws of nature, we simultaneously transcend nature with technology. We live in a state of 'homelessness', being the only animal which does not feel at home in nature. We cannot go back to a prehuman state of harmony in nature and we do not know where we will arrive if we go forward. The sense of disequilibrium varies from person to person, depending on the differential between the individual's instincts and their self-awareness. This existential conflict produces 'certain psychic needs common to all' (Fromm 1973). It is as necessary to fulfil these drives as it is to fulfil the organic drives that keep us alive. As Eric Fromm writes '... resolution of this conflict involves people searching for ever-new solutions for the contradictions in their existence, trying to find ever-higher forms of unity with nature'.

We require nature contact at a personal level to maintain bodily health. Gardens and pets are necessary for our physical and mental health. And we need contact with plants, because plants *do* have 'feelings'.

⊚ Plants have feelings ⊚

To those who play music or talk to their plants, the question 'Do plants have feelings?' does not even need to be asked. To the sceptic, the idea that plants have feelings is ridiculous, but if the proposition that plants do have feelings is true, the link between plants and human health may be clearer.

After reading Charles Darwin's *The Variation of Animals and Plants under Domestication* (1868), the horticulturalist Luther Burbank became interested in the idea that organisms vary when removed from their natural conditions. Burbank talked to his plants, although he was not sure that they understood him. He aimed to create a vibration of love when he carried out his horticultural experiments, and attributed around 20 sensory perceptions to plants. George Washington Carver, another brilliant horticulturist, wrote: '... all flowers talk to me and so do hundreds of little living things in the woods. I learn what I want to know by watching and loving everything' (Tompkins and Bird 1974).

Sir Jagadis Chandra Bose spent a lifetime researching the environmental responses of plants. He concentrated on the issue of whether plants are sentient organisms, and if so, whether their feelings could be measured. Bose established that plants react to the attitude with which they are nurtured.

Bose's theory of organic development, which preceded Darwin's, was not appreciated at the time. It was based on his invention of many delicate and sensitive instruments, including the crescograph, that measured the responses of plants to many types of stimuli, such as food and drugs.

In the late 1700s and early 1800s, the German writer and natural philospher, Johann Goethe, searched for the spiritual essence that lay behind the material form of plants. Long before particle physics was even understood, he held that atoms were 'centres of pure energy and the lowest elements in a spiritual hierarchy' (Tompkins and Bird 1974).

This concept is very similar to those of occult philosophers who appeared in the latter part of the 19th century. They held that the connection between the plant and animal kingdom can be found in the etheric matter that underlies all the universe and all living and so-called non-living things.

⊚ Plant response to music and vibration ⊚

When Doctor T.C. Singh experimented with the effect of musical sound on the growth rate of plants, he found that balsam plants accelerated by 20 per cent

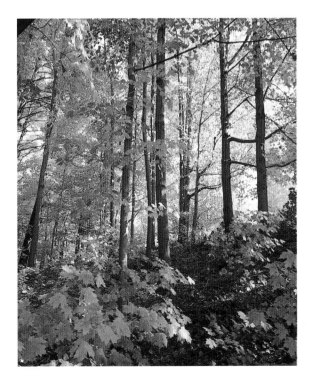

Autumn at Walden Pond, USA
'... pure twilight is become the precincts of heaven. Yet so equable and calm ... that you could not tell whether it was morning or noon or evening' (Henry Thoreau's *Journal*, July 5 1945, 1:13)

in height and 72 per cent in biomass when exposed to music (Singh 1962). Later experiments led him to conclude that *raga* music (a type of music that improvises on a set of rhythms and notes) played on flute, violin, harmonium and an Indian instrument, the *reena*, had the same effect.

Singh repeated his experiments with field crops using a particular type of *raga* played through a gramophone and loudspeakers. The size of crops increased to between 25 to 60 per cent above the regional average. In another experiment, he observed the effect of the vibrations caused by bare-footed dancing, the *Bharata-Natyam*, India's most ancient dance style which has no musical accompaniment, on Michaelmas daisies, marigolds and petunias. They flowered 2 weeks earlier than the control specimens. In the agricultural community of Normal, Illinois, in the United States, the stems of maize and soybeans were found to grow thicker, greener and tougher when played *Rhapsody in Blue* (Tompkins and Bird 1974).

In an experiment conducted in Denver in the United States by Dorothy Retallack (1973), a student of Professor Francis Broman, one group of plants was played the note F for an 8 hour period, a second group was exposed to the same note for 3 hours, while a third control group remained in silence. The first group died within 2 weeks, while the second was much healthier than the control group. Other students then experimented with squash crops which grew towards, and entwined themselves around, a speaker playing Haydn, Beethoven, Brahms and Schubert. Another group of squash plants grew away from a speaker broadcasting rock music, and even tried to climb a glass-walled enclosure in what appeared to be an attempt to get away from the sounds. Retallack replicated the experiment with a variety of plants, observing that the rock music resulted in abnormal vertical growth and small leaves. The rock music caused the same damage as that resulting from excessive uptake of water, causing marigolds to die within 2 weeks. Plants leaned away from the source of acid-rock music, no matter which way they were turned.

Human beings can consciously perceive only a minute fraction of the vibrational world around them. The link between humans and plants could be related to mutual responses to sound frequencies although this seems too simplistic. Sound makes up a very limited band of frequencies in the electromagnetic radiation spectrum. Such radiation, in the form of sound, provides a link between humans and plants. Experiments have been conducted in this area since the 1700s, as has research into force fields on humans and plants. In the 1960s, experimental work began in earnest, and the underlying pattern shown by these experiments is exemplified by the work of Warren Meyer (1973) which demonstrates that plants have the power to communicate. Some people maintain that they are even endowed with personalities.

Many of the principles of *feng shui* are related to the tenuous link that exists between plants and people. This link can be vitalised by adopting the correct attitude to Gaia and all living things, including rocks, crystals and metals. Not only do we need other people for our emotional, mental and spiritual health, we also need plants and nature contact to remain healthy at all levels.

TREES, VEGETATION AND A HEALTHY ENVIRONMENT

Each year tropical forests are disappearing at the rate of 142,000 square kilometres per year (54,831 square miles). That is 0.3 square kilometres (74 acres) every minute (Myers 1990). Fifty five per cent of the Earth's vegetation consists of tropical forests, which are threatened by logging and clearing. Twenty one per cent consists of temperate forests, which are threatened by increasing soil acidity and overcropping.

Yet we depend upon the Earth's forests, which store vast stocks of carbon and constantly take in carbon dioxide from the atmosphere and release oxygen. Rather than referring to the forests as the 'lungs' of the planet, they would be better described as a flywheel that stores kinetic energy and stabilises a system in the same way that the carbon cycle sustains a balanced flow of carbon in the soil, living things, oceans and the atmosphere. Forests also play a major role in stabilising the water cycle.

What is needed is an immediate response at the individual level. Support those groups campaigning against deforestation, and plant your own group of trees, or mini-forest. With careful planning it will create a pleasant microclimate around your home.

The mini-forest

Is there any family that has not suffered the impact of asthma or allergy? The air that enters our houses can bring pollution, dust and pollen with it. To protect your family from allergic reactions and asthma, you could use mechanical filtration to remove these irritants, but natural solutions are much better. Vegetation functions as a very effective air filter. If greenbelts were established throughout cities and towns, along with mini-forests in housing developments, containing forest-sized trees and their associated plant communities, every house could become a centre for the restoration of the forest biomass of the Earth. It all begins with you.

How many trees?

Plants are essential for our survival. The oxygen we rely on comprises about half of the total mass of all matter on Earth. Free oxygen in air and water is present because plants absorb carbon dioxide and give out oxygen during the process of photosynthesis; our lungs absorb this oxygen, and release carbon dioxide. How many trees and how much vegetation should be used just to supply enough oxygen for, say, a family of five? A surface area of 25 square metres (269 square feet) of vegetation (including a small evergreen tree, shrubs and groundcovers) will emit enough oxygen on a sunny day to fulfil one person's requirements during the same period (Bernatzky 1966). Photosynthesis does not occur at night, so you would need to allow extra leaf surface area in order to supply enough oxygen for the full 24 hour period. Between 30 and 40 square metres (323–431 square feet) of vegetation is needed per person, so a family of five would require around 200 square metres (2155 square feet) of vegetation. This would take up an area slightly smaller than a tennis court. On the level of the whole city, the oxygen generated by the vegetation in parks, nature reserves and suburbs helps to counteract the excessive levels of carbon dioxide emitted by vehicles, aircraft and industry.

In addition to regulating oxygen and carbon dioxide levels in the air, vegetation helps control air pollution, in both gaseous and particulate forms (Geiger 1966). Plants also modify odours caused by pollution, and control air temperature, movement and moisture. Our mini-forests, plus privately owned shrubs and lawns, wash and filter incoming air.

Shelterbelts

A shelterbelt is made up of between one and five rows of trees and shrubs, and is designed to control winds and the temperature around a building. Shelterbelt design has become very refined over the years through the use of wind tunnel testing on various combinations of small and tall trees and shrubs. As the need for such planting can vary from a single house to a farm or an entire suburb, the number of trees used varies widely. Belts of two or three layers of vegetation are often used.

WIND CONTROL

The design of shelterbelts for wind control is primarily based on deflecting the wind flow gently upwards, creating as little turbulence as possible. Once deflected upwards, the wind continues to flow parallel to the ground until ultimately returning to ground level. Diverting the wind in this way creates a zone of reduced velocity in the lee of the belt, and this zone extends a considerable distance downwind. To protect occupants from strong and unpleasant winds, the building, landscape courtyard and other useful outside areas need to be located within the protected zone.

At some time of the year most places are exposed to unpleasant winds or weather. By carefully constructing shelterbelts of vegetation around the building, undesirable winds, for example hot and dry, can be deflected away, and their velocity decreased, while desirable winds, like cooling breezes in summer, can be channelled towards the building.

A low density shelterbelt is the most efficient as it allows some breeze to come through, easing turbulence. Although a low density shelterbelt which is relatively penetrable by the wind does not slow the wind speed as much as impenetrable vegetation does, its slowing-down effect extends for a greater distance downwind behind the belt of trees. The optimum permeability for a shelterbelt is between 45 and 55 per cent.

The permeability of the canopy of a particular species can be approximately assessed by photographing a specimen of your preferred tree. Photograph the tree against a bright sky, with the light settings of the camera set to the sky rather than the tree; this will produce a silhouette photograph of the tree. Now estimate the proportion of light areas to dark in the tree canopy by laying over the photograph a sheet of tracing paper divided into small squares. Add up the number of

Figure 7.1: The Manx-cross
pattern for a shelterbelt with
winds coming from various
directions

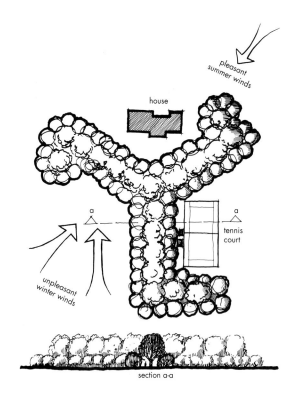

section a-a

light squares, divide by the number of dark squares and multiply the result by 100 to produce the percentage of permeability. For example, if there are 80 light squares and 90 dark ones: $\frac{80}{90} \times \frac{100}{1} =$ a permeability of 89 per cent. The canopy of this species would produce too much turbulence and be inefficient. At lower permeability, for example 15 to 20 per cent, a closed loop of wind occurs on the lee side of the barrier, which means that sand or snow may accumulate.

Where unpleasant winds come from various directions, a technique like the Manx-cross pattern may be useful. It is employed on the Isle of Man, which is exposed to Atlantic gales, and provides several protected outdoor areas to locate cattle and buildings.

AIR TEMPERATURE REGULATION

In the previous chapter we saw how it is possible to use the thermal mass of the floor and walls on the sunny side of a house for storing winter warmth. What happens, though, to heat lost from the building on the shady side? When conditions are windy, heat loss is accelerated, hence wind protection from sheltering trees and shrubs that create a still-air condition near the wall will slow down heat loss. The rate of thermo-dynamic exchange between air outside the shelterbelt and air inside the building is low, because of the still air on the lee side of the shelterbelt. This allows higher temperatures to prevail in the protected zone.

CONTROLLING FIRES

When a building is threatened by an approaching fire front, pushed along by a strong wind, a shelterbelt can deflect the fire over the building. While shelterbelts constructed of 10 or 12 rows provide optimum protection, five or seven row designs have been found, by wind tunnel tests, to be almost as efficient (White 1954; Baggs 1991).

As well as shelterbelts of species that do not ignite easily, landscaping walls can also be used on the windward sides of a building to function as radiant shields. They need to be relatively close to the building in such cases as they are not as efficient as tree shelterbelts in producing a leeward stilling effect on the air flow.

◎ Concealed fencing ◎

The 'ha-ha' is a type of sunken fence or ditch, originally designed in the 18th century to provide uninterrupted views of the landscape, while acting as a barrier to wandering cattle. It is an effective method of unobtrusively defining the boundaries of a property, and can be used in the landscaping around a house to fence off areas within the site, or at site boundaries if the neighbours agree. Instead of a fence, the ditch may contain a wall which retains one side of the grass-covered ditch. A combination of a ha-ha and a hedge would be just as effective, and more visually appealing, than an ordinary fence.

◎ Using vegetation to control air quality ◎

Plants are responsible for improving the quality of our air by negating some of the effects of air pollution. When fresh, oxygen-rich air given off by plants is mixed with air polluted by gases, dirt, dust, smoke, fumes, pollens, chemicals and odours, the polluted air is diluted by the oxygen-rich air. Plants actively cleanse the air when the fine hairs on their leaves and stems trap airborne particles which are then washed into the soil by rain or garden sprinklers. Water is constantly evaporating from trees, cleansing the air around them. We calculated that an orchard around a house releases some 2300 litres (506 gallons) of water into the air each day, while eucalypts (with their canopies touching) at the front and back of a hectare-sized (10,764 square feet) block wash the air with at least 876 tonnes (862 tons) of water each year. When shrubs are added, the mini-forest can move around 1000 tonnes (984 tons) of water, humidifying and washing the surrounding air.

In addition to the effect of fragrant plants which create pleasant odours, all plants have the ability to metabolise odours. The presence of vegetation also causes air to be deflected into low turbulence zones, where the air is relatively still. The air pressure consequently drops, causing particulates, like dust, to fall out of the air stream. Tall, broad-leafed trees are more efficient at filtering the air than shorter, narrow-leafed trees.

IMPROVING AIR IONISATION

Fresh air should ideally contain negions and posions in the ratio of approximately 5:4 (see Chapter 1). Such conditions are only present at the top of high mountains, at large waterfalls, at the base of large glaciers and in wilderness forests. In other areas, pollution and hot, drying winds disturb the balance of ions in the air, causing discomfort and ill health. Balance in air ionisation can be restored by using certain landscaping strategies, such as a mini-forest, or a large pool with a fountain or waterfall.

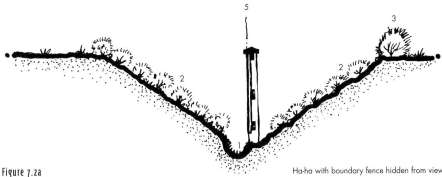

Figure 7.2a

Ha-ha with boundary fence hidden from view

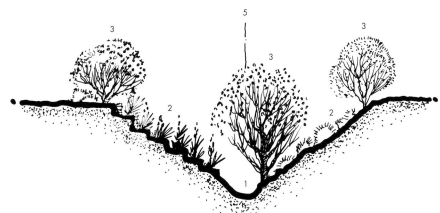

Figure 7.2b

Ha-ha with barrier plants (thornbush) on boundary

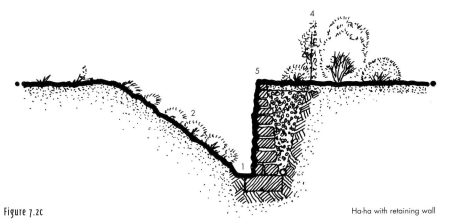

Figure 7.2c

Ha-ha with retaining wall

1. table drain; 2. erosion-control planting to embankment/cutting; 3. barrier planting; 4. vine-concealed mesh fence; 5. property boundary

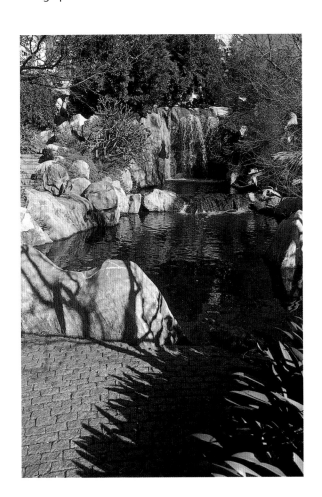

◎ Reducing noise with vegetation ◎

Constant background noise can cause health degradation, but can be reduced by planting vegetation. When the source of the noise is screened from view by planting, the noise level is perceived as being significantly lower than when the source is visible. This psychological effect can be enhanced by utilising landscape elements such as fountains, cascades and small streams. The 'white' noise created by moving, splashing water cancels out many other sound frequencies.

Figure 7.2: A ha-ha to conceal a fence or wall

Left: Use of a pool and waterfall in landscaping improves air ionisation. Guangdong Chinese garden, Sydney, NSW, Aust.

Certain plants are better at attenuating sound frequencies than others. Large-leafed plants (such as the Moreton Bay Fig, *Ficus macrophylla*) are better sound absorbers than those with small leaves (such as Hill's Weeping Fig, *Ficus hillii*). Almost all shelterbelt planting results in some noise reduction, the most satisfactory results being produced by belts 6–15 metres (20–49 feet) in depth (Robinette 1970).

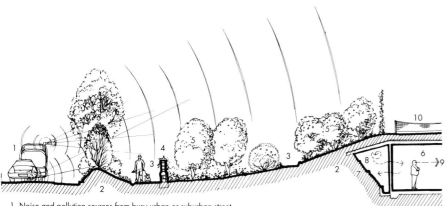

1. Noise and pollution sources from busy urban or suburban street
2. Earth berms absorb incident sound waves
3. Paths
4. Thick front, garden wall
5. Vegetation shelterbelts deaden noise and filter air polluted by traffic
6. An earth-sheltered house with both energy-efficient and 'breathing' capabilities
7. Stabilised embankment
8. Heat exchange duct also used for air exchange at times when outside air temperature and moisture content are appropriate (connected to wind scoop with heat and moisture sensors)
9. Sunlight and view out of building
10. Roof garden (for tennis court, etc)

Figure 7.3: Noise from traffic on a nearby road can be reduced in its impact by earth berms and by using 6–15 m (20–49 ft) of front garden shelterbelts of dense vegetation. This also helps to filter dust and pollution. An earth-sheltered house is the ideal 'quiet house' provided vibration-damping cork (VDC) is used in the wall construction.

◎ Controlling bush and forest fires ◎

Bush and forest fires are a savage reality in countries which have hot, dry summers and receive a reasonable rainfall in the growing season. The intensity of a fire depends on the quantity and type of fuel it has to feed on, the wind speed and direction and the landforms it has to traverse.

In extended periods of low humidity, the moisture content of the finer fuels, such as grass, leaves and twigs, drops. When this is followed by a drying out of coarser fuels such as branches and tree limbs, conditions are right for a fire outbreak. As a drying wind accelerates the rate at which fuel dries out, this process can be controlled to some extent by reducing the wind velocity with shelterbelts. Any means of raising the relative humidity of the air also helps to resist an outbreak and trees — as we have seen previously — do exactly this.

Plants with a high volatile oil content, such as cypress, olive, pine, citrus, rosemary, lavender and eucalyptus, should be planted well away from buildings as they tend to explode into fireballs. Choose smooth-barked trees and succulent groundcovers. Avoid mulching with loose hay or straw; use well-composted materials or groundcovers which act as mulches, such as lucerne, sweet potato, clover, comfrey and nasturtium. Compost and mulch should always be kept moist. For the pergola, you should choose fire-retardant vine species such as passionfruit, kiwi fruit or grape.

Most fruit trees are fire-retardant, consequently any orchard can serve as a firebreak. To protect the orchard itself use shelterbelts of fire-resistant species. All plants will ultimately burn but those with high moisture, ash or salt content and with a low oil content will take longer to ignite and will then burn slowly. Exotic deciduous trees are particularly efficient at retarding the spread of fire. Species to look for are listed in Appendix H.

Maintenance must be ongoing to control the risk of bush and forest fire to your house. Trees and bushes need to be pruned and dead vegetation cleared away from fences, from under houses, out of gutters and around walls. Ground litter should be continuously removed to disrupt the potential path of a fire between the roof and tree canopies. If trees and shrubs that form part of your windbreak die, plant replacements as soon as possible. Any damage to or wear of heat shielding structures such as garden walls, sheet metal fences, screens and outbuildings need to be repaired. Mowing the grass is an essential fire-control task. Consider keeping sheep, goats, cows or horses if the task proves too arduous.

If your site is located in a closed woodland where the tree canopies join together to form a stratum, the continuity of fire fuel can form a natural fire path. The danger can be significantly reduced by providing firebreaks, or disconnections in the upper strata of the woodland.

Some fires, like the bushfires which threatened suburbs of Sydney, Australia, in January 1994, break all the rules. Fanned by fierce drying winds, a fire front may have so much momentum that it leaps across firebreaks, wide roads and major rivers. Yet even in such circumstances, the home that has been prepared and maintained correctly will be a much safer home than one where no precautions have been taken.

GARDEN WATER SUPPLY

Water is a precious resource, so make the most of it by installing tanks to collect roof water — obtain permission from your local authority first. Install another tank to collect grey water that has been used for bathing, washing and cooking. Recycled grey water is suitable for garden sprinklers, so long as biodegradable detergents and washing powders have been used. Grey water is not suitable for use in trickle irrigation, as it may block very fine nozzles.

Pool and stream water should be drawn from an existing stream, or recirculated using a solar pump driven by a bank of photovoltaic cells. The use of chlorine should be avoided in swimming pools and ponds, as it releases the carcinogenic compound chloroform and the gas ozone.

One way around using toxic chemicals in swimming pools is installing a reed-bed containing species of *Juncea* and *Phragmytes* species. Sympodia bamboo (*Bambusa sympodia*), from northern Australia, would also be suitable, and is currently being used in place of trees to form wetlands in South Australia. It does not decline as trees do and does not spread like many species of bamboo; paper can also be made from it without the necessity of bleaching. Water falls out of the reed-bed and is oxygenated by a figure-of-eight vortex as it passes down a cascade of 'flowforms', imparting it with life energy. Designed to resemble a river where you cannot see the river bed, the pool is a total contrast to the 'dead' system of normal pool construction, which costs more than twice the amount of a natural, healthy pool. Craig Pattinson, a designer of such pools, recommends that they be topped up with roof water catchment to counteract evaporation. Evaporation could also be minimised by planting overhanging trees.

The venturesome may choose to use a pool to raise fish or crayfish (yabby or crawfish). Extreme care needs to taken when selecting fish species because if they escape into local waterways during floods, they may cause damage to indigenous species.

Water supply for fire-fighting

A separate water supply should be accessible for fire-fighting purposes. This supply may be connected to hand-held hoses, sprinkler systems and the fire-fighters' portable appliances. When a fire approaches, it is necessary to wet down ignitable wall materials such as weatherboard and cladding. However, if brick walls are hosed and then subjected to sudden intense heat they can spall, just as stones can fragment when water is poured over a campfire. If heated walls are hosed down after or during a fire, bricks can fracture and pieces drop away or fly off.

Large buildings and major subdivisions are required by law to have a separate water supply for fire-fighting. In the case of a single house it is still preferable to have one's own separate supply, particularly if the local water supply is unreliable. For instance, in the bushfires around Sydney, Australia in 1994, water supplies were unable to meet the demand, and in some cases, failed because pumping stations were destroyed. Your independent fire-fighting water supply needs to provide enough head of pressure for hoses to be used or for an external sprinkler system to function, otherwise a pump will be needed. If a pump is necessary, it should be motorised and preferably run on diesel, as the petrol in petrol-driven engines can vaporise and the supply of electricity can be disrupted during a fire. The pump must be able to function for 2 hours under fire conditions. To provide water for a typical external sprinkler protection system for 2 to 3 hours, you will need 10,000 litres (2641 gallons) of water, and must be able to augment your supply with a further 20,000 litres (5283 gallons) of water — swimming pools and rainwater collection tanks that hold a reserve of 30,000 litres (7923 gallons) are obvious resources for these additional water supplies.

The major weakness of an external sprinkler system is that it needs someone to turn it on. Also, during the high winds that usually accompany fires, roof-mounted sprinkler-spray can easily be blown away. Professional help is needed in the design of such a system so that it functions to its best advantage. Sprinkler heads can be designed and located to combat adverse conditions. Ground level sprinklers have dual nozzles, one of which can be directed up to the roof and the other to the walls of the building, unless they are concrete or brick. These sprinklers can be adapted for garden use. Sprinklers can be controlled by fusible links (when heat builds up the links melt, causing water to flow) or a heat-sensor system (which detects infra-red). The reliability of these remote warning systems is reduced in wildfire conditions, which can instantly destroy the whole system if the heat is intense enough.

Figure 7.5: The Arbor system of
sewage effluent disposal (after
Mollinson 1992)

SEWAGE DISPOSAL

◎ Evapo-transpiration beds ◎

Sewage wastes are a large cause of the pollution
affecting our beaches, streams and ground water,
however it is possible to use a sealed lagoon or pond
(an evapo-transpiration bed) to purify liquid wastes
naturally, and avoid them being returned to the
ground water or soil. Sewage effluent is piped to an
open, gravel evapo-transpiration bed. A leach field is a
pit which allows water to move through soil to sieve
out particles from the water. Bill Mollison, a designer of
such systems, recommends that for a single house, a
leach field recessed pit, which is 25 square metres (270
square feet) in surface area and about 0.5 metre (1 foot
7 inches) deep at the highest point, be dug (see Figure
7.4). The bottom of the recess in the ground needs to
slope at 1 in 12 away (about a 4 degree fall) from the
pipe outlet servicing the pit from the sewage effluent
source. It should be covered with a layer of cardboard
and about 18 centimetres (7 inches) of straw, into
which crop plants should be established. The gravel or
crushed rock infill should be graded in size from 6
centimetres (2½ inches) at the bottom to 2 centimetres

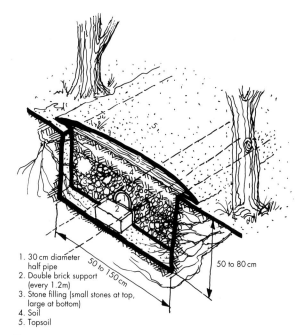

1. 30 cm diameter
   half pipe
2. Double brick support
   (every 1.2m)
3. Stone filling (small stones at top,
   large at bottom)
4. Soil
5. Topsoil

50 to 150 cm

50 to 80 cm

Figure 7.5

(¾ inch) at the top (see Figure 7.4). Plant trees,
preferably fruit trees, around the pit. (Mollison 1992)

The Arbor system, on the other hand, employs
a trench which is 0.5–0.8 metre (1 foot 8 inches–2 feet
8 inches) deep and 0.5–1 metre (1 foot 8 inches–3 feet
4 inches) wide. Inside the trench are half pipes 30
centimetres (12 inches) in diameter, supported by two
bricks every 1.2 metres (4 feet). The trench should be
equipped with cross-bracing (diagonal struts to
support the soil sides) approximately every 1.2 metres.
Topsoil is restored to the top of the trench section
above the gravel. The effluent then enters the half-pipe
system and flows along the bottom of the trench (see
Figure 7.5). The half-pipe keeps a conduit permanently
open after stone, earth and tree roots have established
themselves over time (Mollison 1992).

◎ Reed-bed treatment ◎

For the past 25 years Professor Kickuth of Kassel
University in Germany has been developing what he
calls root zone biotechnology, utilising reeds that
usually grow in association with bullrush (*Scirpetum
validi*) and cattail (*Typhetum*). The reeds absorb
oxygen from the air through their pores above
ground, and transport the oxygen to the root zone,
where it enters the soil. In so doing, the system
extracts nitrates, hydrocarbons, phenols, phosphates,
mineral waste and bacteria that are harmful to health.
The system is in use in several countries in Europe and
is being developed in the United Kingdom.

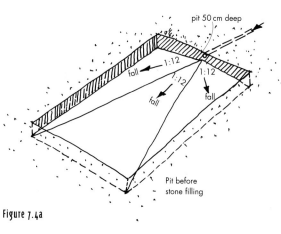

Figure 7.4a

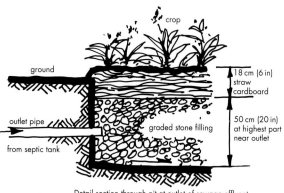

Figure 7.4b

Detail section through pit at outlet of sewage effluent

Figure 7.4: Leach field for
evapo-transpiration bed to
receive sewage effluent (after
Mollinson 1992)

Similar systems have been in existence since 1963, experimenting with 'living filters' in agricultural and forest land. Over a 20-year test period, waste water has been used to irrigate forests and agricultural crops. The system utilises degradation by microorganisms, chemical precipitation, biological transformation, ion exchange and nutrient uptake by the plants' root systems. Using living plants to biologically purify impure water, the 'living filter' system established by Pennsylvania State University has removed the need to haul effluent 330 kilometres (205 miles) to the Atlantic Ocean, and avoids pollution of a natural spring on the sewage treatment land. Over a 20-year period, the water of the spring was monitored and the seven major trace elements all registered very low concentrations while a pH of 7.5 was also maintained. Such a good result in pollution treatment is very unusual. Local ground water supplies are also replenished by the field inundation system and adjoining housing estates alongside Pennsylvania University are now irrigated by the end product of waste water processing.

SURFACE WATER DRAINAGE

The ground contours of your site should be designed to carry surface water run-off away from the building into storm water drains. The least obtrusive measure is to construct 'swale' drains, which are V-shaped and have strong, sloping sides cut at an angle that will support grass. They should be formed within the landscaping, uphill of the building.

Considering drainage from a Gaian viewpoint, our guiding principle is that all surface drainage should be managed naturally, as it was before development occurred. Hard concrete, bitumen and other sealed surfaces for housing developments and landscaping need to be replaced with porous paving materials that allow water to pass through them to the water table. Engineer-designed paths and roads, with their concrete kerbs and gutters that channel storm water into concrete drains and into natural creeks have a disastrous effect on the environment. The high-velocity run-off erodes the banks of creeks, scouring and removing soil and depositing it on beaches or at river deltas and harbours that silt up as a result.

There are alternatives to concrete paving. By changing sealed areas of bitumen and concrete to porous paving, we can cooperate with Gaia, rather than creating problems. Solutions include using modular paving blocks set on a gravel or sand base, or the porous bituminous paving that is now used for airstrips and expressways (standard bitumen is not porous). A porous surface allows rain to filter through the paving into the soil beneath, where it joins the ground water and follows the drainage patterns as they were before we changed them.

The following strategies would help lessen the impact of new housing developments. Use house designs that eliminate roof gutters and downpipes, except where the rainwater is to be stored in tanks. Plan narrow streets and retain natural vegetation already adapted to the soils of the district. Use porous pavements on gravel bases which can be constructed to take loadings for either light or heavy use. Eliminate concrete gutters, sumps and pipelines that normally take the run-off from pavements, and use gravel soakage drains and sumps instead.

Where existing sealed surfaces cannot be replaced, for example in car parks and road drainage systems, silt settlement ponds can be installed to catch initial high-velocity run-off. This water could then be released gradually from the pond to avoid the erosion of creeks and silting of river deltas. The soil type of the area should always be considered when adopting a strategy for a new development.

Trees, shrubs and groundcovers provide the leafy umbrellas that normally absorb most of the impact of rain. When a land surface does not have that protection, rain splash erosion occurs. Both directly and indirectly, rain splash erosion is the major cause of topsoil and subsoil removal. Maintain vegetation groundcovers, particularly on the uphill side of a house, as their vigorous root systems will hold the soil, and their leaf cover will absorb rain splash energy, reducing erosion.

A HEALTHY GARDEN – BUT NOT WITH UNHEALTHY PLANTS

◎ Poisonous plants ◎

We take the trouble to lock chemicals and poisons away from children but who has ever seen a death's head symbol on oleanders or laburnum to indicate their poisonous nature? You cannot tell from a plant's appearance whether it is poisonous or not. In some cases, only part of the plant is poisonous: the leaves but not the stem of rhubarb is poisonous, as are the leaves of the tomato plant. Many plants also lose their toxicity when cooked. Cassava (*Manihot*) contains cyanide yet it is a staple food in some tropical countries, after it has been rigorously washed to remove the poison. Although few deaths are recorded, sickness is common when children eat poisonous plants, as are allergic reactions. The rhus tree, for example, causes skin rashes and blisters at the slightest contact.

No garden should contain a castor-oil plant (*Ricinus communis*) which is very poisonous. In general, brightly coloured berries, stored spring bulbs, fungi and mushrooms of all kinds need to be kept away from children and pets. Some plant families contain more poison than others (see Appendix G).

In 1981 a three year old girl was playing beneath a yellow oleander (*Thevetia peruviana*) in her home in Brisbane, Queensland, Australia. A little later she began vomiting, complaining of a stomach ache. Several hours later her pulse was fast and she was shaking and sweating. It seemed like a case of influenza, but she died of a heart attack on the way to hospital ('Pretty but dangerous' 1983). Fortunately nature protects children to some extent by making the attractively coloured leaves and berries of poisonous plants bitter. Some are even vile tasting and burn the mouth, hence they are not often eaten.

The first botanical gardens in Padua, Italy, from which many European species were exported to the United States and Australasia, without consideration of their allergic or toxic properties

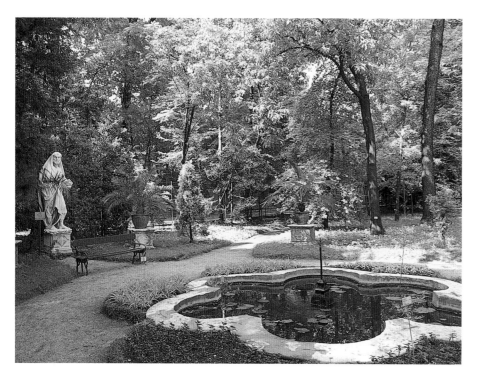

◉ T r e e s   w i t h o u t   s n e e z e ◉

The key to landscaping around a healthy house is to choose garden plants that do not affect your family's health. Pollens can result in bodily reactions such as hay fever, irritated eyes, rhinitis, asthma and extreme fatigue. To a certain extent, this is dependent on geography and climate. For example, in the wide and windy savanna or the hot, dry, semi-arid plains, grasses and wind-pollinated plants tend to predominate, causing a high level of allergies.

Many wind-borne pollens only travel short distances, so controlling the pollen sources in your own garden is very important, especially near windows. Obviously you cannot control the pollen that arrives during rain storms, or that is blown in on hot, dry, dusty winds. It is best to stay inside under such conditions. On hot, still days, when pollen remains suspended in the air, it is best to stay away from the garden. The best time for the soul and the sinuses is the morning, before the heat builds up and breezes begin, as well as cool, cloudy days.

From the allergy point of view, plants can be categorised according to their mode of pollination: those that spread their pollen on the wind are allergens, while those that make use of birds and insects are nonallergens. In allergenic plants the pollen is small enough to enter the nose and attach to the hairs that filter the air flow, but in nonallergenic plants, the pollen is generally too large to be entrapped. Appendix F contains a list of nonallergenic and allergenic trees and shrubs. Your local nursery can give you more detailed advice about low allergy plants.

Choose a grass that produces a low level of pollen and does not have to be mown too often. Avoid freshly mown grass. If you use a lawnmower or edgecutter, wear a mask and goggles to prevent pollen and mould spores from contacting your nose, skin and eyes. Weeds produce a lot of pollen, so suppress their growth by using mulch on the garden, and pebbles and gravel on drives. Groundcovers also reduce the need for organic mulch and keep the weed growth down. Use lightly scented plants, as strong perfumes can cause irritation to sensitised nasal tissues. If you are allergic to mould, do not turn the compost heap over or carry compost to the garden. Handling compost can cause asthma, and nasal, eye, and skin irritation.

Designing the Healthy Garden — Eastern and Western Principles

◉ The joy of gardens ◉

We have spent years photographing and imbibing the spirit of great landscape gardening on the European continent, in the United Kingdom, Russia, Japan, China and North America. We have immersed ourselves in the disciplined hedonism of the Alhambra in Spain, marvelled at the bold scale and detailing in the designs of La Notre, including Vaux-le-Vicomte, the prototype of the elaborate garden of the Sun King at Versailles, France and searched with an anglophile's eagerness for topiarism in England, as at Levens Hall and the original runnels and drains in the garden of Rousham House by William Kent. Gardens have been a great joy.

But what is the spirit of a garden? What is it about a successful garden that makes it able to encourage health, wellbeing and a sense of joy?

Gardens are 'man's idealised view of the world [and] cannot be considered in detachment from the people who made them' (Clifford 1966). Everyone has a different concept of their ideal garden. The ideal garden in England, America, Japan, China, Australasia and so on, will vary as much from person to person as it will from culture to culture. What then do all gardens have in common? The garden is a place which not so much provides an escape from reality, but one where reality has a different meaning.

The garden of your healthy house is not just a setting for the building. It should be an experience that will elevate the spirit, satisfy the mind and senses, quieten the emotions and nourish the body. Moving through such a garden is to experience changes in vista, as one does when walking from room to room in a home. Light, texture, colour and perfume are the design components used to create outdoor rooms, each of which contains something that nourishes the body, soul and spirit.

The choice of an appropriate landscape concept for a healthy garden depends on the location of the site. If it is in an inner urban or suburban area where air pollution is a problem, your primary need will be for plants to control pollution, so the mini-forest approach may be appropriate. For the purpose of filtering the air and encouraging carbon dioxide and oxygen exchange, you should maximise the gross leaf count by choosing evergreen species with an abundance of leaves.

Sites, such as our case study site, which are located in outer suburban or country areas, provide the potential for you to apply the principles of *feng shui* to the design of a healthy garden. The design for such a site can also integrate the cultivation of food plants with *feng shui* design principles.

◉ Feng shui landscaping ◉

The function of a Chinese *feng shui* garden is to provide a setting in which to philosophise. Through a combination of subtle features it creates an unhurried atmosphere. Paths meander from one view and mood to the next. Bridges curve upwards in an arc over the water to encourage you to pause and contemplate the reflections.

The *feng shui* garden avoids the use of the straight 'desire line', a direct path from one place to another, and instead contains paths with subtle S-curves. This not only makes the appearance of the paths more interesting but eradicates the straight-lined path of *sha ch'i* (negative *ch'i*). The curved or zig-zagged bridge fulfils the same function. Unlike a western garden in which rocks are placed in a rockery then covered by plants, the *feng shui* garden emphasises the beauty of the rocks themselves — rugged rocks (*yang*) are placed in a serene (*yin*) setting. Rocks, along with all the other elements of the garden, are used symbolically throughout the zones of the garden. Permanent specimen plants are chosen and located in order to achieve the appropriate *feng shui* form for the garden. It is quite possible to substitute species indigenous to your area for the traditional Chinese *feng shui* plants. For instance, where a water symbol such as a willow is called for, a person in Australia could substitute it with the indigenous willow myrtle (*Agonis flexuosa*) as it has a distinctive *yin*, curved and trailing habit.

The introduction of abundant vegetation helps to balance the *yang* quality of urban landscapes. The use of an interior courtyard garden within a building, a traditional element in Chinese architecture, promotes beneficial *ch'i*. The features described in Table 7.1 (overleaf) are worth including in our garden design.

ELEMENT	FORM	FENG SHUI SYMBOLISM AND ASSOCIATION
Small stream	Meandering in layout. Bridges and stepping stones also meander. Usually to east of gardens and water-flow is north to south	Wealth and health
Fountain	Rounded plan-shape preferred	Generates ch'i and accelerates business (mental vitality and good fortune)
Pond	Ideal shape is circular in external outline and appearing to embrace the building. Used on the south side of the building. Must be clean, ideally containing carp**, tortoises and lotus plants	Water dragon and referred to as the 'mirror of brightness' or *Ming T'ang*
Rocks and boulders	Shape is naturalistic and weatherworn (combine with waterfall if practical on north side of garden). Rocks represent hills and mountains and are used on natural bedding strata (not vertical as in Japanese gardens)	Protection from ill fortune
Plants		Active growth and expansion
Flowers		Happiness and Goodwill
Trees	Not to be used on front-entrance side of buildings	Strength and integrity. When used at rear of building, they are protective
Natural shapes (topiary can also be used)	Triangular (Fire): pine; Deliquescent (Water): willow; Horizontal (Earth): box or yew hedge; Vertical (Wood): poplar, cypress; Hemispherical or domed (Metal): fig tree (*Ficus benjaminii*)	
Garden Walls	Not over 2m (6.7ft) high for a single-storey building. Gate to be proportional to building. Many openings in walls are not good *feng shui* design	Creates feeling of balance and continuity. Square and round openings symbolise Earth and heaven respectively
Paving	Pebble paving paths are best in western part of garden. Should be meandering in pattern	Symbolises the alternating duality of *yin* and *yang*
Pavilions	Usually placed in NE or SW. These are miniaturised in small gardens. Summer-house designs can be substituted in other than Asian contexts. Plan shapes: square (Earth symbol); pentagon (Five elements); hexagon (Wealth); octagon (Prosperity)	Placed at NE and SW 'gates', to guard against 'evil' influences

* Lip, 1990b; Too, 1993
**Carp should only be used where they cannot escape into local waterways during floods

Table 7.1: Landscape elements, shape and symbolic meaning*

Roof-garden house combining underground and aboveground aspects. Castle Hill, NSW, Aust. (Architects: ECA Space Design Pty Ltd; Landscape Designer: S. Baggs)

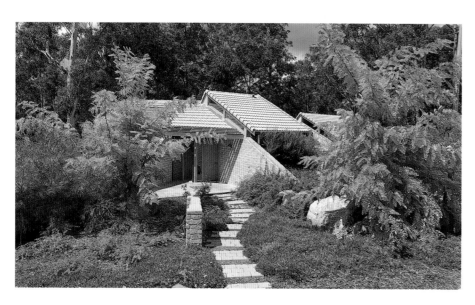

The design of the garden needs to be settled upon at the outset, and adhered to over time. Though it may take years to reach fruition, the original concept must be maintained in its broad outline, allowing for flexibility in minor details. The most important factor is that the garden design should echo nature, be beautiful, light in tone, and meaningful, with contrasts of strength and gentleness. There should be no formal flower beds, or grouped and regulated flowering plants or riotous colour schemes. Colours need to be grouped into supplementary schemes, offset by foliage and used as focal points in neutral backgrounds of foliage massings. Other colours used in the design of landscape elements should endeavour to use the colours and hues of the local environment, that is the soils, rocks, sand and natural vegetation of the area. The house pictured below left was designed using local soil with compressed earth bricks; the wood trims echo the colour of the bark of the local eucalypts, while the roof tiles are the colour of the eucalypt leaves.

Using indigenous plants where appropriate, the landscape design should follow modern principles and be based on accepted landscape design concepts of massing and grouping similar species. Evergreen trees are usually preferred to deciduous.

English style cottage garden planting is inappropriate. The design should be simple and avoid overcrowding: a 'single, common, wild plant, carefully placed in an appropriate setting, will be worthy of contemplation' (Walters 1988). A simple planting scheme can emphasise spaciousness in a small garden.

A single specimen plant may be used to represent many plants. The Dragon, Bird, Tiger and Tortoise may be included as sculptural features (or stones suggesting these forms) in the east, south, west and north sectors respectively. Trellis structures are used to deflect malevolent *sha ch'i* from adjoining environmental elements. By paying careful attention to the shapes of walls, wall openings, rocks, water bodies, paths and garden beds, you can create a *feng shui* garden within the constraints of suburban space.

WATER

A *feng shui* garden is incomplete without water. Flat ground will need ponds and hilly ground will need streams or rivulets. The depth of the water is irrelevant, but the surface needs to be reflective and the shape sinuous. The sound of running water is an important acoustic element in the design. Stepping stones across water are best located at a lower height than the banks of the pond or stream, as this gives a sense of walking near the surface of the water.

In dry climates and where authorities require, water may have to be conserved and recirculated. In areas of poor drainage, a subsoil drainage system will need to be designed and installed.

Remember that when you alter the natural landscape of a site you may disrupt the flow of *ch'i*. When making any excavations on your site, or installing things like pools and watercourses, it is vital that the *ch'i* of the site be taken into consideration. After major excavation work, the landscape should be restored to the original, or improved, levels of *ch'i*.

THE OUTDOOR ROOM

In some traditional *feng shui* gardens, screens and walls divide the garden space into a series of experiences. This creation of outdoor rooms gives containment and human scale to the garden. Such a garden is known as a mobile garden. The static garden, another type of *feng shui* garden design, is based on a fixed viewpoint from, say, a window of the building. In the mobile garden, the visitor strolls from one experience to another, an experience that can be likened to the unfurling of a Chinese scroll painting, revealing one scene after the other (Walters 1988). Some gardens combine characteristics of both the static and mobile garden, while poorly designed gardens contain neither.

Some aspect of the distant scenery should be preserved and unsuitable views should be screened or walled out of sight. Tops of distant hills and mountains are good features to preserve, while their bases should be hidden from view. The same principle applies to artificial features in the environment: roofs should be revealed, while the bases of buildings should be screened. Even in industrial environments, it is possible to select and preserve certain views. For instance, if the Wood element is appropriate in the garden, a distant tower framed by a gateway may provide depth and interest.

CONFLICTING DESIGN PHILOSOPHIES

As we begin to design our garden it will become apparent that a conflict exists between the philosophies of eastern design and western, Gaian design. If we were to follow the philosophical

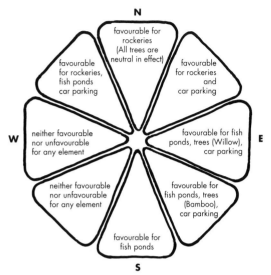

Figure 7.6: Site sector diagram. Most favoured locations of garden elements in *feng shui*. When the four elements: fish ponds, trees, rockeries and car parking are not mentioned, their use is unfavourable (after Lip 1990b)

COMMON NAME OF PLANT	SYMBOL	YIN or YANG status
Pine	longevity	
Willow	grace	yang
Plum	beauty and youth	
Pear	longevity	yin
Cypress	royalty	
Acacia	stability	yang
Pomegranate	fertility	
Tangerine	wealth	
Camellia	evergreen	
Loquat	wealth	
Peony	wealth	
Bamboo	youth	yang
Peach	friendship	yang
Jasmine	friendship	
Rose	beauty	
Narcissus	rejuvenation	
Orchid	endurance	
Peony		yang
Chrysanthemum		yang
Date		yang
Persimmon		yang
Cherry		yang
Maple		yang
Camphor		yang
Banana		yin
Grape		yin
Papaya		yin
Blackwood		yin
Eucalypt (gum tree)		yin

*Lip 1990b

Table 7.2: Symbolic meaning of plants and *yin/yang* polarity*

principle 'to tread lightly on the Earth', we would undertake companion planting to avoid the use of chemical pesticides, and would grow organic vegetables, fruits, grains and nuts. A mixed jungle of plants would result, contrasting with the simplicity of a *feng shui* garden.

Yet it is possible to combine the two philosophies. The jungle effect can be avoided in any zone of the site by keeping the trees to a limited number of species, grouping shrubs within the same height range, limiting groundcover plants to one, two or three species, and growing trees, shrubs and groundcovers in two or three associated groups. A path, wall or stream, garden furniture or even a single common plant species can become the coordinating element from one association, or precinct, to the next. Simplicity and coordinated landscape design themes are needed, perhaps varying from one precinct to another.

◎ The landscape site survey plan ◎

For the purposes of designing a simple, residential garden, much of the site information that you gathered in the initial process of choosing your site (see Chapter 2) can be used to make a single survey drawing on which all the natural features, buildings on neighbouring properties, prominent landforms and trees that may cast shadows on your site are recorded.

The next step is to apply *feng shui* principles (see Figure 7.6 on the previous page) to the survey plan, noting which landscape elements are appropriate for each sector. For the case study family discussed in Chapters 5 and 6, from a *feng shui* viewpoint, pavilions are best located in the southwestern or northwestern sectors of their site. The topography, as well as the distant view available from the highest point of this site (the northeastern corner) favours the location of a gazebo or pavilion in that sector. As the design develops, it may become clear that other little pavilions are also appropriate to optimise views within the site. The carport or garage should be located last of all. It should be located in the northeastern, eastern or southeastern sectors of the garden. An eastern location is preferable, as it would provide a useful screen for a drying area on the sunny side of that building. The most appropriate place for an access drive to the garage and a visitor parking area is the southeastern sector.

WATER AND SURFACE RUN-OFF

The surface flow of run-off is plotted by setting out equal divisions along the highest contour on your survey drawing. One centimetre (½ inch) is a workable distance between the divisions. At each division, draw a line at 90 degrees to that contour and then slowly curve the line until it meets, at a 90 degree angle, the next contour below it. Repeat this step for each division. Now begin the process again, working from the points where your lines intersect with the second contour line. Draw lines, at 90 degree angles, from the second contour line down so that they reach the third contour line at 90 degree angles. Continue this process until you have worked through each contour line on your survey drawing. The pattern which emerges where the lines are closest together will indicate where surface run-off will accumulate. Some control of surface silt carried by run-off may be necessary if conditions are extreme. This can be done by excavating a stilling pond which will cause the surface flow to slow down and give the silt time to settle.

In our case study site, a 'turkey-nest' dam was already in existence to conserve surface water. In the new plan for the garden, it will be replaced with a stilling pond to overflow into a new pond and stream system. The water in this system will be continuously filtered and recycled, with the assistance of solar-driven pumps. Surface run-off flow from the garden areas can be intercepted by using a stream and cascade as a diversion drain. The *Ming T'ang* pool, traditionally in the south, is at the entrance to the building and will contain a silt trap to collect silt from the stream system. This trap will require continuous maintenance.

The case study family's design would need a higher than average investment in landscaping. Water flows from the waterfall (the Tortoise direction) down the Tiger side of the site and across the south-facing entrance side. The entrance porch bridges to an island in the centre of a *Ming T'ang*. In this way *ch'i* flows around the building and slows as it pools in the *Ming T'ang*, allowing beneficial *ch'i* to accumulate. *Ch'i* then exits to the Dragon side of the site via a hidden outlet grating and pipe which leads underground to the natural filtration tanks and water-filtration pump housing. Photovoltaic cell panels collect solar energy to run the pumps.

PLANTING CONCEPT AND PRACTICAL STRATEGIES

The case study's landscape survey plan shows that the site is exposed to hot summer and cold winter winds from the west. A shelterbelt of vegetation is required all year round, so evergreen species will have to be chosen.

Some of the species on the leeward side of the shelterbelt can be of a fragrant type. We would choose the evergreen *Elaeagnus pungens*, a rather prickly, fast-growing hedge which grows to around 4 metres (13 feet). The westerly winds, their velocity reduced by the shelterbelt, will carry fragrance to the remainder of the garden and the house. Species of plants must then be chosen for the rest of the planting beds in the layout, keeping in mind the needs of the family.

As a way of bridging the purely aesthetic and the practical and healthy garden, we suggest that the texture, scale and colour characteristics of vegetable, nut and fruit plants be explored and a companion planting procedure be adopted. Plants not commonly associated with *feng shui* gardens can be combined with traditional *feng shui* species if this will produce a garden which avoids chemically based pest and disease control techniques.

The local knowledge of gardeners, nurserymen and horticulturalists in the district where you intend to live will be an invaluable resource when choosing species for your site. They will be able to recommend companion plants that will work for your climate and soil, and will also give advice about indigenous species, the texture of different plants, their leaf size and habits, colour and fruiting seasons. Combine local, native plants with food-producing plants and a few key exotic plants to suit the theme of the garden. Group your selection of plants with regard for their companion planting characteristics, using contrasting sizes only for emphasis. Try to achieve a unified appearance by placing your plants according to their height and leaf size. The aim is to achieve an overall unity of size and scale.

COMPANION PLANTING

When planting a healthy garden, you should remember that in nature, all plants grow in communities and often help sustain one another. For the past 10,000 years, western agriculture has gradually developed monoculture, the cultivation of one crop at a time. The machinery, fertiliser and pesticides employed in this type of agriculture have destroyed much of the animal and insect life formerly present in the soil, reducing it to a lifeless medium. The use of chemical fertilisers and pesticides, combined with inappropriate cropping and cultivation procedures, have caused the soils of the world to become impoverished.

Companion planting is a method of gardening based on the mutual support and interaction found in natural communities, which benefit each plant. Companion planting has developed from the observations of many gardeners over time and many practices have become almost universal. Much more research is needed, however, to give it a scientific basis. It is a successful form of cultivation because a diverse selection of plants produces flowers with varying blooming periods, supplying nectar to beneficial insects such as bees, wasps and flies throughout the year. The food supply for particular plant-feeding insects and their larvae is not as plentiful as it would be if single species were grown in the normal manner. This keeps insect population numbers down.

Some plants exude substances from their roots that adversely affect the microorganisms that produce diseases in other plants. One type of plant may release from its root system large quantities of various organic compounds, including proteins and sugars. Bacteria feed on these compounds and their populations cluster around the roots. Some of these bacteria produce compounds that slow or prevent growth of other microorganisms. Root exudates can also act in a detrimental way, inhibiting the growth of other plants, so it is essential to know the effects of one plant on another.

Combining plants attracts various species of insects. No single species of insect dominates, so no single type of plant is exposed on its own to insect attack. It is essential to adapt the system to suit indigenous insect species. A good local nurseryman, or the agricultural department, can guide you on this.

If you plant a citrus tree, thrip, aphids, scale and other insects proliferate. Planting a variety of plants helps to solve this problem. For instance, broad beans will draw aphids away from the citrus. In addition, like most leguminous plants, broad beans have nodules in their roots which store nitrogen, then make it available to neighbouring plants via the soil.

A good general rule is to combine deep- and shallow-rooting species. Comfrey (*Symphytum officinale*) has a long taproot which raises nutrients, particularly potassium, from deep levels in the soil and makes it available to surface-rooting plants. All plants from the mint (*Mentha*) species are excellent for companion planting, as they repel white butterfly and aphids, and improve the flavour and health of several types of vegetables. Marigolds (*Calendula officianalis*) and all plants from the family Asteraceae (including daisies, dahlias and chrysanthemums) guard against aphids by attracting hover flies and lace wings, which eat the aphids. All mint and marigolds also attract parasitic wasps which feed on other insects.

Check with your agricultural department when populations of insects are at their greatest, then consult your local nursery and find a plant species that fruits earlier or later than that time. In this way the conflict of your needs with those of pest insects can be avoided. If you want to find out what pests are in your area, take a yellow bowl, fill it with water and place it in your garden. After a few days, you will find specimens of the main insect species floating in it.

To attract bees, plant borage (*Borago officinalis*). Try to provide a variety of habitats, grow only small stands of particular crops, avoid using pesticides and include plenty of flowering plants. Also use composting techniques and recycle sullage or grey water. Be careful what detergents you use, as very few are compatible with plants. Introduce a wide variety of local native plants to achieve a composite of many plant species.

COMPANION PLANTS FOR FRUITS AND VEGETABLES

The following companion combinations are successful in controlling pests on fruit and vegetables:

Apples grow well with nasturtiums, which control woolly aphids, and combined with chives, control scale. Asparagus grows well with tomatoes, but not with basil and parsley. Beans grow well with nasturtiums, dill and sage, and with the brassica group of vegetables, which includes cabbage, cauliflower, broccoli, Brussels sprouts, kohl rabi, radishes and turnips. The brassicas, in turn, grow well with peas, potatoes, garlic, cucumbers, tomatoes and bush beans (those with a bushy growth habit). Candytuft (*Iberis amara*), a summer annual often mistaken for a large form of Sweet Alice, is useful to control small beetles.

Hyssop (*Hyssopus officinalis*) which has pink, blue, purple and white flowers, will act as a decoy to caterpillars. Beets grow well in the company of bush beans, onions, lettuce and the brassicas. Beans that grow on a single stalk (pole beans) do not grow well in the company of mustard plants. If white flowering daisies are planted with cabbages, the cabbage moths mistake the white flowers for other moths and as they are territorial, they fly away. Carrots grow well with leek, lettuce, peas, onions, garlic, tomatoes and salsify (*Tragopogan porrifolisu*), also known as the 'vegetable oyster'.

Chives deter insects that attack the carrot root. Flax and sage are also useful. Celery grows well in companionship with brassicas, beans, leek and tomatoes. Cucumber grows with the legumes (clovers, retches, lupins, beans, etc, all of which vary in their capacity to fix nitrogen in their roots) and radishes, with corn (maize) and sunflowers for support. Lettuce grows well with carrots, radishes, cucumbers and strawberries. Onions grow with lettuce, tomatoes and leek. Peas grow well with beans, carrots, cucumbers, radishes, potatoes and corn (maize) as companion plants but keep them well away from onions and garlic. Potatoes grow well with legumes, brassicas and corn (maize). Radishes prefer cucumbers, peas and lettuce for company.

Strawberries grow well with beans, lettuce and spinach. Capsicum or sweet pepper (*Capsicum frutescens gross*) grows well with eggplant (aubergine). Basil can be used to decoy aphids but it prefers not to be near brassicas. Tomatoes grow well with asparagus (because this helps deter tomato root nematodes) as well as with carrots, onions, garlic and radishes. French marigold will deter a wide range of white fly. Borage can be used to build resistance to insects in tomatoes. Sagebrush (*Artemesia tridenta*) stimulates tomatoes to produce high levels of a natural chemical pest deterrent. When rhubarb is planted with angelica it tends to be less tart in flavour. When camomile is planted with lemon thyme (*Thymus citriodorus*) fungal diseases are deterred. Because both grow as groundcovers they help to control weeds. Stinging nettles deter fungal diseases and stimulate oil production in herbs, increasing the rate of ripening and the length of time that they can be stored. The young leaves can be eaten much as you would spinach.

NATURAL INSECT CONTROLS

Home-made, organic pest control is slower than chemical pest control and needs more diligence in application and repetition, but it is worth it. To avoid chemical pesticides use plants that are lemon scented; they contain citronella, which helps control mosquitoes.

Tomato leaves and stems, and rhubarb leaves contain toxins. When the leaves and stems are boiled in water and strained, the liquid makes a good natural insecticide for spraying. This is a 17th century recipe which works well: boil tomato stems and leaves, strain, and when cold, spray over plants attacked by aphids (Jane 1987).

Sucking insects and caterpillars can be controlled with various organic sprays, applied as many times as necessary. Garlic spray can be made by soaking 85 grams (3 ounces) of crushed garlic in 50 millilitres (1¾ fluid ounces) of liquid paraffin for 1–2 days. During that time, gradually add 600 millilitres (1 pint) of water in which 28 grams (1 ounce) of pure soap have been dissolved. (To melt soap, grate and add to boiling water. Stir while simmering until dissolved.) Strain the garlic liquid and store in plastic or glass containers.

Another solution to the problem of sucking insects and caterpillars is to combine in a blender either hot chillies or capsicum (washed thoroughly) with an equal amount of water to which a teaspoon of liquid dishwashing detergent has been added. Rhubarb spray is made from 2 kilograms (4 pounds 6 ounces) of rhubarb leaves boiled for 30 minutes in 3.5 litres (7 pints) of water. Strain, add 28 grams (1 ounce) of pure soap. Dilute with equal quantities of water before using.

Wood ash (not coal ash) can be spread over the soil to add potassium and phosphorus and control pests. There are also several teas which can be made that do not harm ladybirds, bees and other beneficial insects, yet deter pests. Tea made from wormwood deters slugs and other soft-bodied insects. Pick the leaves early in the morning and dry in a shaded, airy place until crumbly. Put the leaves in a saucepan, cover with water and bring to the boil. Strain and dilute with four parts of water, and stir for 10 minutes. Horseradish tea, which can be prepared in the same way as the wormwood tea, slows the spread of fruit tree fungus if painted or sprayed on when the fungus first develops.

Not all chemicals are nasty. For example, the product Dipel™ kills caterpillars by causing parasites to grow inside them. It operates selectively and causes harm to nothing but the pest itself.

However, despite the widely held belief that they are harmless, plant-based pesticides such as the pyrethrin from pyrethrum flowers and derris dust from the root of the derris tree *are* dangerous to humans. Pyrethrin can damage eyes and pyrethroids (synthetic pyrethrin) are absorbed through the skin and accumulate in the body, causing dizziness, headaches, fatigue, loss of appetite and abnormal facial sensations (Short 1994). Derris dust is also cumulative in its effect on the body (Jane 1987). You should always protect your skin with clothing and use a mask during spraying and dusting.

COMPOSTING

Composting makes the best use of organic wastes by creating conditions for their rapid breakdown into homogenous material which can form part of the soil system. All organic waste can be converted to a fertiliser and soil improver. Composting is a natural process, good for the soil and ideal for improving your results in the garden. It reduces or eliminates the need for using fertiliser and automatically reduces waste collection, disposal and the impact of landfill or incineration on the environment. The compost bin is best sited on the sunny side of the garden. In our case study garden, it has been located in the service and drying yard.

At the bottom of the compost bin use a layer of coarse, organic waste and previously composted material or soil, 15–20 centimetres (6–8 inches) deep. A handful of lime or dolomite is spread over this layer, which is then covered with 2.5 centimetres (1 inch) of soil. Add organic material to the bin and leave it for 10 to 12 weeks, turning regularly. Use a variety of organic matter, including animal and poultry manure, but do not include woody branches and prunings, thorny branches, oily or waxy plants, large bones or fat, diseased plants, plants contaminated with chemicals, weeds with tough stems and root systems that can survive heat or those that reproduce from corms or bulbs. Such weeds can be recycled by placing them in a drum, covering them with water and letting them decay. They can then be used to water the garden and pot plants.

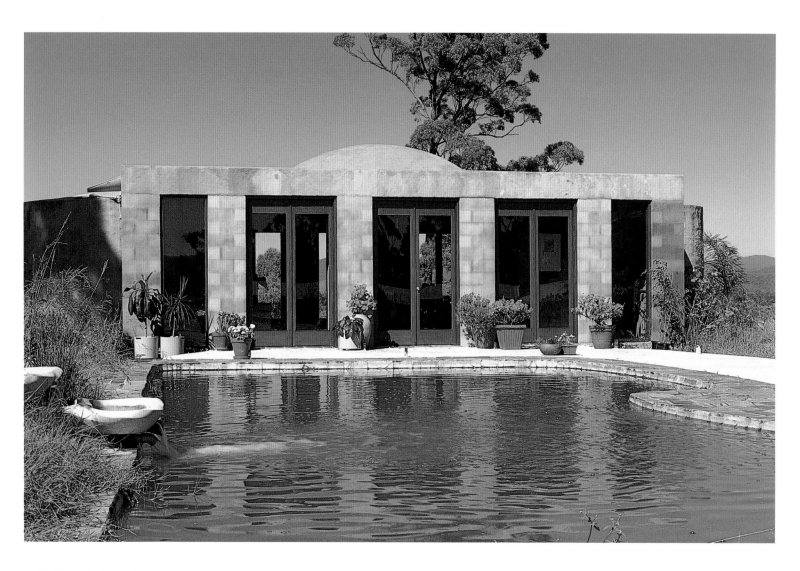

Tank building and cabana with pool-water pumped and treated by reed-bed filtering. (Architect: C. Pattinson, Arcoessence Pty Ltd)

It is acceptable to add general kitchen waste such as cooking oil, food scraps, fruit, vegetable peelings, tea leaves and bags and coffee grounds, along with lawn cuttings, most weeds and leaves, cereal products, the contents of the vacuum cleaner, wood ash, shredded rags and paper and egg shells. The shredding of materials accelerates decomposition. When mature, the compost should resemble and smell like good topsoil, and can be used as a mulch or fertiliser. It can also be sieved and used to dress lawns, but keep it approximately 0.5 metre (20 inches) away from the trunks of fruit trees.

⊛ Aquatic garden resources ⊛

Our case study garden design has incorporated large areas of pond and rivulets. This system utilises a natural reed bed ecosystem which, in itself, is a water purifying and filtering system operating entirely by natural means. The concept can be expanded to include an aquaculture system, where the water resources are used to cultivate freshwater organisms for food. We are not suggesting intensive farming, rather aquaculture at a level to satisfy the needs of family and friends.

An aquaculture system can be very productive, perhaps exceeding the land-based companion plant system in terms of food production. It may contain fish, yabbies (freshwater crayfish), waterfowl, freshwater snails, water lilies (for both flowers and edible roots), fish eggs, eels, water chestnuts, wild rice and domestic watercress. Frogs should be present to control pests. Ducks can also be included, but they need a waterside, overnight pen for protection against foxes, cats and dogs. Ducks control green algae and water weed as well as fertilising the water for fish and eel production. They eat insects, slugs and garden snails and they do not scratch or eat mature vegetable greens. However, they can trample young plants and have to be fenced out of such areas until the plants develop. Muscovy ducks should be avoided in the garden as they are vegetation eaters and forage mainly on grasses.

The herb garden

A walled, kitchen herb garden with fragrant shrubs in pots can be such a delightful place, with its perfumes and stimuli for the family cook, that in our case study design it has been located in the atrium or central courtyard of the house (see Figure 7.9 on page 119).

The pyramid form of the atrium, said to develop a solitron (standing columnar wave) stimulates plant growth, possibly due to the effects of morphic resonance. In hot climates, shade mesh is utilised as the covering for the atrium to create an aviary and reduce incoming solar radiation. In cooler climates, only bird mesh is necessary, while in tropical climates it is advisable to use mosquito-proof mesh.

A herb garden is best located in the atrium or very near the kitchen door for maximum convenience. It needs to be compact and to have easy, paved access as, to allow the herbs to be picked, the bed can be no wider than arm's reach.

The kitchen garden

Located as near as possible to the kitchen door, this garden uses miniature fruit trees to give protection from the sun in summer, nursery beds, and perennials for decorating the house. The kitchen area in our case study house has reasonable northern sun and is well sheltered by the shelterbelt on the western side.

The first set of beds in the kitchen garden should be narrow, follow the meandering path of the *feng shui* garden and contain vegetables that have already been raised as seedlings. While following companion planting principles, select vegetables that can be cropped for months on end, like broccoli, silver beet (Swiss chard), zucchini (courgettes), capsicum (peppers), Brussels sprouts, celery, onions, beans, tomatoes, carrots, peas, eggplant (aubergine), broad beans, fennel and so on. Easy path access to these narrow beds is essential for transplanting, moving plants, accessing seed when plants have run to seed for the following year's crop, and for picking herbs such as camomile, cumin, chervil and caraway. Remember that tomatoes need to be surrounded by a small shelterbelt of broad beans or Jerusalem artichokes.

In the broader garden beds, plants should be closely spaced, and companion planted in large masses. Recommended crops include corn (maize), leeks, turnips, swedes, beetroot, various melons, onions and potatoes.

JAPANESE GARDEN DESIGN

We have concentrated on Chinese *feng shui* garden design principles, but it is also worth considering a closely related style of garden: the Japanese garden. The link between Japanese and Chinese garden design is strong, originating between the 6th and 8th centuries AD. Based on a veneration of nature, it has its roots in the Taoist nature-mysticism of China. Later reinforced by the philosophies and practices of Zen Buddhism, the Japanese garden emphasises quiet meditation. If a Japanese style garden appeals to you, it is possible to design one while still utilising some of the *feng shui* principles discussed, given its links with Chinese garden design.

The Japanese style of garden design prescribes groupings of three, five or seven of landscape elements such as stones of carefully related shapes and sizes. It also advocates the installation of a partially obscured waterfall and the use of a tall guardian stone in the foreground of a set scene. Traditional Japanese garden design contrasts passive and dynamic forms in compositions of quiet restraint. There are three main approaches in Japanese design: the flat garden, the dry garden and the lake-and-island or hill-and-water garden.

The flat garden can be constructed in the smallest urban garden courtyard. The ground should be covered with raked sand, or gravel and rock. Plants and ornaments need to be carefully grouped, for example, a lantern can be used as a recumbent form, a flat stone as a prostrate form and bamboo as a

Below: Temple garden in autumn where space flows from inside to outside. The quality of the Japanese garden contrasts to the systematic and geometric character of the Italian and French garden

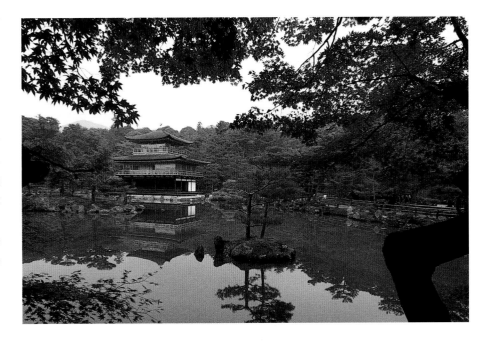

vertical form to complete the whole picture. The dry garden contains mounds of earth formed into hills, while water is symbolised by white gravel, and land by stones (in Chinese garden design, a few carefully placed rugged rocks can symbolise great mountains, emphasising the beauty of the rocks themselves). The hill-and-water garden contains grouped hills, a stream, foreground rocks and plants such as the recumbent, rounded forms of azalea and dwarf conifer. These elements are balanced by the wind-worn pine and the verticality of bamboo.

Texture is more important in Japanese gardens than in any other type. Indigenous species, which encourage bird life, can be used, while still employing the Japanese sense of balance, evocative shapes and an economy of materials. The association between house and garden is particularly close in Japanese garden design, the two spaces merging in an organic flow.

The Tea Garden, a later development, with its focus on the tea ceremony and elements such as stepping stones, stone lanterns and water basins, has determined modern Japanese garden design. There are three principal characteristics of the Japanese garden: naturalism, an amalgamation of natural and artificial forms and the absence of symmetry. Nature is abstracted and natural materials are used. Another essential characteristic of the Japanese garden is the subjective Buddhist experience of the oneness and unity of all natural things.

THE LIFE JOURNEY

Let us assume that the design and construction of our case study garden are complete. We are now free to wander the paths, undertaking the 'journey' which is the goal of Chinese *feng shui* garden design.

Figure 7.7: The southern approach to the case study family's house is in the right foreground. One crosses a bridge over the Ming T'ang *entrance pool*

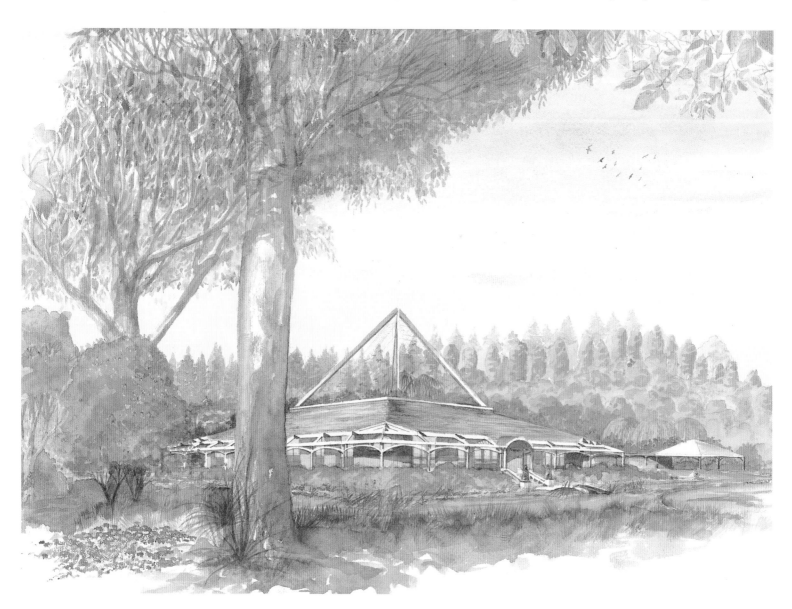

The visitor first crosses the *Ming T'ang* guarded by two symbolic lions, the female and cub on the left and male on the right, and enters the porch of the Red Bird of the south (Figure 7.7, opposite page).

The carved entrance doors open and we move into the entrance vestibule; ahead, the central fragrance court or atrium, containing fragrant herbs and flowers, is visible (Figure 7.9, below). We enter a cloistered walkway around the court. On the far side of the court are the living and dining rooms, facing the sun.

From the living room there is a view of the lake with rising rock shelves from an old quarry forming a low barrier to the Tortoise of the North. The foliage of trailing plants drapes over the rocks, the plateaus of which are filled with deep soil to form rockery beds. A shelterbelt of various pine species retains the *ch'i* accumulating around the pool, integrating with the pine forest to the north of the site. (Pine is also the tree of the Tortoise of the North.) The garden is designed to restore our contact with wild nature. Wild places are symbolised by the rising ground in the northeast corner, a mountain with a forest of *Prunus* species on the slopes, a stream and a waterfall. The natural landscape elements are reduced in size to suit the site and are integrated into the setting of the garden. This allows the occupants of the house to experience the wild without having to negotiate slippery mountain paths or raging rivers. Mountains and rivers were potent symbols in the philosophy of ancient China, linking human beings with nature. The streams are the arteries of the dragon, and the dragon and tiger are conjugating in the forms of the symbolic mountain. The garden represents the Earth's body: mountains are the skeleton and plants are the skin and muscle.

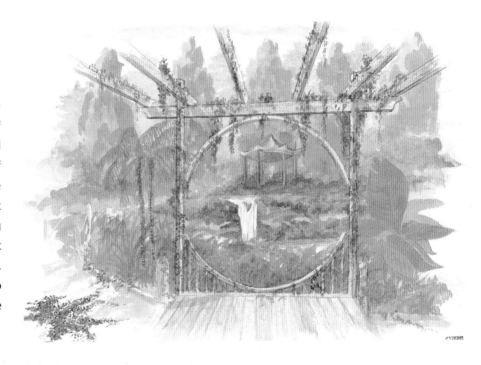

Figure 7.8 (above): On the black tortoise shore of the pond the waterfall and pavilion create an atmosphere for relaxed contemplation

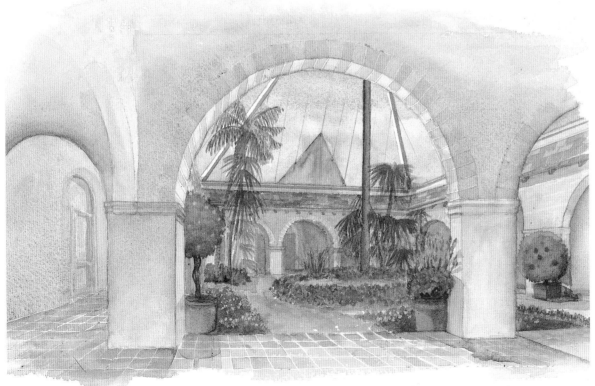

Figure 7.9 (left): The central fragrance atrium courtyard

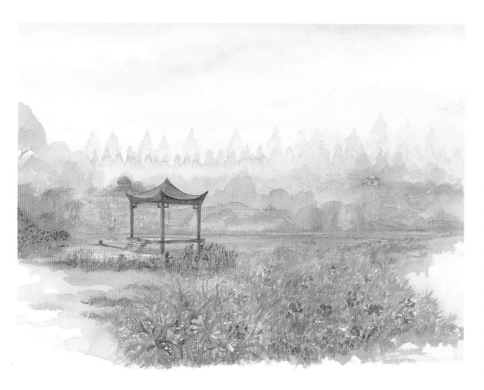

Figure 7.10: The water platform on the northern edge of the fragrant sun garden

Figure 7.11 (opposite page, top): The sunset pavilion with its high view beyond the site to the mountains beyond

Figure 7.12 (opposite page, bottom): Moon gate and *yin/yang* conversation area. The Heaven mound is in the middle ground, the waterfall in the distance

We pass through the portals of the garden into both confined and open spaces, and zones of various characters. Stepping out of the house we enter the fragrant sun terrace, which is flanked on the northern edge by a platform built over the pond (see Figure 7.10).

Here we see reflections of the opposite side of the pond; the rockery 'mountains' and a small gazebo or pavilion in the distance, our first goal as we begin the journey. As we pass by the garden wall, supporting a covered walk from house to garage, the aromas of fragrant herbs and flowers surround us. Abelia (*Abelia floribunda*), with its drooping clusters of pink-mauve flowers, climbs up the warm sunny wall; borders of abelia and boronia (*Boronia ledifolia*), which has large, pink, bell flowers and an aromatic fragrance, enclose the edges of the gravelled terrace. The gravel path leading from the terrace wanders beside the pond and around the mock orange (*Murraya paniculata*) hedge, which has leaves that smell powerfully of spice and can be used in curries, and flowers that smell like jasmine. The path is flanked with Australian myrtle (*Baeckia camphorosmae*) which releases a camphor-like odour when the walker brushes against it.

Now we reach a small bower for contemplating the reflections of the sky on the pond, and the ducks and carp. At this bower, a curved pergola is encased in clematis (*Clematis afoliata*), a soft and sweetly scented, daphne-like climber. The garden seat in the pergola is protected from wind by a low hedge of daphne (*Daphne odora*) planted in rich humus soil. Growing around 2 metres (6½ feet) tall, the clematis surrounds the bower with white flowers that have a spicy aroma.

Wandering further along the path through the various companion-planted vegetables that are natural groundcovers, we come to a narrow inlet leading to the reed-bed filtration pond for water treatment, on the far western boundary of the site. Crossing a small, arched wooden bridge we ascend the 'mountain' path. We pass through a forest of ornamental, flowering fruit trees (*Prunus* spp.) which can grow to 6 metres (20 feet) high. The forest contains both evergreen and deciduous trees, some of which have aromatic leaves and flowers. Flowering almond, peach, nectarine, apricot and cherry all give spring blossoms and coloured foliage to form a base for the rockery mountain. They create the reflections and textures which we viewed from the house and sun terrace on the opposite side of the pond.

The dappled shade of the *Prunus* forest creates ideal conditions for the companion planting of vegetables and other plant species. Reaching the mountain top, we may rest in a small pavilion, around which entwines hardy, fragrant honeysuckle. Here we can watch the sun set (Figure 7.11, opposite page).

Leaving the little pavilion, we take a path that skirts the drop to the lake below, with the pine forest in the distance and our pine shelterbelt on the right. Eventually we come to a small pavilion and waterfall. The water for this small waterfall is filtered and purified in the reed-bed and lifted by solar-activated pumps to the head of the fall. As the water tumbles down the rock ledges it produces negatively ionised particles conducive to health and relaxation. A winding gravel path then leads towards the northwestern corner of the site, into a thicket of black-stem bamboo (a type which does not have an aggressive root system). The bamboo thicket opens onto a bower of evergreen native wisteria (*Milletia* (or *Wisteria*) *megasperma*) and shade tolerant honeysuckle (*Lonicera* × *telmanniana*) which form a shady tunnel of green along the western boundary of the site, where the shelterbelt gives protection from unpleasant winds at all times of the year. This path skirts the edge of the rockery. Below, in the microclimate created by the enclosing rocks and the moist air, temperate rainforest plants create an exotic pocket of greenery.

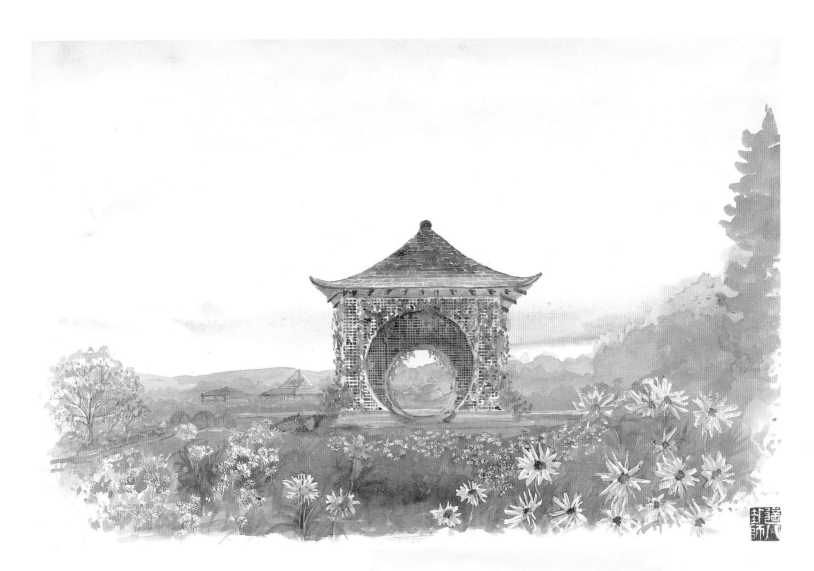

As we descend to the pond level, staggered flagstones lead to a simple timber bridge across a stream. At the other side of the stream, we find an open-air room formed by a pergola-pavilion which contains a reading niche. Looking at the view of the distant shore of the pond through a moon gate in the wall, one can reflect on the life journey, now reaching completion (see Figure 7.12, at right).

Passing through the moon gate we ascend a small mound winding around a serpentine pilgrim's path, to reach a little meditation pavilion at its summit. Here we sit, symbolically in the 'heaven life' and reflect on the vista of the life's journey we have just taken. Descending from the mound, we return home, closer to our loved ones than we were before.

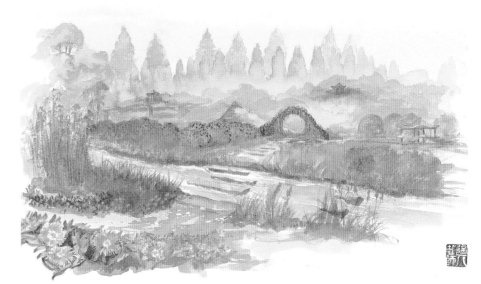

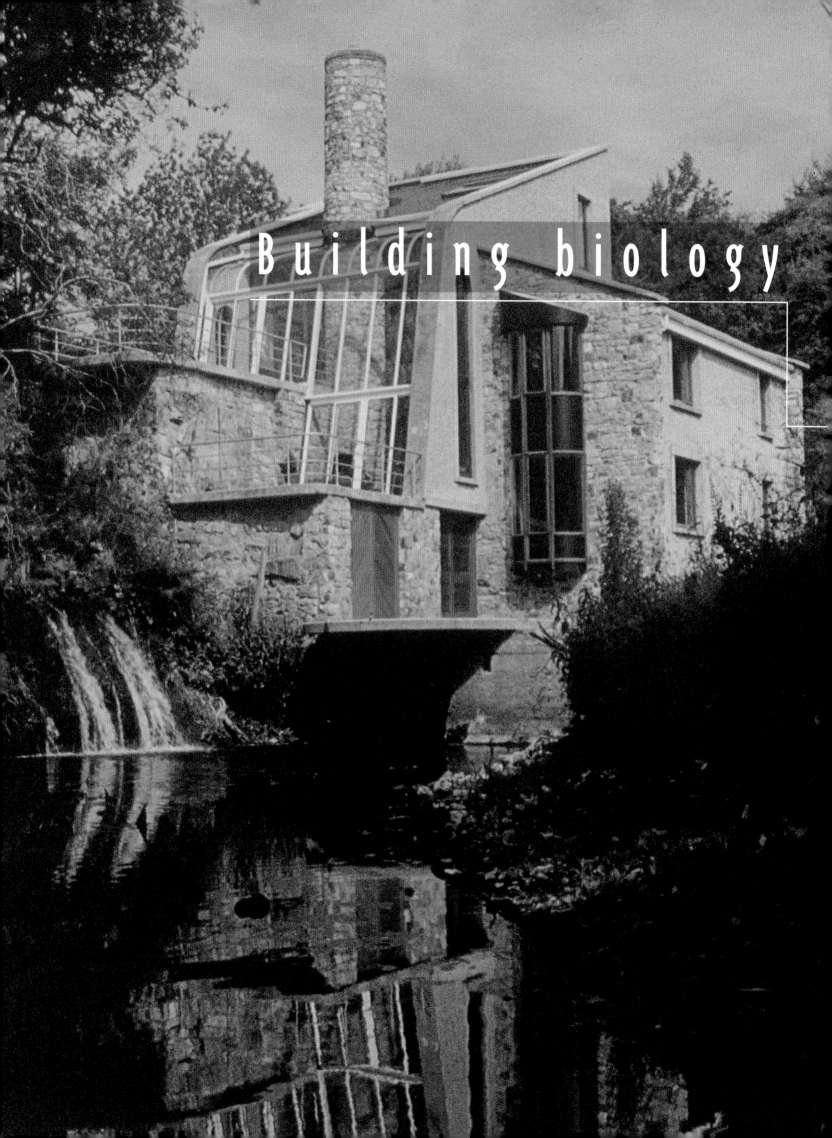

Building biology

and ecology

building biology is an interdisciplinary science — and art — which integrates the creativity of the design process with the holistic study of the interactions between all living things and their natural and built environments. It involves the study of the impact of built environments upon the health and wellbeing of people and animals. The goal of building biology is to holistically integrate human construction with the life sciences.

The Building Biology and Ecology, or Baubiologie™, movement, which developed the practice of building biology, began in Germany in 1975 and now has institutes in New Zealand, Austria, Switzerland, The Netherlands, the countries of Scandinavia, and the United States. The teachings of the movement have also been termed 'bioharmonics' by Reinhard Kanuka-Fuchs, the director of the Building Biology and Ecology Institute of New Zealand, and 'Gaian architecture' by the Gaia movement. We use the term 'bioenergetic' to describe architecture that is designed with an understanding of the energy and radiation relationships produced by living things. In the next three chapters we look at the differences between standard and bioenergetic building construction.

The way to create a truly healthy home is to incorporate the life sciences into our design principles. We need more than a knowledge of building and architecture – we need to understand biology and ecology as well.

BUILDING BIOLOGY, CULTURE AND TECHNOLOGY

Biology, culture and technology should form a balanced trio of causes which together produce an appropriate building or development. The balance is often distorted because of the inadequate education in

Page 122: Built from the ruins of
an old mill, this house runs
almost autonomously with the
help of a water turbine and
passive-solar features.
Kenstown, Meath, Ireland
(Architect: P. Leech, Gaia
Associates; Photograph: P.
Leech)

holistic matters — or even arrogant disdain — of the professionals responsible for the design and construction of buildings. The effects on humans arising from an overemphasis on technology in the trio of causes may be seen in the psychological aberrations of modern city populations. People have lost their sense of being related to nature and in many cases are suffering physically from the deprivation. The modern lack of contact with natural things is similar in its effect to a lack of vitamins on the human organism. In both cases the body is weakened and the psyche suffers. Nature contact is a basic human need. Building biology supplies the key to resolving the overemphasis on modern technology at the expense of culture and biology.

◎ Building biology and ecology ◎

The addition of the concept of ecology to the original term of 'building biology' is the key to the wider application of these concepts in the planning sphere. Ecology is the study of the niches, habitats and environments of all animals. The planning of human settlements should take ecological principles into consideration; our buildings should be planned and constructed with an understanding of *human* ecology.

The entrenched building establishment is unlikely to appreciate, or act for, change. It is for enlightened individuals to show the way, providing habitats fit for the new generation of individuals who have a heightened awareness of these issues. We are privileged to have seen such radical changes in human consciousness occur in our lifetime, now suitable shelter has to be provided to nurture these evolutionary changes.

THE ENVIRONMENTAL CRISIS AND BUILDING MATERIALS

The building materials we use, our building practices, and attitudes to technology and science need reconsideration, taking into account ethical concerns for human and social welfare, and for all natural systems. Natural, hygroscopic (breathing) building materials absorb and release moisture readily, filtering out air pollution and releasing clear air in the transaction. Such materials should replace synthetic materials and fresh air systems replace mechanical ventilation and air conditioning. Chemicals from nature should replace those synthesised by science.

Buildings should be sited with an understanding of natural terrestrial radiation so that areas affected by ionised radiation can be avoided. Terrestrial magnetism needs to be mapped, anomalies avoided and building systems used that will not destroy the natural electromagnetic field. Building materials that allow cosmic and gamma rays from deep space to pass into the building's interior unchanged are preferable.

Sites and building materials need to be chosen according to how well they minimise stress from noise. Planning of settlements should integrate low density housing with open space for recreation, Permaculture, indigenous vegetation, shelterbelts, areas of companion planting, and areas devoted to fish and livestock.

All building products and systems should be in concert with human biology and natural ecology. The bioclimate (living climate) within a building should positively affect human health and wellbeing.

THE BIOCLIMATE WITHIN A HEALTHY BUILDING

'Bioclimate' is a term coined by Professor Anton Schneider to describe the meteorological conditions of the interior air, as they relate to human health and comfort (physical, emotional and mental). The visual, tactile and acoustic qualities of an interior affect the air moisture, temperature and airspeed that define the bioclimate of a building. The effects of a balanced bioclimate upon human beings who occupy a building are: improved physical and mental health, a sense of wellbeing, a cosy and harmonic atmosphere, a positive attitude to work, easy respiration, ion-exchange appropriate to good health, improved oxygenation, balanced metabolism, raised immunity and stimulated blood supply to the skin.

The effects of an inadequate bioclimate are: colds, asthma, catarrh, rheumatism, allergic reactions and heightened sensitivity, sleeping difficulties, tiredness, irritability, a sense of unease, depression, disturbed blood pressure levels, kidney and bladder dysfunction, epidemics occurring in groups of buildings, hot skin flushes, breathing difficulties, eye inflammation and irritation, dry and chapped skin, growth problems, unpleasant body odours, lack of thermal diversity and hence bodily stimulation, accelerated aging, infertility, food consumption difficulties, deteriorated physical and mental performance, toxic gas poisoning, nervousness and a lack of muscle tone which affects the organs of the body.

Natural materials in animal and human shelters

Structures made by animals, unlike the majority of those made by humans, show a direct response to climatic factors. Termites use orientation to the sun and the Earth's thermal mass to control the temperature inside the termite mound. Moles use the infinite thermal mass of the Earth to delay seasonal impacts in the burrow. They also use 'stack-effect' ventilation: the differential between air pressure at the top of the mound and air pressure deep down in their hole causes cool air to circulate. In summer, wombats dig 1–1.5 metres (3–5 feet) into the exceptionally hot Nullarbor Plain in Australia, delaying the summer heat for 2½–5 months.

Desert birds like the South African weaver bird and cold-climate birds such as the penduline tit of west-coast Canada and Europe suspend an intricate woven nest from a branch. The desert nest is porous and open, so air becomes trapped in its pores, providing ideal insulation against the heat. The penduline tit's nest is tightly woven and lined with soft plant down, forming dense thermal protection against the cold. Sociable weaver birds achieve even better results. Rather than each pair building a single nest, a group of weaver birds constructs a compact agglomeration of nests which can reach 5 metres (16½ feet) in diameter. This is ideal in hot climates as it presents minimum surface area to the desert heat, while housing a maximum volume of nests. The form of the nests of weaver birds is typical of climate-responsive design. Egyptian villages also respond successfully to the climate as their compact layout and narrow, shaded streets provide minimum surface area for maximum accommodation.

Traditional construction, proven methods and indigenous materials produce the useful vernacular dwellings of Asia, Europe, the Mediterranean area, America and Africa. The clay bricks used in Egypt, Greece, Italy and Mesopotamia, the mud bricks and rammed earth used in China and the timber and thatch used in southeast Asia are all a response to the climate and availability of natural materials. Up until the early part of this century, neutral materials such as clay, bricks, stone and timber were used in the construction of buildings. Today, buildings are constructed principally of synthetic materials such as concrete, steel, glass and plastic. This rapid change has produced bioclimatic problems. The artificially derived interior climates of modern buildings have effects beyond present scientific knowledge, of which the Sick Building Syndrome is only the beginning.

The effects of temperature and humidity on health and comfort

Personal differences in preferred indoor temperature vary considerably. To maintain strength and vigour, you should create significant temperature differences throughout the building by allocating various temperature zones. Differences in temperature act as stimuli to human metabolism. For study, writing and strenuous intellectual activity, 18 degrees Celsius (64 degrees Fahrenheit) is the maximum. A good combination for intellectual work is an air temperature of 10 degrees Celsius (50 degrees Fahrenheit) and a floor temperature of 18–20 degrees Celsius (64–68 degrees Fahrenheit), as occurs with an earth-coupled concrete floor that shares the steady temperature of the earth beneath. However, you can begin to feel cold at 16 degrees Celsius (61 degrees Fahrenheit), leading to restlessness and lack of concentration unless warm clothes are used to balance the need for body warmth against the need for brain coolness. The optimum temperature for bedroom air is 10 degrees Celsius (50 degrees Fahrenheit), as low temperatures enhance deep breathing during sleep, with bedcovers being used to blanket the body in a pocket of still air at a comfortable body temperature.

ABSOLUTE AND RELATIVE HUMIDITY

At a specific temperature, there is a maximum level of moisture that a body of air can hold — this is called its saturation point. Relative humidity is an expression, in the form of a percentage, of how much water vapour is present in the air at a given temperature, compared to how much water vapour would be present in the air (at the same temperature) if it was completely saturated. Absolute humidity is measured in grams of water per cubic metre of air and is a reading of the *actual* moisture content of the air. Dew point is the temperature at which air is *just* saturated. Humidity increases when air temperature increases, thus relative

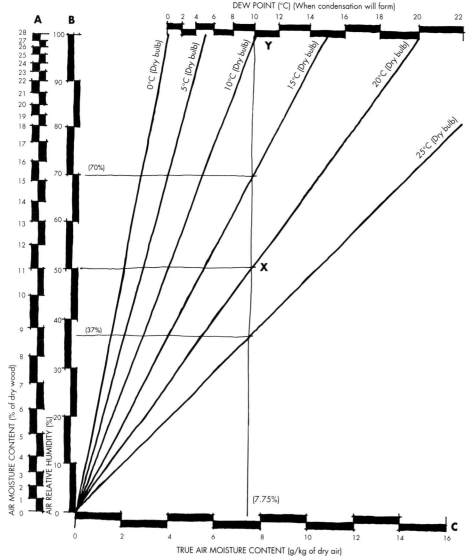

Note that 'dry bulb' is an ordinary mercury or alcohol thermometer while relative humidity is measured with a psychrometer (see Resources Directory) (Redrawn and adapted from Richardson 1991)

Figure 8.1: How air-moisture content can remain constant while relative humidity and temperature fluctuate.

humidity is lower in winter than in summer. However, if the air temperature drops below dew point, condensation occurs and dew or mist is formed. This tends to happen in still, humid conditions, or when warm, humid air comes into contact with cool surfaces.

If the temperature rises while the air-moisture content remains constant, the relative humidity drops. Conversely, if the temperature drops, to say 10 degrees Celsius (18 degrees Fahrenheit) and the air-moisture content remains constant, the relative humidity becomes 100 per cent because the dew point has been reached.

How can we estimate the average relative humidity of the air inside a building — and how do we know whether the moisture it contains will create a healthy environment in which to live? The average moisture content of any wood in a building that is away from rising damp or obvious moisture pene-

tration sources is a record of the average relative humidity in that building. The moisture content of wood can be measured using a hygrometer. By constructing a graph which relates the average relative humidity to the average air temperature, the moisture content of the air and the dew point can be plotted.

To calculate whether a house has a healthy air-moisture content, refer to Figure 8.1.

Step 1. Using a protimeter (see Resources List), measure the moisture content of a typical piece of wood in the house (say it is 9 per cent). Plot this on Scale A. Draw a horizontal line across the graph (note that it intersects Scale B at around 37 per cent).

Step 2. Measure the dry bulb air temperature with a thermometer (say it is 20 degrees Celsius). Now extend your horizontal line until it hits the 20 degrees Celsius oblique line. Mark this meeting point as X.

Step 3. Draw a vertical line at X. The intersection with Scale C will tell you the true (not relative) moisture content of the air (in this case, 7.75 per cent).

Step 4. Follow the vertical line upwards. In this case, air moisture increases as the temperature drops. It reaches 100 per cent at 10 degrees Celsius. While the relative humidity averages about 37 per cent, if the temperature drops below 10 degrees Celsius, condensation will form on cold surfaces, mould will grow in cupboards and allergies will proliferate.

Air outside and air inside always have the same absolute humidity, or moisture content — when a temporary imbalance occurs pressure differentials cause air to flow from one space to the other until equilibrium prevails. The breath exhaled by the occupants of a building, their perspiration and the hot water they use cause the moisture content inside the building to rise, thereby increasing the water vapour pressure. This causes the water vapour to diffuse towards the outside walls. If the outside air is already saturated with water vapour, condensation will form when the interior air approaches the outside air. The condensation may cause fungal infections to develop in wood. In cold conditions, condensation is also likely to form on glass or on walls which have little or no insulation, when the moisture content of the air is particularly high, for example in the bathroom or kitchen. Wardrobes or beds placed against cold walls function as thermal insulators, and if the movement of air in the room is minimal, they will encourage condensation to form. Curtains against windows have the same insulating effect.

FACTORS AFFECTING INDOOR HUMIDITY

When air passes over the surface of our lungs as we breathe, it becomes humidified. When the air is cool and of low relative humidity, more water vapour can be absorbed by breathing. Our bodies also emit water vapour, which takes toxins with it. The amount of water vapour we lose depends upon the relative humidity of the air. According to medical opinion, the optimum relative humidity is 40–50 per cent. In buildings, the relative humidity should not fall below 40 per cent or exceed 70 per cent. The relative humidity in cold climates and hot/dry climates can drop to 15–35 per cent. Such low levels of relative humidity result in throat irritations, dry chests, colds, nervous complaints, headaches, eye complaints, tiredness, higher incidence of illness, and loss of efficiency. An electrostatic charge develops and the dust content of the air also increases. The sweeping movement of the cilia (the small hairs on the epithelium of our respiratory passages), which normally clears away mucous, is restricted. Consequently, our respiratory passages are not self-cleansed of dust and bacteria, and illness can result.

As human sensitivity can not detect relative humidity with any accuracy, it is best to trust instrument measurements only. The most fundamental way to control the relative humidity of a building is to use a high proportion of hygroscopic materials in its construction. The use of such materials leads to less fluctuation in the air-moisture content and greater independence from the relative humidity fluctuations that accompany movements of air. In climates with a relatively high air-moisture content, hygroscopic materials are essential to minimise condensation and keep relative humidity levels below 70 per cent. The factors affecting the water vapour content of air are:

- temperature of room air and room surfaces;
- hygroscopicity of building materials, furniture and furnishings;
- ratio of room size to number of occupants;
- type of activity undertaken in a room; and
- whether the heating system operates by convection or radiation.

Another factor affecting indoor humidity is the mode of construction of the building. Dry modes of construction, such as the use of precast concrete modules, are preferable to building with wet concrete and brickwork, which take a long time to dry out as they contain tens of tonnes of water.

THE TROUBLE WITH AIR CONDITIONING

Low relative humidity is the core problem of what we know as the Sick Building Syndrome, which produces 'dry symptoms' like running or blocked nasal passages, dry throats, thirst, breathing difficulties and a feeling of tightness in the throat. In a poorly designed house, in winter, draughts introduce a wind-chill factor into what could be conditions of tolerable coolness. As a consequence, heating is used, reducing the relative humidity and making the interior air dry. Improperly designed mechanical ventilation and air conditioning systems are also major causes of low relative humidity.

Air conditioning is the process of altering the temperature and moisture content of the air so that the occupants of a building are comfortable. Thus, moisture should be removed from the air when it is too humid for comfort, and added when it is too dry. Forty years ago, to be called an air conditioner, a system had to include humidifying as well as dehumidifying functions. Time passed, standards slipped. Today, most air conditioners simply aim to deliver cool air, without regard for its moisture content. In the cooling and reverse cycle heating processes, they deliver air which is often too dry for comfort. Similarly, when such systems are used to heat the building, they again supply dry air. The situation is further exacerbated by the 'stripping out' of negions. Other symptoms associated with air conditioning are headaches and lethargy caused by an imbalance in the level of carbon dioxide in the air.

Wet air conditioning systems, which use cooling towers with running water, require constant professional maintenance, cleaning and testing to detect the presence of fungal spores, viruses and bacteria in the water. If these precautions are not taken, allergic reactions to the presence of spores in the air processed by them, as well as serious infections and toxic reactions to airborne viruses and bacteria can result. For economic reasons, a high proportion of stale air is often recirculated in the air conditioning system, introducing new viruses and bacteria in the process. In poorly maintained wet air conditioning systems, the Legionnaire's disease bacterium, *Legionella pneumophili*, becomes a problem. This organism flourishes in the warm iron-rich water and organic substrate found in cooling towers and evaporative condensers, as well as spas and large hot water systems. It can spread where tepid water, dust and soil are found. Early symptoms of the disease include high temperature, coughing, muscle aches, chills, chest and stomach pains, and diarrhoea. More than 50 varieties of the organism exist, some milder than others. Death can occur in 24 to 48 hours in susceptible people but healthy people usually survive the disease. Heavy smokers and drinkers are most vulnerable, as are those with chronic respiratory diseases and damaged immune systems. Control and maintenance programs are essential for the cooling towers of air conditioning systems. (Legionnaire's disease can also be contracted by handling contaminated dry plant-potting mix, so it is recommended that water be added to the mixture prior to handling and that a face mask be worn to prevent the inhalation of contaminated dust.)

There is also a risk in air conditioned buildings that the air could be contaminated by other pathogenic microorganisms such as *Protens* and *Pseudomonas*, coliforms, viruses, and protozoa. A great variety of organisms proliferate in the slime on the baffle plates of air conditioners carrying recirculated water. When these air conditioners are open to the wind, such organisms may be carried elsewhere, as happened in a cluster of occurrences of Legionnaire's disease in Western Sydney, Australia in 1995. Manufacturers of new air conditioning towers should be compelled to undertake independent measurements to make sure that their equipment complies with relevant standards. Local authorities should reject applications to install such systems until evidence of compliance is given. Fortunately, air conditioning systems have now been invented that avoid the use of cooling towers entirely.

HEALTH PROBLEMS AND HIGH AIR HUMIDITY
The residents of any temperate or tropical coastal region will be familiar with the mould that appears in unventilated spaces such as wardrobes and shower recesses. Shoes and handbags bear the evidence and have to be brushed off, wiped with a vinegar-soaked rag and sterilised by the sunshine. Is this just a nuisance, or something more serious?

Mould and and other fungi are the main allergens that cause sickness in sensitive people. In damp conditions, fungal spores and dust mites proliferate, causing allergic reactions. Some fungi that develop under humid conditions are capable of decomposing a wide range of materials, producing toxic gases in the process. Polyurethane (often used in acoustic false ceilings, furniture and office partitions) can yield cyanates; urea (used in glues) can generate phenol; and melamine formaldehyde polymers (such as the laminates used in kitchens) can produce formaldehyde.

The experimental work of Doctor Barry Richardson, a research scientist who specialises in the study of the deterioration of structural materials and associated health problems, has raised our understanding of the problems connected with the high and low humidity environments to which we are subjected in contemporary buildings. He has raised doubts about the use of heavily plasticised polyvinyl-chloride (PVC) products such as mattress covers, as they degrade under certain conditions of humidity and temperature. He is also concerned about the effects of pigments and preservative systems containing arsenic compounds.

In the late 19th century, a spate of mysterious illnesses and deaths were recorded. It was later discovered that these illnesses were caused by exposure to arsenic pigments used at that time in wallpaper. Size, which is a thin sealer that equalises the porosity of wall surfaces before they are covered with wallpaper or plaster, caused similar problems. Size contained gelatine, produced by boiling horses' hoofs. Consequently, it had a high protein content, which encouraged the development of a specific fungus, *Scopulariopsis brevicaulis*. The fungus growing on the arsenic-based pigments in the wallpaper as well as on the size generated the toxic compound arsine. The presence of arsine in the interior environment caused significant health problems. The fungus develops in humid conditions, in deteriorating milk, cheese and meat, and in the wardrobe in leather and damp wool. It first begins to grow in a white membranous form which eventually becomes tan and powdery, with a folded appearance. It can convert relatively innocuous compounds into extremely toxic gases, like tryhydride and phosphine, as well as arsine and stibine from any phosphorus, arsenic or antimony compounds that it accesses.

Scientists have subsequently developed wood preservatives containing copper, which prevent the development of the fungus that converts arsenic compounds into the problem substance, arsine. However, Richardson is concerned that those designing new wood preservatives may not have a grasp of the history of the use of arsenic compounds and the need to include additional fungicides in their formulations. He has reservations about Australia's wide use of arsenic compounds, particularly in relation to controlling Powder Post Beetle. So *caveat emptor* — let the buyer beware! Richardson has also pointed to a potential link between Sudden Infant Death Syndrome (SIDS, or cot death) and the gases phosphine and stibine, which are similar in effect to arsine. The antimony compounds and phosphorus commonly used in fire-retardant treatments can generate phosphine and stibine which could be inhaled by a sleeping infant (Craig 1986).

Doctor Richardson hypothesises that local concentrations of humidity caused by a sleeping child breathing into any woollen products in its crib, and by pockets of body warmth and perspiration, permit the development of the fungus *Scopulariopsis brevicaulis*. He asserts that all babies are at risk of SIDS because arsine can be generated under such circumstances. He postulates that more active babies may avoid death if the gases cause headaches and irritability so that the baby moves and disperses the gas.

AN IMMEDIATE SOLUTION: VENTILATION

A significant increase in ventilation is required to counteract the humidity problems caused by still air. Any sub-floor or roof space, false floor beneath kitchen cupboards or wardrobes, bathrooms and toilets should either incorporate extra ventilation openings with insect-proof, wire mesh covers, or ventilation fans, connected to light switches. Meshed ventilators are available for installation in the space beneath the ground floor. You must approach the ventilation of your building carefully though, because too much ventilation can cause a wind-chill effect in winter. Heating the internal air to counteract the wind-chill effect can cause the opposite problem of low humidity.

WET AND DRY ROT FUNGI

In poorly constructed buildings, damp can rise up from the ground, water can diffuse from a wet area to a dry one, or rainwater can enter the interior. These conditions can cause the moisture content of the wood to rise to a level where it can support wet rot fungi and dry rot fungi (so called because of the condition the wood is reduced to after attack). The fungal strands (the hyphae) of brown rot fungus (*Serpula lacrymans*) and wet rot fungus (*Coniophora puteara*) infiltrate timber and draw on the cellulose for

food. The fungi release microscopic spores into the air, and these can produce severe skin and respiratory reactions. A fatal asthma attack may result if someone who is highly sensitive to this allergen comes into contact with it. Brown rot fungus thrives in wood that has a moisture content of 25 per cent, but can survive at a level of 18 per cent. While damp conditions will sustain development of wet rot fungus, it also needs to be saturated continuously. When leaks occur due to faulty construction, for example, in a shower recess, the extra water allows wet rot fungus to thrive.

Creating a healthy bioclimate

The heating of buildings causes more health problems than any other factor in building design. Whether from the drying-out of air by heat, the introduction of fumes into indoor spaces, the creation of pathogenic conditions due to rogue electromagnetic fields, or because of the distortion of cosmic and terrestrial radiation, heating of interior air is a major design problem. The creation of comfortable indoor climates involves:

• maintaining air humidity at 45–70 per cent;

• the use of radiated rather than convected heat (if convection heaters are used, they should incorporate wet filters to remove dust);

• hygroscopic building materials and furnishings;

• natural ventilation through pervious building materials to filter air with low water vapour loss; and

• the use of radiant heating which creates a room air temperature of around 18 degrees Celsius (64 degrees Fahrenheit) and higher wall temperatures (preferably around 20 degrees Celsius (68 degrees Fahrenheit)).

For a building to be truly healthy, it must be constructed using materials that store heat and provide thermal insulation. This equalises temperature and creates a high surface temperature, particularly on floors. These materials need to provide excellent hygroscopic potential to regulate the air humidity in the room. Building materials should help avoid condensation and be electrically neutral, especially in regard to electrostatic charges. They have to be pervious to air, as permeability and diffusibility allow continuous breathing and gaseous exchange with the outside air. It is essential that they are absorptive so that they bond chemically with, and neutralise, gaseous pollutants. They need to have a neutral odour.

They should not conduct electricity, thereby creating EMFs, distortions and anomalies, and they should not alter the natural terrestrial and cosmic microwave radiation. Any of the microflora and microfauna which are supported by the material must be benign and favourable to human health, and they should be of a colour that suits the climate and orientation of the building.

A common error when selecting building materials is to choose those without thermal storage or insulation qualities, and that are airtight, impermeable and non-diffusible. Materials that do not absorb gaseous air pollutants are often used, as are materials that have strong odours and outgas toxic chemicals. Hard, impervious surfaces encourage condensation, so harmful microflora and microfauna are encouraged to proliferate. Many materials accumulate dust and are difficult to clean without using chemicals and consequently, house dust mite infestation can become a problem. People often choose particular materials in order to copy architectural styles or mannerisms of other periods, without regard to climatic suitability.

Many of the materials used widely in modern construction are electrically conductive and accumulate rogue electromagnetic fields, affecting the health of the building's inhabitants. Synthetic materials hold electrostatic charges, while natural terrestrial and cosmic microwave radiation can be affected by metal roofing, wall claddings and reinforcement in concrete slabs. Electrical installations create electromagnetic and electrostatic fields. This can be avoided by following the procedures outlined in Chapter 9 regarding electrical systems.

Building materials can be conductive (steel), partially conductive (reinforced concrete) or nonconductive (wood and insulation). Thus all materials will influence the electroclimate of a building's interior, affecting:

- the electrostatic charge inside the building;
- electrical fields in the interior air;
- the positive or negative polarity of a charge, and direction and strength of electrostatic (direct current) fields in a room;
- the ratio of posions to negions in an interior;
- the transmission (or non-transmission) into a space of low and high frequency vibrations;

- the extent to which the interior of a building remains under the influence of natural environmental electric fields and to which it neutralises or exaggerates the influences of harmful pulsed electromagnetic fields from outside electrical sources, such as high voltage electrical transmission lines, transformers, sub-stations, microwave antennae and television towers;
- the formation of rogue alternating current (AC) fields, created by electrical installation; and
- the induction of an electric charge, magnetism or current by reason of the equipment's or wiring's proximity to similarly energised components or elements of an electrical system.

The physical body is controlled internally and externally by radiation, electromagnetic and geomagnetic fields, and ions produced by electrical currents. Typical modern built environments provide the cells of the body with their first experience of a totally artificial environment since human evolution began. Not only are they subjected to synthetic chemicals, but the electroclimate in which these cells evolved has been significantly altered by modern building materials and electrical appliances, systems and installations.

Ideally, building materials should be electrically neutral, so that they do not disturb the natural electrical influences to which our bodies should be exposed. Wood is an excellent material, as long as it has a moisture content of between 8 and 12 per cent, which will prevail if long-term relative humidity remains in the range of 40 to 65 per cent at an average of 20 degrees Celsius (68 degrees Fahrenheit). When wood has a moisture content of less than 8 per cent it becomes an insulator and carries an electrostatic charge. When it has a moisture content of above 12 per cent, it becomes more electrically conductive, and at high moisture contents it is as conductive as water. In their natural state, cork, bark, straw, woodwool, sisal, peat and hemp are all ideal building materials.

Although little research has been undertaken into the electroclimates of modern building interiors, it is recognised that materials such as plastics, chemical paints, varnishes, adhesives, artificial floor coverings, glues, furnishings, upholstery, curtains and clothing change the polarity and strength of interior electrostatic fields.

Conductive materials, particularly those that are inorganic, have definite effects upon the electroclimate of a building's interior. Metals, in particular, form induction fields, transferring electrical or magnetic charges from one body to another without needing to actually be in contact with them. Conductors, or materials that carry positive or negative charges, distort the ratio of posions to negions. For example, in a duct carrying dry air, the negions are 'stripped' off from the air flow, becoming attached to the duct itself. The air which is delivered to the building's interior consequently has a high proportion of posions, which can affect health and wellbeing.

Climatic conditions such as temperature, humidity, air movement and air exchange also produce changes in the interior electroclimate, so these factors must also be considered. One example of an environment that creates a healthy electroclimate is the log cabin with timber shingle roof, unsealed surfaces, furniture and furnishings made from natural materials, and heating that produces the recommended relative humidity of 40–70 per cent. In such a structure the direct current (DC) field would be similar in rhythm and polarity to the natural DC field of the locality, with a positive charge nearer the ceiling and a negative charge nearer the floor. It would create no distortions of the electrical charge on large gaseous air ions. Natural ELF microwaves and high frequency microwaves would enter the building undistorted, or only moderately reduced. The oxygen ions would be negatively charged, which is physiologically ideal, small electrostatic charges would prevail, and there would be no induced currents from electrical installations and other potential sources.

Cosmic and artificial microwaves

The effects of microwave radiation on living cells vary from athermal (non-heating) at the low frequency end of its range to thermal at the high end of its range. The issue of the effect of microwaves upon human beings revolves around the differences between thermal and athermal effects and whether the radiation, instead of being in a continuous wave, has a modulated or pulsed waveform. Athermalists believe that pulsed and modulated waveforms are more biologically active than those from thermal sources,

which invalidates the commonly accepted notion that only thermal microwave radiation is harmful to cells. Electromagnetic radiation, of which microwave radiation is one type, not only permeates the environment but is in the same band as the natural ELF field of the human body.

Cosmic radiation has a marked effect on the endocrine systems of organisms, which include the pituitary, thyroid, parathyroid and adrenal glands, the ovaries, testes, placenta and part of the pancreas (Endros, in Schneider 1988). As microwave radiation passes through a material, the spectral structure changes so that desirable, low frequency microwave radiation is weakened and undesirable, high frequency radiation is increased.

ELFs and building materials

The most permeable type of construction in relation to atmospheric electrical fields within the ELF range is the brick house. The least permeable is a reinforced concrete structure. Concrete-block houses are, on average, twice as permeable as those made from reinforced concrete. A wood-framed house has reasonable permeability. Permeability also varies depending on the size and disposition of window and door openings in a building.

Areas not yet researched include the impact of solar collectors and photovoltaic panels on permeability. Rogue fields from high voltage power lines, train and telephone lines, various types of antennae, plumbing and electrical installation and other transmitters all complicate such research.

AIR MOISTURE AND HYGROSCOPIC MATERIALS

One of the key factors in the choice of healthy materials is their capacity to absorb water vapour out of the air and release it again, that is, their hygroscopic quality. Given appropriate air conditions, naturally hygroscopic materials, like timber and other products of plant origin, dry out more easily than other materials. As this moisture exchange takes place, a building material will gradually develop a degree of stability or equilibrium in its moisture content.

Large areas of hygroscopic materials ensure a levelling out of fluctuations in air humidity inside a building. Healthy, hygroscopic materials should have air moisture contents of between 40 and 60 per cent. In arid climates, new buildings may have air humidity as low as 20 to 30 per cent because of air conditioning systems and the use of interior materials that lack hygroscopicity. Materials that are hygroscopic include: unsealed timber; timber, such as softwoods, finished with a pervious treatment; porous plasters finished with porous, natural paints or seals; paper-based wallpapers; and furnishings made from natural fibres. The more of these materials that are used the better. Hygroscopic materials should not be tightly sealed as this reduces their level of hygroscopicity. Use porous finishes only.

Wool and timber are particularly permeable materials, air passing through them as humidity or dampness increases. However, the spaces in the weave of both cotton and silk close under increasingly humid conditions, reducing the rate of diffusion. This effect is even worse in synthetics. A fibre reaches saturation point when it has taken in so much moisture vapour that its moisture content is equal to that of the air in the room. Wood has a high saturation point — 1 cubic metre (35 cubic feet) of wood is capable of absorbing 197 litres (43 gallons) of water over a prolonged period (Schneider 1988).

The taking in of moisture lowers the insulation value of nonhygroscopic materials. Hygroscopic materials, however, release water back into the air if the relative humidity of the air drops into the unhealthy range. Timber is particularly useful in areas of high humidity, such as in bathrooms and kitchens, or in coastal regions. It is necessary to have a good natural or forced ventilation system which dries out the timber. Pervious sealants must always be used on wood, or mould can grow beneath the film.

The most permeable bricks are pressed earth bricks, followed by kiln-baked commons (moulded). The least healthy are the relatively impermeable kiln-baked extruded bricks. Most of the diffusion in a brick wall occurs through its joints; the presence of lime in the mortar assists diffusion. For every square metre (10¾ square feet) of an unplastered, solid brick wall, 36.5 centimetres (14 inches) thick, with mortar joints, there is an air flow of 3 cubic metres (106 cubic feet) every hour. In a brick wall of the same dimensions which does not have mortar joints, there is only an air flow of 0.00074 cubic metres (¹⁄₄₀ of a cubic foot) per hour (Schneider 1988). It follows that the diffusion rate is improved when comparatively small bricks or blocks are used, and when the joints between them are numerous.

Harder, less porous materials may not be suitable for use in the home. Remember too that wet construction methods not only cause a drop in the rate of diffusion, but in thermal insulation values as well. For an increase of 2 per cent in the moisture content of a concrete wall, for example, there is a corresponding 25 per cent lowering of the wall's thermal insulation value.

When choosing insulation materials, avoid mineral and glass fibre insulation which, apart from other health issues, are poorly hygroscopic, as are exploded or expanded, lightweight aggregates and expanded-bead, plastic insulation materials. They do not breathe, so do not contribute to the moisture-balancing of the air, which is essential to the health of the building's occupants.

Air moisture and new buildings

Moisture in buildings is an ongoing problem, requiring careful selection of materials and well-designed ventilation to avoid condensation and mould. A new house with reinforced concrete floors and brick and plaster walls contains thousands of litres of construction water which has to dry out before the building reaches its optimum air moisture level and is fit for occupancy. The amount of drying-out time varies greatly depending on whether wet (concrete, plaster, render) or dry (precast concrete or steel-framed walls with hardboard linings) construction techniques were used. It is advisable to accelerate the

Table 8.1: Relative hygroscopic quality of various building materials*

FINISH MATERIAL	BASE MATERIAL	WATER STORED, IN G/M² (OZ/FT²)
Paper wallpaper	Lime plaster	34
Whitewash	Lime plaster	17
No finish	Lime plaster	13
Latex paint	Lime plaster	9
Emulsion paint	Lime plaster	3
Oil-based paint	Lime plaster	2
Wallpaper	Tempered hardboard	44
Wallpaper	Plasterboard	80
Vinyl wallpaper	Irrelevant	2·7
Carpet	100 % animal hair	61
	100% coconut fibre	58
	100% wool	52
	100% synthetic fibre	26

* Adapted from data in Schneider (1988)

drying-out process of a building's interior by using a dehumidifier for the first year or so of occupancy. Dehumidifiers can be hired. In hot, dry climates, a similar drying-out effect can be achieved by leaving the windows and doors open regularly. After the drying-out period, the air inside the building will contain a healthy level of moisture, so long as:

• materials were selected according to their hygroscopic quality;

• appropriate air-exchange rates are maintained, remembering that the usual approach to energy efficiency (using tight seals around doors and windows) means that they must be opened regularly for the exchange of large volumes of air, when the temperature and relative humidity are appropriate;

• air moisture tests are conducted regularly in spaces like wardrobes, cupboards and kitchens on a regular basis, and ventilation rates adjusted if necessary; and

• all sources of internal moisture production such as bathrooms, laundries and food-preparation areas are serviced by exhaust systems which send moisture-laden air outside.

In general terms, a 13 centimetre (5 inch) thick reinforced concrete slab with no waterproofing dries out under good conditions (ventilated on both sides) in about 9 months. An ordinary earth-brick wall dries out in around 6 months. Hence, taking into account the additive effect of building elements that release water into a typical room with a suspended concrete floor and earth-brick walls, you would need to hire a dehumidifier for about 12 months to dry the space properly.

◎ Air moisture and old buildings ◎

All the issues relating to moisture content of materials apply equally to existing buildings when wet construction techniques are used during the renovation process, or when uncontrolled condensation has formed due to improper ventilation, leaks or rising damp.

To test for moisture content, use your hygrometer on the architraves, skirting boards or interior door frames of the building. To keep track of the drying-out process it is wise to also monitor both the temperature and humidity inside the building, using a simple, pocket-sized, combined thermometer and hygrometer (see Resources List).

◎ Diffusible materials and air exchange ◎

An ongoing exchange of gases occurs between the air inside and outside a building, through diffusible wall, ceiling and floor surfaces. The interior air is renewed with outside air, and the higher concentrations of outgassed, interior pollution are exchanged with the lower concentrations in the outside air. The result is a dilution of interior pollution. This process, which is assisted by the cycles of high and low barometric pressures in the weather patterns outside, is equivalent to breathing. In appropriate climates, windows and doors can be part of this air-exchange process.

The diffusion resistance factor (DRF) of a material is a useful indicator of its capacity to resist the intake and release of water vapour and diffusion from the interior air to the exterior. It is also a measure of the amount of exterior oxygen that can be taken in by a material to oxygenate a room of stale air.

The sponge-like labyrinths of capillary systems within hygroscopic and diffusible building materials can regenerate interior air by absorbing water vapour, gaseous pollution, odours and dust. They release water vapour and stabilise the interior air moisture content when the relative humidity drops. This creates an air moisture balance suitable for human health. Through physically bonding with molecules or by absorbing them, hygroscopic materials cleanse the air in a chemical fusion process similar to that of natural vegetation.

The moisture contained in hygroscopic materials can later be released when the relative humidity of the room air needs to be increased, or can be stored within the permeable material when the level of moisture in the air needs to be lowered. An exchange of stale internal air for fresh, outside air should take place one to three times per hour in a healthy room. The rate of air exchange is lower in buildings that have been designed with tightly sealed surfaces in order to be energy efficient. In such houses it is vital to the health of the occupants that permeable materials like adobe, mud-brick and earth-brick be used.

Most modern, concrete-block, reinforced concrete and lightweight buildings achieve two to four air-exchanges per hour. According to research undertaken in Germany by Professor Lotz, this is an acceptable air-exchange rate in cold climates, and will occur automatically through cracks and gaps in the building (Schneider 1988). However, in temperate climates the rate needs to be increased to six changes per hour. The use of timber floors helps greatly in air-exchange, though it brings problems in the form of heat loss and gain, and potential radon ingress. Using air conditioning as a way of achieving higher air-exchange rates is a backward step, as it can cause an imbalance in the relative humidity and the gaseous ions in the air.

Following is a comparison of the DRFs of a variety of building materials. The higher the DRF, the less acceptable it is for the healthy house.

ADHESIVES, VARNISHES AND MOISTURE-BARRIER MATERIALS: Moisture-barrier materials include bitumen papers or foil thermal insulation. Such materials, and adhesives and varnishes, are impermeable and hence unacceptable. Manufacturers of aluminium foil insulation have responded with a compromise in the form of needle-punctured foil insulation.

ADOBE, EARTH-BRICK OR PISE WALLS: Walls made from various types of earth have acceptable air-exchange rates (DRF = 10). Mud and straw block walls have a DRF of 2 while straw-bale walls have a DRF of 2–10.

BRICK WALLS: Fired clay brick walls have a low air-exchange capacity which can be offset by using a porous mortar, like lime. (DRF = 10)

CONCRETE: The effect of concrete walls, floors and ceilings is almost equivalent to that of a vapour barrier, a barrier which obstructs the natural breathing process of a building. When finishes are added to the surface, concrete becomes impermeable. This can be offset with natural ventilation, but if you are looking for a diffusive building material capable of reducing indoor air pollution, concrete is not a wise choice. (DRF = 35-40)

SOLID TIMBER: Solid timber is an excellent diffusible building material. In regard to moisture retention, 100 square metres (1076 square feet) of solid timber, 13 millimetres (½ inch) thick, can hold approximately 8 litres (1¾ gallons) of water if the temperature of the room air is 20 degrees Celsius (68 degrees Fahrenheit) and the relative humidity is 80 per cent. Solid board-finishes need to be treated with wax or natural paints to allow diffusion to occur freely and avoid chemical outgassing. (DRF < 5)

STONE AND GLASS: Stone walls are similar to concrete in their impermeability, unless constructed of porous stone such as sandstone or limestone. Structures made of stone should be serviced with good ventilation, although using lime and mortar joints between the stones would help. Glass is a totally impermeable material.

WALLBOARDS: Plywood, chipboard, particle board, wallboard and tempered wallboard are all relatively impermeable unless they are used with a multiplicity of joints. Wallboards contain chemicals that could be toxic, so if they must be used, treat the surface with wax (not varnish) or oil-based paint. (Plywood DRF = 50–200; chipboard DRF = 50–110; tempered, coated hardboard DRF = 1390)

VAPOUR BARRIERS: Vapour diffusion occurs when water vapour penetrates through a building's roof, ceilings and walls. The rate of vapour diffusion is dependent on the permeability of the building materials, the air temperature, the relative humidity of the air, and vapour pressure differences. When a material becomes damp on one side and dry on the other, vapour diffusion will cause the material's moisture content to equalise so it dries out consistently. This cannot happen, however, if the diffusion is blocked by vapour barriers such as aluminium foil or tightly sealed paint or varnish films. If a concrete sub-floor has not dried out sufficiently prior to the laying of a timber floor, which has been sealed with paint or varnish, the timber may rot because the moisture cannot diffuse out. A similar problem occurs when timber window or door frames are exposed to the weather, not given sufficient time to dry out, then sealed with paint or varnish. Similar damage can also occur to walls which have been exposed to the weather and sealed with films that do not breathe.

The problems created by vapour barriers are numerous and it is better to use construction methods and materials that avoid their use, rather than to incur the difficulties they cause. Alternatively, by using a material with a relatively high surface temperature, you can prevent the problem of condensation. However, this does not necessarily avoid some of the other problems caused by vapour barriers. When vapour barriers are used, all the harmful pollutants generated within a building are retained. This effect can be ameliorated by a conscious increase in air-exchange rates, for example, by opening windows when outdoor temperatures permit. Vapour barriers also reduce, or even prevent, gaseous air-exchange. The electrostatic fields in the house increase, electrostatic discharges increase, and charge polarities are reversed.

The DRF of vapour barriers is very high: aluminium foil, DRF = 70,000; polyethylene foil, DRF = 24,000; bitumen, DRF = 800–1200; glass and foam glass, DRF = infinite; linseed oil-based paints, DRF = 9800–24,000. For the purposes of comparison, limewash paint and natural paint have a DRF of only 180–215.

◉ Relative humidity and odours ◉

Our sense of smell can quickly become tired, or less acute. For example, cooking smells may be unnoticeable to the cook, but to a newcomer they may be overpowering; a strong perfume may overpower the natural odour of the person using it. It was found that the relative humidity of the air defines the threshold of perception of an odour. Thus by using hygroscopic materials to control the relative humidity of a room, you can also control the level of odours.

STIMULATED NATURAL VENTILATION

◉ The traditional wind tower ◉

Wind towers and cooling towers have been used for hundreds, possibly thousands, of years in a hot, arid band just north of the Tropic of Cancer, including Pakistan, Iran, Saudi Arabia, Egypt and North Africa. Traditional wind tower structures use either the 'stack effect' principle of encouraging air to move from the inside to the outside of a building, or more commonly, they evaporatively cool the incoming air and release it via leeward openings. The wind tower reaches up into the relatively uninterrupted wind stream and scoops air down into the building, from whence it is released so that air movement, and hence cooling, occurs.

The construction of a wind tower depends upon the wind-directional characteristics of the terrain. On the River Nile in Egypt, the coolest wind blows mainly from the river and the Mediterranean Sea. Consequently, the wind catchers on top of the wind towers face towards the river or the sea and

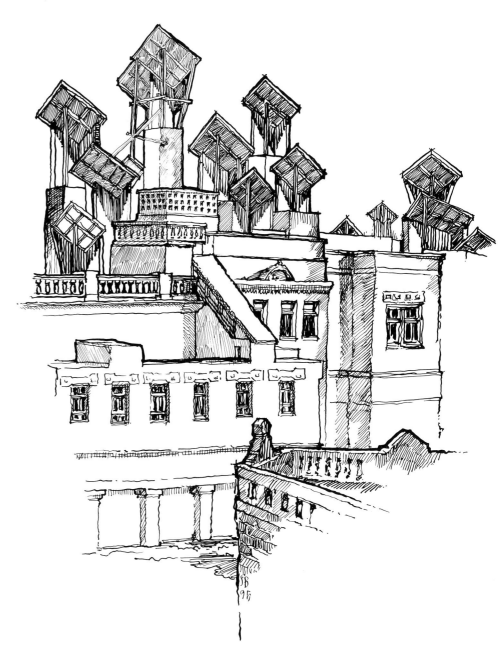

away from the desert. Along the Arabian Sea and the Gulf coasts the wind can blow from the four points of the compass, therefore the wind catcher must be multidirectional. This is achieved by using four baffles within the intake. These baffles are constructed to form an 'X' shape in the wind catcher, providing four triangular intakes in the vertical shaft. In Iran, around Esfahan and Yazd, wind directions vary both in strength and direction. Large towers are used with openings on four sides; various small shafts lead from each opening, facilitating the greatest intake of air from the principal wind directions and less from minor ones. During desert winters, wind catchers are usually blocked with timber covers.

Figure 8.2: Wind towers with wind catchers in Hyderabad, Pakistan (after Thompson, O'Brien and Editors of *Life*, 1966)

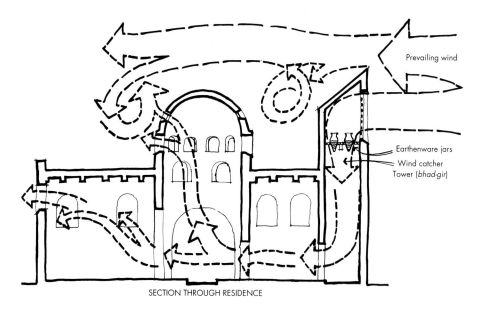

SECTION THROUGH RESIDENCE

Prevailing wind

Earthenware jars
Wind catcher
Tower (*bhad-gir*)

Figure 8.3 A traditional middle-eastern building where a wind catcher (top right) channels wind through porous clay jars of water in the wind tower, thus cooling the interior. Hot air is released through high windows

The 'stack', or chimney, effect

When a room communicates with the outdoor air by having two openings at different levels, and there is a temperature difference between the outdoor and indoor air, the stack effect operates. This is the same principle by which a chimney and fireplace work. Once the air at the base of a chimney flue has been warmed by the fireplace, the air rises because its density decreases once heated. That small volume of air is pushed up the chimney by the cold air from the room rushing into the space it leaves as it rises, just as, in weather terms, a cell of high pressure rushes in to replace a rising cell of low pressure. Once the effect has begun, the stimulated flow continues, providing the fire continues to supply the warm air needed to sustain the upwards flow. Imagine then, that the room itself is the chimney stack and the outlet and inlet are two openings in the room, at different levels. These openings function similarly to the traditional wind tower.

The intake and exhaust of air by a wind tower depend upon the pressure differential between the exterior and interior air, and on the two temperatures. The wind catcher and the building it serves function in combination as a self-regulating system. When the outside air is still and warm, and the interior air is cool, the interior air pressure is higher than that outside. The denser, higher-pressure interior air prevents the less dense exterior air from entering. As the interior air warms, its pressure lessens in comparison to the air outside, so the cooler external air enters the wind catcher and flows down the shaft, cooling the house.

The air which enters the wind tunnel when the wind is blowing has a low air moisture content. The occupants of the house place unglazed earthenware pots full of water, or sheets of water-soaked cloth, near the air inlet, so that incoming air is cooled as the water evaporates. This evaporative cooling process is a completely free source of energy in hot, arid countries. The water jars are also used as a source of cool drinking water and for the storing of food.

In climates with high daytime temperatures and low night-time temperatures, the stack effect can be achieved by using energy-efficient building strategies that utilise the delay caused by the low rate of heat transfer of walls which slows down the effect of hot daytime temperatures until night-time cooling takes effect. Table 8.2 gives an idea of the capacities of various wall materials to give this slowing-down effect.

Where the indoor temperature is equal to the outdoor temperature however, some form of stimulus is needed to achieve a reasonable rate of air-exchange. Historically, this stimulation was achieved by a simple cowl and self-trimming vane, where the vent is trimmed into the wind; a pressure drop across the outlet of the vent stimulates the exhaust of heated air from below.

The house pictured on the opposite page is ventilated via a large wind scoop in the ceiling. The wind scoop was designed to run on a circular track and have a self-trimming vane which, like a weather cock, always keeps the wind scoop trimmed so that its intake points downwind. This creates an air pressure drop on the leeward side to stimulate the normal stack effect in the room below. This procedure is used in temperate and hot, humid climates. Once this wind scoop system is further developed, it may be used to design a city-scale system that would remove the need for mechanical ventilation. In the future, it may produce a completely energy-efficient method of interior ventilation and pollution control in city buildings.

Table 8.2: The ability of wall materials to slow down daytime heat transfer

Material	Thickness	Time lag
Concrete	25 cm (8½ in)	6.9 hr
Cavity double brick	25 cm (8½ in)	6.2 hr
Adobe	25 cm (8½ in)	9.2 hr
Rammed earth	25 cm (8½ in)	10.3 hr
Compressed earth-bricks	25 cm (8½ in)	10.5 hr
Mud-brick (sandy loam)	100 cm (39 in)	30 days

The thorough evacuation of all interior air is essential for keeping building interiors free of radon and chemicals which have been outgassed by materials inside the building. Preferably, a thorough airing should take place every day, when temperature and wind conditions are appropriate, or at least every second day.

In hot, dry climates the wind tower can be combined with evaporative cooling devices by trimming the intake cowl so that it points upwind. If the prevailing wind blows very reliably from one direction, the intake can be fixed in place. Most sites receive winds from several directions; to accommodate this variability, a multidirectional or tracking wind scoop is appropriate.

A high wind tower stimulates higher rates of air-exchange in the building, because the pressure differential between the interior and exterior air is greater. Six to 12 metres (20–39 feet) is an excellent range (Wright 1978), depending on the roughness of the area to the windward side of the building. When land is rough, the drag in the air stream at ground level increases, while air at higher levels, such as at the top of the shaft, stays at relatively undiminished velocity. This increases the pressure difference, and hence the rate of air-exchange. Correctly proportioned ducts can supply intake air to all rooms; exhaust openings must also be provided to release this air.

To avoid excessive intake of hot air into the interior, and to reduce the dust content of the air taken in, the wind scoop should be installed at the top of the shaft to catch prevailing winds and direct them downwards into the building interior. For extra cooling, the air flow can pass over evaporative cooling tanks of water, through water sprays or water-saturated masonry shafts (Figure 8.5, overleaf).

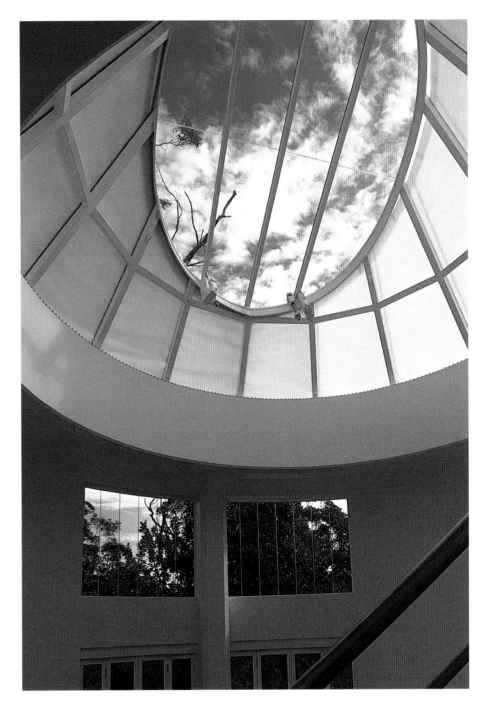

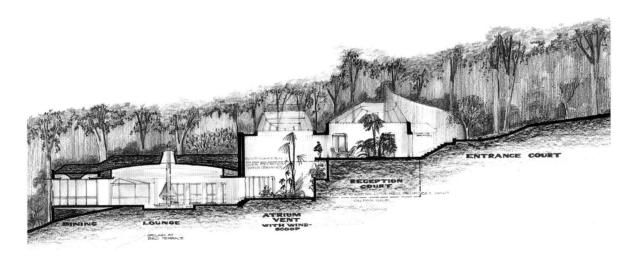

Above: Wind scoop ventilator to residence (see Figure 8.4, below) (Architects: ECA Space Design Pty Ltd)

Figure 8.4: An earth-sheltered residence with a wind scoop that functions as a thermal chimney. Sydney, NSW, Aust. (Architects: ECA Space Design Pty Ltd)

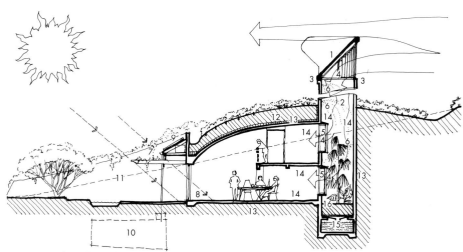

1. Rotating intake cowl with self-trimming vane and skylight sloped roof; 2. Wind-tower atrium (cylindrical in plan) with mist sprays for evaporative cooling and support of rainforest plants; 3. Roller track; 4. Air-intake to atrium court. Direction of air-flow reverses at night when cowl can be locked and stack-effect ventilation occurs; 5. Folding windows; 6. Mist-spray nozzles; 7. Sun-control pergola with deciduous vines; 8. Winter sun heats concrete floor to reradiate at night; 9. Photovoltaic and solar-collection panels (and rainwater collection); 10. Underground storage of potable water; 11. Natural ground line; 12. Earth-cover to roof; 13. Egg-crate type hydraulic pressure-release against all surfaces in contact with soil to allow 'breathing' to occur; 14. Bioconcrete building envelope; 15. Filtered soil-water sump for recirculation to mist-sprays (submersible pump); 16. Soil and plant species selected for pollution control

Figure 8.5: Semi-arid region earth-sheltered house combining several passive strategies for interior climate control

◎ Solar chimneys for forced ventilation ◎

Another forced ventilation system is the non-mechanical, solar chimney which avoids the use of a cowl intake or exhaust structure. With a solar chimney, ventilation can be stimulated even when the air is still. This ordinary-looking chimney is equipped with a heating element (usually solar) and creates a natural draft as the heated air in it rises. Solar chimneys are very effective at removing stale and hot air from a building. In its simplest form, it is a chimney covered on the outside with black metal which

Figure 8.6: A roof fleche (decorative roof ventilation structure) is used to house a solar chimney; as day heat increases in the daytime, the chimney becomes hotter and air exchange is stimulated

FLECHE (decorative roof ventilation structure)

1. incoming solar radiation; 2. glass traps heat into 3. cavity; 4. black metal (or high-density black material for thermal mass storage overnight); 5. radiant heat; 6. stimulated air updraught ventilates room; 7. in cold, draughty conditions, insulated hatch is lowered (with rod or line and pulleys).

absorbs solar heat. As the temperature increases in the chimney, convection draws the interior air up and out of the chimney. As the day becomes hotter the solar chimney improves in efficiency. Its effectiveness can be increased by lining the chimney with glass and thermal-mass materials so that even after the sun has set, the chimney continues to function on stored heat. In many cases, a west-facing chimney may help counteract the excessive heat problems presented by afternoon summer sun.

◎ Solar induction (trombe) walls ◎

The solar induction wall is useful for both convection cooling in summer and warming in winter. It is a wall version of the solar chimney. Air is brought into a building through a system such as a wind tower. To stimulate the exhaust of unwanted stale air, a solar induction wall adjoins it. The solar induction wall is made up of an exterior, glass wall which is separated by a cavity from an interior wall of high thermal mass material, such as earth-brick, with very efficient insulation. Interior air is drawn in at the bottom of the cavity and is pulled up by heated air reradiated from the wall and trapped within the cavity between the glass and the wall. The warm air then rises up the wind tower and is exhausted into the outside air. Air flow dampers and one-way air flow flaps are necessary to avoid unwanted down-draughting, or back-pressure effects, where the system is connected to the outside air.

◎ Earth-tube air-cooling ◎

This system is based upon the cooling effect of pipes leading into rockbeds. After air has been passing over these rockbeds and through these pipes for years, a mould or mildew problem may develop. Consequently, pipes and rockbeds should lead to a drainage point where non-toxic, antifungicidal and antibacterial sluicing can take place and any condensates can drain away. This process is difficult to monitor, and the chemicals needed to eradicate the problem are to be avoided in the healthy house. For this reason the earth-tube cannot be recommended as an appropriate system to use in a healthy house. We will, however, briefly describe it because of the increasing interest in this type of system.

In hot climates the temperature of the air delivered into a building can be considerably reduced if the air intake shaft is elongated so that it passes through the earth mass, preferably through soil outside the building, to avoid the building's temperature influencing the soil around the pipes. Such a system is known as an earth-cooling tube or earth-tube. In dry climates the air is passed across an airlocked volume of water in an underground storage tank, so long as the average ground temperature at depth is considerably less than the desired temperature within the building. Tubes should be given at least 3 metres (approximately 9 feet) of soil cover and laid in a serpentine pattern, away from the main volume of the house. Another type of earth-tube passes air through heat-exchange chambers which wind in a serpentine shape through a rockbed cooled by evaporation. These systems can be constructed of various materials, such as clay pipes of large diameter or spiral-bound, circular aluminium ducting.

AIR POLLUTION FROM BUILDING MATERIALS AND FINISHES

Dilution (introducing air from outside) is an inadequate solution to pollution, so you must not only provide adequate ventilation, but also choose your building materials wisely. Indoor pollution can be controlled by the selection of appropriate materials during the design stage, before construction or renovation. Materials should be judged on the basis of their chemical composition, how natural they are, and the quantity of volatile or gaseous substances they emit. For hypersensitive individuals, even the slightest contact with volatile materials can cause problems. The greatest health risks exist in newly completed or renovated buildings, which have, on average, 10 times the level of organic vapours normally found in old buildings.

There is a vast range of products available, and research into their health effects has never been undertaken systematically, however some product manufacturers are beginning to understand the market's demand for such data. Some products are advertised as 'environmentally safe' or 'non-toxic', but these claims need to be supported by published test results. Consumer pressure should be brought to bear to force manufacturers to test the health effects of their building products.

Some of the outgassing from formaldehyde and other volatile organic compounds (VOC) is only recognisable as a strong smell while some acts as a toxic assault on the immune system. The ratio of the level of total volatile organic compounds (TVOC) in interior air to the exterior air is expressed as a percentage. Baldwin and Farrant (1990) report that on the first day of painting a renovated office building with proprietary paints, the level of TVOC was 734 per cent, while on the second day, it had risen to 897 per cent. It was only after 6 months with no construction taking place that the ratio returned to normal.

Setting standards for outgassing and emissions

In an attempt to promote the sale of paints and varnishes with low solvent and pollutant content, in 1980 the Federal Environment Agency in Germany created a special award and designed a symbol to make these products more recognisable. For a product to display the environmental symbol, it must not contain heavy metals, or anything that can produce mutagenic, carcinogenic or other chronic effects. The TVOC content must not exceed 15 per cent of the product's weight; some products contain as little as 0.5 per cent. These low solvent paints and varnishes have been shown to be of equal quality to conventional products. By 1989, the sales of low-solvent paint had risen from 1 per cent of total paint sales to 20 per cent (Plehn 1990). Germany has become the major manufacturer of low-solvent paints, establishing markets worldwide. In Australia the price is also competitive with the toxic paints on the market.

In the United States, Washington State is the leader in setting environmental standards. Tenderers for the construction of new buildings are required to submit data on the emission levels of the products they intend to use (Tucker 1988).

How to deal with chemical emissions in old buildings

The older a material is, the fewer substances it outgasses into the surrounding air, so the older furniture is, the greater its place in a healthy interior. Antiques epitomise healthy furniture, providing they have not recently been renovated or coated with a plastic finish, and that any dust mite problems in covers and padding have been eradicated.

In order to artificially age materials and reduce the level of outgassing that occurs, a process referred to as bake-out has been developed. By raising the interior temperature, troublesome emissions are driven out of the materials. In California, it has been proposed that all new public buildings be subjected to bake-out. The process involves the application of convection heaters and infrared heating to buildings with natural ventilation. Heaters are used and operating temperatures are raised higher than usual in mechanically ventilated buildings so that some of the toxins can be ventilated out to the atmosphere.

Provided there is sufficient ventilation to remove the solvents emitted, raising the temperature by 13 degrees Celsius (24 degrees Fahrenheit) will produce a 200 per cent increase in emission removal. Although the process is still in a developmental stage, it seems that 4–5 days of heating is required, during which time the temperature must be between 32 and 39 degrees Celsius (90 and 102 degrees Fahrenheit) for at least 24 hours (Haghighat and Donnini 1993). To avoid damaging paint finishes, it is important that the bake-out process is not used when paint has just been freshly applied.

◎ Suitable building materials ◎

The concentrations of pollutants in the air inside a building is reduced by a variety of materials, as solid aerosols adhere to their surfaces. A material's permeability controls the efficiency with which it controls air pollution. Interior air pollution can be lowered to 20 per cent of the levels found in the outside air, simply by choosing interior finishes and furnishings that absorb pollutants.

The following list of building materials (in order of most to least favourable) was devised by weighing many factors, including a material's capacity to absorb toxic vapours and gases, its hygroscopicity, diffusion resistance, sound transmission, heat storage capacity, resistance to electrostatic charges, surface temperature and conductivity. We also took into consideration the ecological impact of producing the materials.

1. Beeswax as a surface for wood products
2. Solid timber and cork
3. Woodwool slab (compacted wool shavings)
4. Magnesite (a composition of cement, magnesium compounds, sawdust and sand as a hard, continuous floor finish)
5. Clay and earth bricks
6. Softboard
7. Hardboard (compressed wood fibre), not tempered or sealed
8. Asphalt and bituminous felt
9. Clay brick (baked) and linoleum
10. Lime mortar
11. Veneered board
12. Unglazed, baked ceramic products
13. Lime sandstone
14. Cement mortar
15. Pumice block
16. Fibre cement (wall or ceiling lining)
17. Gypsum plaster
18. Glass
19. Glass fibre
20. Mineral fibre (from slag)
21. Polystyrene
22. Hard polymer PVC products
23. Synthetic resin glues
24. Reinforced concrete
25. Aluminium foil vapour barrier

◎ The weatherisation or tightening of houses ◎

In the 1970s, people began to take seriously the need to conserve fossil fuel resources. In the United States, particularly after the Bay of Pigs incident, people were encouraged to 'weatherise' their houses — to tighten up all the gaps and air pathways between the inside and outside air — to reduce the need for heating. By the 1980s, the government had formalised the procedure by granting tax breaks to those who insulated or weatherised their house.

Weatherisation transforms the conventional 'leaky' building — with its air exchange through wall vents and cavities, ceiling vents, gaps in timber floors, and cracks behind skirtings, around pipes, electricity boxes, doors and windows — into a tightly sealed vessel. Buildings constructed in the conventional way produce up to six complete exchanges of interior air every hour. Weatherised buildings produce only a half, or even less, of an air exchange per hour.

After the upsurge in weatherisation of buildings, something unexpected occurred: people began to feel off-colour, even ill. The synthetics and chemicals found inside these people's homes were producing emissions, resulting in an environmentally induced illness indentified relatively recently: Tight Building Syndrome.

The researchers Thomas Randolph (1970) and Samuel Rodgers (1987) highlighted how the syndrome is spreading and how individual sensitivity to it is growing. According to Laura and Ashton (1991), American research shows that mobile homes, which are becoming more prevalent particularly in the United States, are the 'worst case scenario'.

The key to dealing with this problem is the same as for Sick Building Syndrome, that is, more fresh air, the use of natural materials, the avoidance of the use of synthetics and chemically treated, composite materials, and the introduction of plants to help absorb the outgassing of toxins.

◉ Recommendations for clean air management ◉

Each of us, as individuals, should do what we can towards the development and implementation of control strategies for the 20th century plague: indoor air pollution. The final success or failure of any indoor air quality control program hinges on the behaviour of maintenance staff in commercial, industrial and major residential buildings and on the owners and occupants of houses and small-scale buildings.

We could begin by implementing more effective ways of handing over a building to a new owner. A procedure could be developed something like the current pest inspection certificate often required for the sale or resale of a property. An indoor air quality report could describe the original design specifications in terms of the amount of fresh air intake and recycled air for each space served by an air conditioning system, what areas (if any) are designed as separate air systems for smokers or for toilets to be located, and the level of toxins outgassed by the

furnishings. The ongoing records would be part of the deed of sale when buildings change ownership; the pollution control strategy could be updated as changes are made. New buildings should include the monitoring devices mentioned earlier for all the major organic, chemical pollutants and radon.

Building-related illnesses have only reached courts on a small number of occasions. As with passive smoking, which is now considered an unacceptable risk, perhaps building-related health issues will become part of the legal scene in the future.

Table 8.3: The interior air of a house can be many times more polluted than the outside air. Plants help counteract this pollution

POLLUTANT	PLANT TO COUNTERACT POLLUTANT*	
	COMMON NAME	LATIN NAME
Benzene from fuel exhaust, grain fumigants, dry-cleaning, cigarette smoke, certain foods and water	Gerbera Daisy Chrysanthemum Devil's Ivy (Golden Pothos) Chinese Evergreen Mother-in-Law's Tongue Peace Lilly	Gerbera jamesonii Chrysanthemum morifolium Scindapsus pictus 'Argyraeus' Aglaonema modestum Sansevieria trifasciata Spathiphyllum wallisii
Formaldehyde from chipboard, particle board, plastic bags, vinyl-plastic wall and floor tiles, permanent press clothing, plaster board made from phospho-gypsum, fire-retardant fabrics, plastic foam, polypropylene and polyesters in carpets, some glues and perfumes, dishwashing detergents, copying paper, tobacco smoke, certain foods and water	Chrysanthemum Common corn Devil's Ivy (Golden Pothos) Heartleaf Philodendron Peace Lilly	Chrysthemum morifolium Zea mays Scindapsus pictus 'Argyraeus' Philodendron scandens Spathiphyllum wallisii
Trichloroethylene (chloroform odour), a solvent from paints and degreasing	Devil's Ivy (Golden Pothos) Chrysanthemum Mother-in-Law's Tongue Peace Lilly	Scindapsus pictus 'Argyraeus' Chrysanthemum morifolium Sansevieria trifasciata Spathiphyllum wallisii
1,1,1-Trichloroethane (used in glues and correction fluids)	Peace Lilly	Spathiphyllum wallisii
Carbon monoxide from car fumes, all organic materials when burned, gas stove and fuel stove fumes	Devil's Ivy (Golden Pothos) Spider Plant (Ribbon Plant)	Scindapsus pictus 'Argyraeus' Chlorophytum comosum 'Vittatum'

* Use one or two mature plants to each 10 m² (12 yds²) of floor space
Specific sealed chamber experiment results from Wolverton 1984; Wolverton 1989

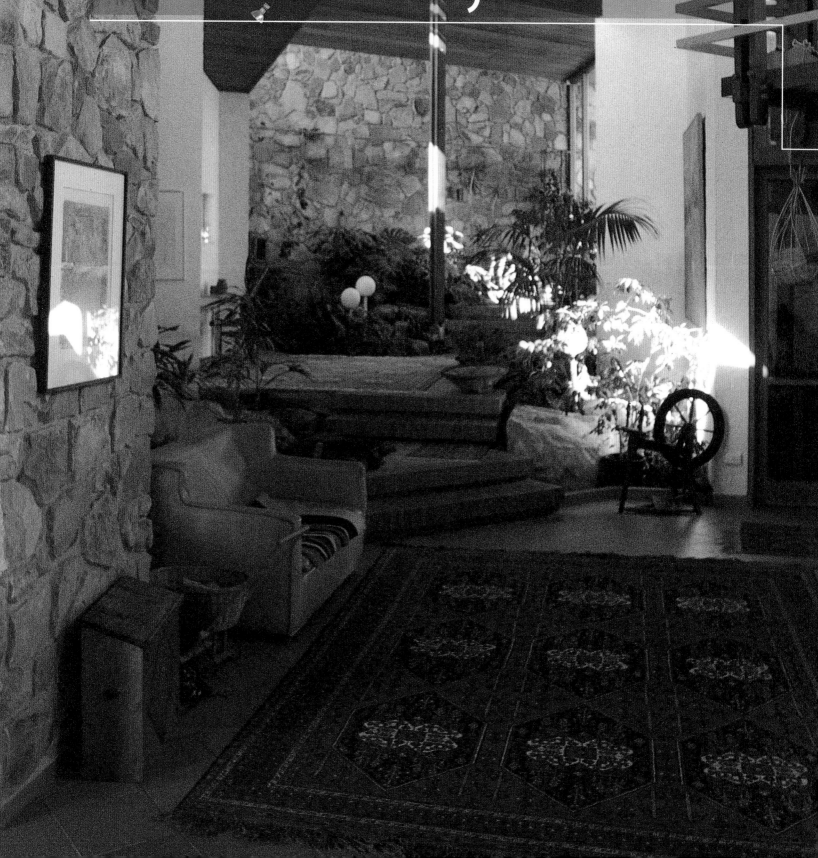

Constructing the safe

and healthy house

In this chapter we look at the actual construction of your building, on a trade by trade basis, discussing only those trades where practices differ from the commonplace in order to produce a healthy house. Where possible, we have avoided technical terms. In some cases, because it is essential that you be able to communicate with your architect or builder in a direct and practical way, certain technical terms have been included.

Select materials and methods carefully, contract tradespeople who understand the principles of building biology and ecology and remain true to your goals. The result will be a healthy living environment for you and your family.

At this point in the process you should have given consideration to those who will assist you in constructing your home. We suggest that you interview all building professionals and tradespeople before committing yourself to using their services. Enquire into the type of projects they have worked on previously and, if possible, visit those projects to see whether they conform to the standards you require and the occupants are satisfied with the work. After viewing the work of several different people, choose which project exemplifies the quality of workmanship, materials and finish that you would wish for your own building. Include references to that project in any contractual arrangement you make with a professional or tradesperson, as this will provide a benchmark standard for your own project.

It is essential to know whether the professionals you are using are familiar with the principles and details outlined in this book. If they are not, you should insist that they master the issues raised here before entering into a contract with them. By asking a few pertinent questions you will find whether they have the requisite

Page 142: Low allergy, passive
solar residence in South
Australia (Architect: G. Schurer;
Photograph: G. Schurer)

knowledge, share your philosophies and are able to interpret the spirit as well as the practice of healthy house construction principles.

You, the informed reader, have control over how your house will be constructed. You are paying for the results, so be firm about your standards. A good quality professional or tradesperson will be grateful to have a client who appreciates their efforts.

DEMOLITION

When preparing to undertake demolition work, consult the authorities who control the supply of gas, water, electricity, telephone, cable television, optical fibre communication networks and other services which are supplied to the demolition site.

The first rule to remember when demolishing a building is that no matter how convenient it may seem, building materials should never be disposed of by burning on-site. The Gaian philosophy requires that as many materials as practicable should be recycled or reused in the new house, but you may be left with some materials that require disposal. Beware of old ceilings, and wall and floor linings that may have been painted with lead primer or contain arsenic-based glues or finishes — be careful of wallpapers of earlier centuries. Lead was also used in roof joints, galvanised piping and for sink, bath and basin waste-traps. The best way to dispose of toxic metal is to sell it to a scrap metal merchant, who will subsequently recycle it.

Asbestos

Asbestos is a general name for a group of fibrous silicate minerals. In the past asbestos was used as a thermal insulation material, in asbestos-cement roofing, wallboards, water pipe insulation, boiler pipe packing, paint and fireproof gloves. Asbestos fibres are smaller than other industrial fibres and single fibres cannot be seen with the naked eye. Over time the fibres age, weather and flake or break. They become airborne and can be inhaled or carried on clothing. All types of asbestos are carcinogenic. The degree of risk depends on the size of the fibre, and hence the type of asbestos present, but there is no agreed minimum level for safety. Asbestos is found where cheap additions or outbuildings have been constructed. Fibres from a demolished building that contained asbestos can often be found in the soil of the site.

Demolition and removal of asbestos is a job for an expert. The removal of asbestos is dangerous and hence expensive, so its presence may be a critical factor in whether you decide to purchase a property. In Australia, a property owner can be fined if asbestos drifts into a neighbour's property during demolition.

The most dangerous type of asbestos is Category 1, once used as insulation around furnaces and pipes, but all types must be correctly handled. Category 2 is found as corrugated roofing, shingles, flat wallboards, rainwater gutters and downpipes. There is an encapsulating sealant which controls the release of asbestos fibres into the atmosphere, but it is a chemical and chemical outgassing should always be avoided.

Asbestos should only be removed using these precautions:

- If the asbestos is external, close all doors and windows while work is ongoing.
- Seal all asbestos-cement sheets with PVA paint or wet with water.
- Use a complete industrial 'space-suit' when removing Category 1 asbestos and an approved disposable respirator (with a cartridge approved for asbestos dust). Better still, have it removed by a professional. Use overalls for full cover when removing Category 2 asbestos.
- Clean gutters with water and collect any loose asbestos fibres for disposal.
- Avoid breaking any material containing asbestos by lowering, not dropping, the material.
- Stack all materials on very thick, industrial-standard PVC sheeting, wrap, seal and promptly remove from the site.
- Vacuum clean all affected areas.
- Keep all demolition waste wet, wrapped in plastic sheeting, or in lined bins or covered vehicles.
- Dispose only at approved toxic waste sites (usually designated for Categories 1 and 2 asbestos). Consult your local environmental protection authority for advice on where to dispose of asbestos. (NSW State News Building Industry Connection 1994b)

EXCAVATION

From the Gaian viewpoint the less excavation needed the better, because excavation has the potential to impact on the geomagnetic field. It is difficult to quantify this impact, but as a general guideline it is wise to minimise cutting and filling. Your general aim should be to maintain the site's integrity. If excavation is unavoidable, when the project is completed, restore the site as close as possible to its original profile.

◎ Preserving valuable topsoil ◎

Topsoil is a virtually irreplaceable natural resource. During the building of a house, topsoil should be stockpiled. This ensures that the soil is not destroyed in structure and texture by the compaction that would occur if building operations were carried out on top of it or if it was mixed with subsoil. Before the builder arrives on the site, all trees and shrubs that are to be retained should have protection barriers erected around them. A delivery access track should be marked out to minimise destruction of plants and traffic compaction of the soil around tree roots, which usually extend just beyond the edge of the tree canopy. Areas should be set aside for the topsoil stockpile. Barriers should be erected around them, and all tradespeople warned off by clear and durable notices, as builder's lime, cement and heavy boots will alter the topsoil's texture, porosity and chemical balance. If you have the space on-site, stockpile the topsoil at a depth no greater than 1 metre (3 feet 3 inches), and keep it well weeded and aerated until it can be reused. This provides the perfect opportunity to alter the texture of your soil if need be, for instance by adding sand if the soil is a little heavy.

While the building is in progress make enquiries as to where you can obtain various mulches. Mulches are excellent for retaining soil moisture, keeping soil temperature variations within a reasonable range and protecting plants from the sudden onslaught of winds which dry out the soil and induce water stress so quickly that you may not be able to rescue your plants in time.

SEWAGE AND WASTE WATER

As a community matter, responsibility for treatment and disposal of waste is accepted by a local authority. However, very few authorities treat this valuable resource as a material that can be reused to the benefit of plants or to the building industry, in the manufacturing of building blocks. While such large scale treatment is limited by the presence of heavy metals and toxic materials, it is still worthwhile for us, as individuals, to look at ways of recycling our sewage and waste water.

◎ Composting toilets ◎

In the presence of oxygen and other biological materials, human waste breaks down naturally, however, once the waste is engulfed by water, the breakdown process ceases. Oxygen, chemicals and mechanical systems must then be used. This requires an immense infrastructure and water-storage systems, with all their attendant construction and maintenance costs.

There is an alternative though. A wide variety of composting toilet technology is available, not only for domestic use, but for community and municipal use as well. The composting toilet is often also referred to as a 'waterless' or 'humus' closet. The composting process that this type of toilet employs is the same as in the garden compost bin, utilising a starter mix of worms and soil organisms. It is not completely waterless, as the humus requires some water to help control temperature and circulate oxygen. Animal waste matter introduces relatively high levels of nitrogen, thus a desirable balance of carbon and nitrogen is maintained. Carbon is supplied by plant matter.

Table 9.1: Comparison of on-site waste disposal methods*

ISSUE	COMPOSTING TOILET	SEPTIC TANK TREATMENT	AERATION PLUS CHLORINATION**
Destroys viruses	yes	no	uncertain
Destroys beneficial bacteria	no	no	uncertain but regrow later
Destroys harmful bacteria	yes	no	will regrow later
Destroys parasitic worms, except nematodes (roundworms)	yes	no	no
Destroys nematodes (roundworms) only	unsure	no	no
Destroys protozoan cysts (including Giardia and Entamoeba)	yes	no	unlikely
Reduces phosphorus pollution	yes	no	no
Reduces nitrogen compound pollution	yes	to some degree	yes
Creates carcinogenic trihalomethanes	no	no	yes
Creates residual sludge	yes	no	no
Requires chemicals to be added	no	no	yes
Maintenance-free period	3 months	3 months	constant supervision
Requires de-sludging	15–20 years	1–4 years	6 months–4 years
Health risk if mechanical failure occurs	low	high	medium
Degree of water conservation	high	low	low

* adapted from Pedals 1992; ** Faecham, et al 1990

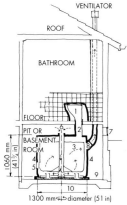

1. Pedestal pan
2. Outlet pipe from pan
3. Receiving container (rotates)
4. Outer container
5. Access hatch
6. Air inlet
7. Ventilators (flyproof)
8. Fan (12 volt from PV panels)
9. Reinforced-concrete floor
10. Insulation
11. Heater (hot water pipe)

Figure 9.1: Cross-section of a Rota-loo system (redrawn from Pedals 1992)

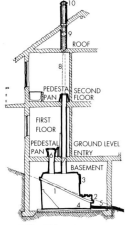

1. Clivus Multrum unit
2. Compost access
3. Access hatch
4. Tank
5. Drainage of liquid effluent
6. Waste pipe to pan (on lower floor)
7. Waste pipe to pan (at upper level)
8. System ventilation pipe
9. Exhaust fan
10. Hood

Figure 9.2: The Clivus Multrum composting system for wastes from toilets and urinals. The system can be varied to include one or many pans (Based on information supplied by Clivus Multrum Australia Pty Ltd)

Cold climates present problems for the installation of composting toilets, as low temperatures can stop the biological processes needed for the breakdown of waste matter. The overriding problem worldwide is that fresh water is becoming scarce and expensive. Consequently, any system that addresses water conservation should be given careful consideration.

THE ROTA-LOO

The operation of this type of toilet is quite straightforward. The container that receives the human waste from the pedestal pan is kept warm to stimulate bacterial growth. The aerobic bacteria digest the excreta, rendering it into compost. Any resultant odours are extracted by a mechanical exhaust fan run by solar or mains power. Over time, at a sufficiently high temperature, all pathogens are destroyed. The Rota-loo pedestal and tanks are made of fibreglass with a thick, white, gelcoat finish. Although the Rota-loo satisfies health criteria, it requires a heating element well beyond the capability of photovoltaic (solar) power. Solar-heated water with some backup heat source is a viable option.

A grease trap is essential when using a composting toilet system to deal with liquid effluent that contains oils and fats. We recommend that a small septic tank be used to provide pre-treatment to the waste water. This tank will need desludging every 20 years or so. The absorption trenches for such a small septic system will have nutrients and water that can be used around the area of the trenches on vegetation with moderate rooting habits.

DOWMUS COMPOSTING TOILET

The composting toilet manufactured by Dowmus Pty Ltd has a fan which runs on 12 volts (from photovoltaic panels if desired). It has a circular reactor chamber made of recycled plastic, and has no moving parts. There is a wet and a dry model. The wet model has a hatch which allows kitchen waste, cardboard and paper as well as garden waste to drop into the chamber below. Moisture percolates to a garden irrigation system or is collected for further treatment and re-use. The wet system maintains a core temperature of 30–35 degrees Celsius (86–95 degrees Fahrenheit). For each person using the system, 80–85 square metres (860–915 square feet) of garden is required to absorb the liquid effluent

produced. The dry system operates at 29–37 degrees Celsius (84–99 degrees Fahrenheit) and requires only 1 square metre (11 square feet) of garden per person.

THE CLIVUS MULTRUM COMPOSTING SYSTEM

This system has the capacity to handle both single residences and multiple dwellings and produces organic compost as its end product. Used throughout the world, it requires no water or chemicals. Toilet wastes are collected in the tank to which carbon rich materials such as lawn cuttings, wood shavings, leaves and sawdust are added. An enclosed, aerated environment accelerates the breakdown process, which eventually leads to decomposition. A small fan, run by solar power, activates a ventilation pipe in the roof to exhaust odours and aerate the waste material. This system is said to eradicate odours in toilet cubicles in all weather conditions.

◎ Septic tanks ◎

While the composting toilet is by far the preferred option in terms of waste disposal, some local authorities remain out of touch with the latest developments and still insist on septic tanks. The water used by a septic tank may comprise some 30–50 per cent of all domestic water used. The effluent from septic tanks contains pathogens from the sewage as well as added nutrients from grey water, in which pathogens multiply rapidly. In theory, septic tanks achieve reasonable levels of effluent quality, but when inadequately maintained, they can cause ground water pollution. Contaminated water from septic tanks can easily enter the ground water when trenches become blocked with fats and oils that have escaped from the grease trap. The polluted water leaches into underground water supplies, and the high levels of nutrients contained in it can cause destructive algal growths in waterways.

The malfunctioning of neglected septic tanks is well documented, with pathogens able to travel 'hundreds of metres through the ground' (Pedals 1992). Consulting engineer, Doctor Terry Lustig has been quoted as saying that concentrations of pathogens in the effluent from a septic tank can exceed by 1000 times the allowed concentration in water for use for public recreation. The effluent is probably in the order of 1,000,000 times the concentration of that in the sludge from a composting toilet (Pedals 1992).

If you have a septic tank with effluent trenches and wish to upgrade it without replacing it entirely, ask your landscape architect to design a miniature wetland system to receive the effluent. Plants will help to counteract possible inadequacies in the system.

EARTH CONSTRUCTION

The use of earth as a construction material began in prehistoric times when sun-dried bricks began to be used for all types of buildings in the Mediterranean region. They continue to be used there in the present day. In China, rammed earth has been used since the third millennium BC and is still being used. In Tongding county, large multi-storey rammed earth buildings up to 50,000 square metres (538,200 square feet) in size exist, some of which have been standing for 500 years.

The advantage of using clay as a building material is principally that it allows heat energy to move slowly from the outside of the building to the inside. In China, where the rammed earth is around 50 centimetres (20 inches) thick, it may take 15 days for heat transfer to occur. This delays the impact on the building's interior of the intense heat of summer or the cold of winter. The adobe type of wall (sun-dried clay brick) provides a lag of only one day in the transfer of heat energy. However, when it is mixed with straw and other organic materials, it becomes a good insulator against heat transfer, while remaining permeable to terrestrial and cosmic radiation. In climates where nights are cool and days are very hot, clay brick walls can be used in living areas so that the impact of daytime heat is slowed, while in sleeping areas, a material with low thermal mass, such as wood, ensures that sleepers benefit from rapid night-time cooling.

Adobe construction has a negligible impact on the broader environment, unlike the vast clay pits and energy-profligate kilns used to mass produce the extruded and baked clay bricks which are the common building materials of many so-called advanced countries. In France, where earth-wall construction is referred to as pisé-de-terre, and also in Germany, buildings of this type have been in use for more than four centuries. Although often hard to identify because of the plaster coating hiding the earth construction, rammed earth churches, homes and castles occur in England, Russia and Spain. Part of the Palace of Versailles in France is even earth-walled.

Not all modern professionals accept the idea of earth-wall construction, perhaps because 'many of today's professionals were trained at a time when Modernism was associated with a few new materials such as glass, concrete and plastics. These are the fruits of a technological age that seemed to forget about the Earth's natural riches' (Vershure, in Armstrong 1988).

High thermal mass

Thermal mass is the capacity of a material to store energy as heat. The highest thermal mass is achieved by a building encased in the surrounding earth. An earth-sheltered building uses the infinite thermal mass of the earth, extracting summer heat and storing it for warmth the following winter, and making use of winter heat loss for cooling the following summer.

On a daily basis, earth-wall construction can absorb daytime heat and release it for night warming or store the cool of the evening for daytime use. Both building types require an understanding of sun-control to permit solar heating to occur only when it is necessary. For this, a specialist solar architect should be consulted.

Testing for soil components

The type of soil available on a site may determine whether rammed-earth, adobe mud-brick or pressed earth-brick technology is appropriate for use in a healthy building.

HAND METHOD OF IDENTIFYING A SOIL TEXTURE TYPE

• Take a sample of soil, small enough to fit comfortably in the palm of the hand. Discard obvious pieces of gravel.

• Moisten the soil with water a little at a time and knead it into a ball. Add more moisture until it just fails to stick to the fingers.

• Inspect the sample to see whether sand is visible; if not, it may still be felt and heard as the sample is worked with the fingers.

• Next, squeeze the sample hard to see whether it will form a cast; if so, determine whether it is durable or falls apart readily.

• Finally, squeeze it out between the thumb and forefinger with a sliding motion; note the length of self-supporting ribbon or bolus that can be formed. (Handreck 1980)

Ribbon (mm)	Ribbon (in)	Field test criteria	Soil texture group	Potential use
up to 10	1/3	Cannot be moulded; single grains stick to fingers; no coherence	Sand	
		Dark stain discolours fingers; fragile casts can just be handled	Loamy sand	Stabilised earth-bricks
		Sticky when wet	Clayey sand	Rammed earth, stablised earth-bricks
10–30	1/3–1 1/5	Very sandy to touch; fine sand heard or can just be felt in some	Sandy loam	Rammed earth, stabilised earth-bricks
		Smooth, greasy if organic matter present	Fine sandy loam	Rammed earth, stabilised earth-bricks
20–30	3/4–1 1/5	Bolus strongly coherent; sandy to touch	Light sandy clay-loam	Rammed earth, stabilised earth-bricks
		Bolus coherent; spongy, no silkiness	Loam	Rammed earth, stabilised earth-bricks
		Bolus coherent; spongy and sandy to touch	Fine sandy loam	Rammed earth, stabilised earth-bricks
		Bolus very smooth and silky; coherent but will crumble	Silt-loam	
40–50	1 1/2–2	Sandy to touch	Sandy clay-loam	
		Bolus plastic, forms coherent cast, spongy feel, smooth to manipulate	Clay-loam	Mud bricks
		Bolus plastic and silky	Silty clay-loam	Mud bricks
		Fine sand felt and heard	Fine sandy clay-loam	Mud bricks
50–80	2–3 1/8	Fine medium sand grains can be felt	Sandy clay	Mud bricks
		Smooth and silky plastic bolus	Silty clay	
		Slight resistance to shearing	Light clay	Mud bricks
80	3 1/8	More resistance to shear than light clay	Light-medium clay	Mud bricks
more than 80	over 3 1/8	Feels like plasticine	Medium clay	Mud bricks
		Feels like stiff plasticine	Heavy clay	Mud bricks

*Sources: Northcote (1965); Handreck (1980)

Table 9.2: Method of field analysis of soil textures*

- Refer to Table 9.2 which analyses the bolus and its 'feel'. Use it as a guide to determine soil texture prior to deciding on the suitability of the soil for the preferred earth construction.

Rammed earth

Rammed earth is a simple mode of wall construction, requiring only locally available subsoil and labour. Moist soil is compacted one layer at a time inside very strong timber forms. When the most recent layer, rammed into place with the ends of poles, is firm and compacted, the forms are immediately dismantled and reassembled for the next layer above or alongside the previous layer. Hence each section is a huge earth-block bonded to the others. This bond can be so tight that the wall is almost monolithic. As time passes, well constructed rammed-earth walls become as durable as sandstone.

Earth-wall construction has to begin with a complete understanding of soil. Clay, sand, silt and gravel are needed in just the right combinations for any kind of rammed or compressed earth-wall construction. Larger-sized grains give strength and clay particles bind the mix together. Laboratory analysis is required to develop an ideal mix for a rammed-earth wall if it is to withstand the rigours of time and weather.

The water content of the mix is critical. The soil should bind together as it is rammed into the forms so that it does not adhere to, or build up on, the pestle or rammer. If a mix contains too much water, when the rammer is thrust into the mud, bulges will appear elsewhere. For David Oliver, an expert in rammed-earth construction, the ideal mix is one that:

> *. . . will result in walling, which, on removal of formwork has even and dense compaction throughout, an even and smooth surface finish showing no signs of segregation prior to any applied finishing and exhibits no cracking and minimal shrinkage on drying. Technically, the granular 'pebbly', 'wavy' surface finishes popular with many rammed-earth contractors are poor, readily prone to erosion and moisture degradation. This is indicative of poor mix particle-distribution and compaction in layers too thick, at often lower than optimum moisture-content.*

The formwork used to construct a rammed-earth wall needs to be moved constantly, so a balance has to be struck between strong, heavy forms that are difficult to move and light forms that are not strong enough to take the pressure, yet are more easily moved. Rolling formwork, which have rollers in the bottom to allow for easy horizontal movement, are easy to use and are most suitable for long, straight walls.

Rammed earth may take 2 years to dry out but it has a correspondingly slow rate of moisture absorption. Even in wet climates, as long as the top and bottom are waterproofed, such walls are very durable. They will accept plaster, render, nails, screws and cladding. Being soil, it is wise to seal rammed earth with a clear, natural sealant to control radon emissions, should higher than normal levels be detected in the soil. Not all soils have this problem, so it is worthwhile testing for excessive radon before beginning construction.

Architect Graham Osborne, a specialist in rammed-earth technology, described the formwork he uses as follows:

The patented climbing rammed-earth formwork aids in improving efficiency in the site manufacture of walls. The climbing formwork and upright supporting system have enough tolerance to allow the shutters to clamp onto the previous rammed earth and when filled, release to slide vertically free of the wall. This process is repeated until the top of the wall is reached. In another form, the upright supporting system can be set up with the stationary forms set on their end, but at right angles (or other angles) with adjoining pieces to form corner nibs. The vertical supporting structure can be set up to align with the ends of the shutters to form infills, sills and lintels.

◎ A d o b e   e a r t h - b l o c k s   o r   m u d - b r i c k s ◎

Adobe blocks are earth-blocks — some say mud-bricks — which are made by hand using a mould. They are usually sun-dried rather than fired or cured. Some 85 per cent of Chinese buildings are constructed of earth-blocks. Such buildings can also be seen throughout Pakistan, India, Eurasia and North Africa as well as in the southwest of the United States. Adobe mud-brick is different to rammed earth in that it has a different proportion of water to earth and reabsorbs water almost as fast as it dries out.

As a technology, adobe has been used for many thousands of years. In Anatolia and Crete archaeological adobe sites date back to 5000 BC, and in Iran to 6000 BC. The equipment used to make blocks varies little worldwide, though the blocks vary greatly in shape: spherical, cylindrical, conical and rectangular. This technique is increasing in popularity as modern architects experiment with traditional dome and vault constructions using mud-bricks.

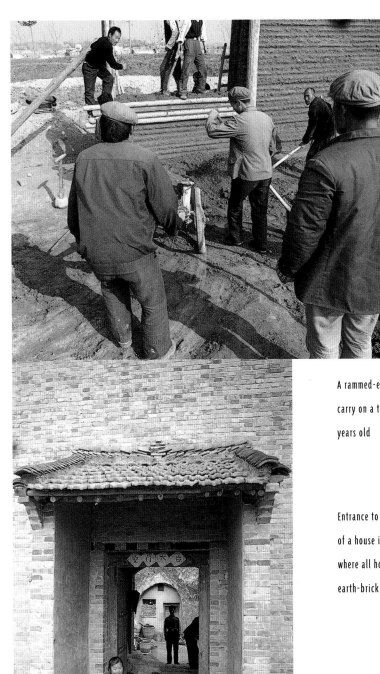

A rammed-earth team in China carry on a tradition thousands of years old

Entrance to the inner courtyard of a house in a Chinese village where all houses are built of earth-brick

Most earths, other than topsoils containing organic matter, are acceptable for the production of adobe blocks. They must contain enough clay to bind the earth particles together without containing so much that the blocks crack because of shrinkage. If the soil available to you has too much clay, it will be unsuitable for making adobe blocks.

The secret of waterproofing adobe is the type of render used. The most common render is chopped

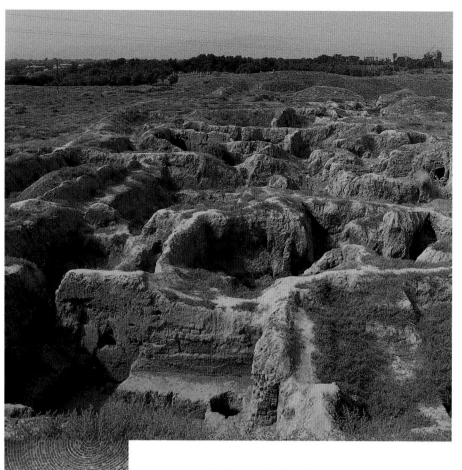

Top: Prehistoric adobe settlement in Samarkand

Above: Ancient mosque dome under restoration, Uzbekistan

Figure 9.3: The relationship between cement content and strength in earth blocks

CINVA (Pressed) earth-bricks

The CINVA is one of the most common types of earth compression machines available. When operated by hand, the CINVA produces bricks 10 centimetres high by 15 centimetres thick by 30 centimetres long (4 inches by 6 inches by 12 inches), as well as tiles. When mechanically operated, it produces bricks of adobe measurement, 11.5 centimetres high by 25 centimetres thick by 37.5 centimetres long (4½ inches by 10 inches by 15 inches). The American version produces bricks 10 centimetres high by 15 centimetres thick by 30 centimetres long (4 inches by 6 inches by 12 inches). The soil particles of a CINVA brick must be very small, as the process does not involve ramming, which would otherwise break up the particles. Cement is added to the sieved subsoil before water is added. A minimum of 35 per cent clay is needed for handling. Water is added and thoroughly mixed in so that the block is firm and does not slump when it is removed from the press.

Compressed earth-bricks

Compressed earth-bricks, virtually blocks of reconstituted sandstone, are made up of clay, sand and loam milled and mixed with cement, which makes up about 10 per cent of the block's mass. According to the industrial designer and architect, Doctor William Lawson, 'compressed earth-brick production uses approximately 25 per cent of the total energy per kilogram (per pound) needed to produce an ordinary clay brick, 35 per cent of that for a concrete block and 20–35 per cent of that for sawn soft and hardwood respectively'.

straw, similar to chaff used as horse feed, mixed with mud and dung. There should be a high proportion of straw in the render, so that it appears as a shiny fleck throughout the mix. It is recommended that the joints between the blocks be kept flush with the block face and the surface plastered to prevent rain from entering any crevices. If plastering is undertaken, the joints should be raked, or recessed, with a special tool to ensure that the plaster bonds to the wall firmly. Water should not be allowed to collect at the base of adobe walls. It is essential to use a roof overhang and in some cases a stronger material than mud-bricks for the base.

The bonds between minute clay particles break down when clay is exposed to water. Clay is an unstable material, swelling when wet and shrinking when dry, yet when it is mixed with larger particles it becomes manageable. It is often added to sand and gravelly soils as a binder. Builders add cement to coarse-particle soils such as laterite. The cement reacts with the soil and its water content to form a hardened material. Lime can also be used to harden clay as it reacts with some of the minerals and the water found in clay. Bitumen can be used in the mix to act as a water repellent.

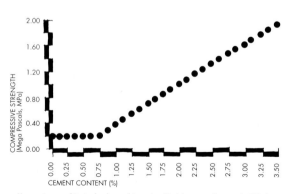

Your engineer, architect or local council inspector will advise you on the strength of block you will need. Find that strength level on the vertical axis, go across till you hit the sloping line, then trace down to the horizontal axis to find what percentage (by volume) of the earth block needs to be in cement.

Figure 9.3

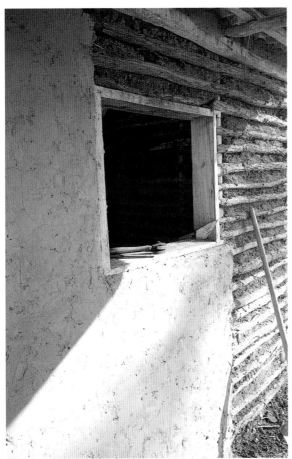

Carpentry

◉ Wood, the ideal biological building material ◉

The useful life of timber extends well beyond that of other materials, at little economic or environmental cost. It can be used again and again, so long as an appropriate species of wood is selected for a particular purpose and correct procedures are followed. Timber is the ideal material for balancing the levels of gas and vapour between interior and exterior air. It can help control air pollution and allows the diffusion of oxygen. Timber is easily worked and its energy input in production is relatively low.

Wood, an electrical semi-conductor, should be used in living areas in lieu of reinforced concrete and metals, as it does not interfere with natural electro-magnetic fields. A structure made predominantly from wood does not create unhealthy patterns of high frequency and microwave radiation. Rogue electro-magnetic fields from alternating currents are not focused and collected by a wooden structure.

◉ Timber for the world ◉

Two hundred million tonnes (197 million tons) of timber are used for pulp in the developed nations every year and 25 million tonnes (over 24 million tons) in the developing nations. Developed nations obtain specialist hardwoods for use in industry from the developing world. Some 59 million cubic metres (2084 million cubic feet) of hardwoods are extracted, and in the forests of southeast Asia 'at least half of the remaining trees are injured beyond recovery' (Myers 1985). Almost all houses in the developing countries use timber for fuel or for simple building poles.

Tropical rainforests have the greatest genetic diversity and are the richest habitats on Earth, covering only 6 per cent of the land surface of the planet yet containing 50–90 per cent of all living species. Tropical rainforest once covered about 16 million square kilometres (6 million square miles) of land, but now only covers 9 million square kilometres (3 million square miles). It is estimated that very little will remain by the end of the century, yet the world continues to use many tropical rainforest species. The timber used in furniture and building joinery comes mainly from southeast Asian forests. Taiwan supplies the greatest amount of timber,

In terms of their cost over the life-cycle of a building, compressed earth-bricks are probably the best commercially available masonry system available. They require little, if any, long-term maintenance. Because of its inherent strength, if the building is to be demolished at the end of its useful life, the material can be reprocessed into a medium-grade, hard-core aggregate for use in other building products. Compressed earth-brick walls are comparable to or better, in terms of their load-bearing capacity, than many commonly used wall blocks and bricks.

Earth-bricks must contain cement to achieve full strength. Below 0.75 per cent by volume of cement, the cement can no longer link the particles of soil together, so the soil itself governs the strength of the mix. Some who use earth-brick machines specify a cement content between 5 and 10 per cent, the strength of the bricks being proportional to the amount of cement used. In a study carried out in 1995 by Ozkan and Al-Herbish, it was found that bricks stabilised with cement are at least twice the strength of those stabilised with lime. A mixture of clayey loam soil with 5 per cent cement is almost as strong as fired clay.

Wattle and daub construction used extensively in the early settlement period in Australia. The walls were made up of twigs plastered with a mixture of clay, water and sometimes straw

around 75 per cent of it coming from rainforests.

The forests of the world maintain climatic balance. They stabilise atmospheric processes by absorbing radiation and solar energy. If the tree cover is removed, the albedo (reflectivity of the land surface) increases and solar heat is reflected back into the atmosphere. This causes convection and wind currents, resulting in changed rainfall patterns. The rate of soil erosion increases and the atmosphere's carbon dioxide balance is altered.

We need to act as a world community for the benefit of all. Not only should commercial fuel-wood plantations be established in tropical regions but each developed nation should review its policies on timber production. Developed nations need to produce more home-grown hardwoods and softwoods and should make paper recycling a major commercial issue. In most developing countries, forestry departments are understaffed and lacking in funds. Each country has to develop its own guidelines to help people choose timbers appropriate to the Gaian philosophy. Old-growth native forest requires protection from exploitation, and governments need to be pressured so that source and species identification marks are placed on timber. Lend your support to 'green' pressure groups that work in the political arena. Only use timber from acceptable sources, avoiding those from exploited countries which obtain their timber from rainforests. Ask your supplier for both the name and source of any wood you intend buying. You can double check their information by telephoning regional advisory services, wilderness societies or the local forestry department.

Alternatively, visit demolition yards and second-hand dealers where you will find a wonderful resource of relatively inexpensive structural and joinery timbers. When you use timber in constructing your house, design the joints and fixings so that nails can easily be removed to enable recycling at a later date; this makes your home a wood bank for the future. Experiment and obtain professional advice on how to bleach wood safely, and stain and finish plantation timbers so they will be as attractive as rainforest timbers.

Some of the many rainforest timbers to avoid are listed at left (common names have been supplied for simplicity, with alternative names in brackets).

Purchasing the timber of Oregon or Douglas fir (*Pseudotsuga menziesii*) can be problematic as suppliers do not state whether it comes from old-growth forest or is plantation timber, hence it is best avoided. Interesting developments are taking place in the use of coconut palm timber from the Pacific Islands, particularly Fiji, but if you use it make sure you are buying plantation timber.

Anyone who is in the building industry will tell you how wonderful Western Red Cedar (*Thuja plicata*) is for all types of building use. Cedar is slow growing, straight-grained and contains natural oils that make it highly weather and decay resistant. (Make sure that aromatic cedar oil is not one of your allergies before you use cedar.) It is only acceptable to use Western Red Cedar when you can be guaranteed that it comes from sustainable, managed regrowth forest.

◎ Recycled wood ◎

From the viewpoint of Gaian philosophy, the most satisfactory wood to use is recycled timber. Using recycled timber reduces waste and helps to preserve rainforest and old-growth forest. Recycled wood has an attractive aged quality and can be economically obtained by approaching demolition crews or second-hand dealers. If you do buy from a second-hand timber yard, try and find wood that has not been stripped and had its nails cut flush with a grinder, as the metal will be almost impossible to remove. To clean the wood, use an electric planing machine to strip dirt and paint but be careful to use gloves, long sleeves and a face mask as old paints were usually lead-based. A metal detector is useful for locating hidden nails and screws.

◎ Flooring — timber frame or concrete? ◎

Disruptions in the natural 'rain' of cosmic and gamma radiation, ultraviolet rays, photons, radio waves and microwaves from outer space may cause health problems in human beings. Until physicists undertake more detailed research, the most sensible decision is to avoid conventional reinforced concrete and steel reinforcement as much as possible, as these can scatter or intensify cosmic rays. Our buildings should not alter the path of the rays entering from outer space.

Concrete can be a very useful energy-saving building material in that it has a high thermal mass, thus stores heat energy for later benefit. In warm climates, a complete earth-coupled concrete floor is appropriate because it shares the steady temperature of the earth, stabilising the air temperature inside the house. It is possible to substitute reinforced concrete with a coarse aggregate of crushed limestone and glass with polypropylene or fibreglass reinforcement mesh.

The best available compromise, which does not disturb the pattern of cosmic rays entering the building, is to combine timber floors with unreinforced concrete thermal pads in the areas of the house where solar gain is possible during winter (usually near the sills of windows designed to take in sunlight).

If using a concrete slab, you need to install a damp-proof membrane, usually made of hard polymer plastics. Such plastics outgas, but if the concrete floor has been correctly designed and laid it should not crack and will stop the fumes from entering the building. The damp-proof membrane should be laid over a thin layer of sand and a drainage bed of hard core (crushed stones) which breathes freely at the edges.

If one tests the soil of a site and finds that radon emissions are high what options are there to seal it off or ventilate it away from a building's interior? As timber is a hygroscopic, or 'breathing' material, radon will be able to enter the interior via a timber floor system. Your decision on whether to use concrete or timber for your floor will depend upon the amount of radon emitted by the soil and rocks of the site. Though natural microwave and other radiation will be less distorted if you use timber, if the amount of radon being emitted by the ground underneath the house is high, it is advisable to use concrete. By using discontinuous steel reinforcement in concrete floors you will avoid the creation of rogue pulsed electric and magnetic fields (discussed later in this chapter).

Wood floors can be sealed to prevent radon ingress if you make the effort to seal the gaps between the floor system and the walls (see Chapter 10). Elevated wood-framed floors can be augmented by combining them with natural insulation materials. This not only reduces the noise transmission and improves the heat transfer qualities of the floor, but also creates a biologically healthy breathing floor system.

CARPENTRY/BUILDING

⊚ The wooden pole house ⊚

The pole house is vulnerable to bushfire and also requires highly termite- and fungi-resistant timber. For the serious follower of Gaian principles, only plantation timber should be used. Much of the pine timber used for pole house construction is currently treated with wood preservatives which the manufacturers claim are not harmful — yet they issue warnings not to inhale the fumes should you burn the wood. The most commonly used preservative contains chromated copper arsenate (CCA) which is made up of salts of arsenic, copper and benign chromium (usually arsenic pentoxide, cupric oxide and chromic acid). When these three metals act together they become toxic.

We all take in an average of a few micrograms per day of arsenic from the environment, but problems can occur when our normal intake is increased by further exposure to CCA. For example, in studies conducted in Canada, the soil up to 10 metres (33 feet) away from playground equipment treated with CCA was found to contain 1.8 to 23.5 times the normal concentration of CCA. The surfaces of the equipment revealed high levels of arsenic, however the main risk came not from skin contact but from children ingesting the contaminated soil (Reidel, et al 1991). As early as 1968, workers were reported as feeling ill from their contact with sawdust from the treated pine logs they were using. In a study carried out over a 3-year period, people who burnt treated logs in fuel stoves showed

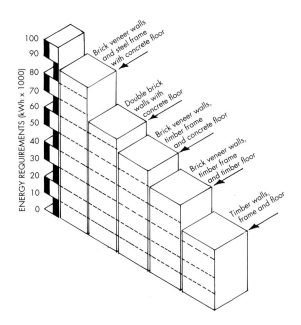

ENERGY REQUIREMENTS (kWh x 1000)

100
90
80
70
60
50
40
30
20
10
0

Brick veneer walls and steel frame with concrete floor

Double brick walls with concrete floor

Brick veneer walls, timber frame and concrete floor

Brick veneer walls, timber frame and timber floor

Timber walls, frame and floor

Figure 9.4: Energy requirements for various types of residential construction (after Pearson 1989)

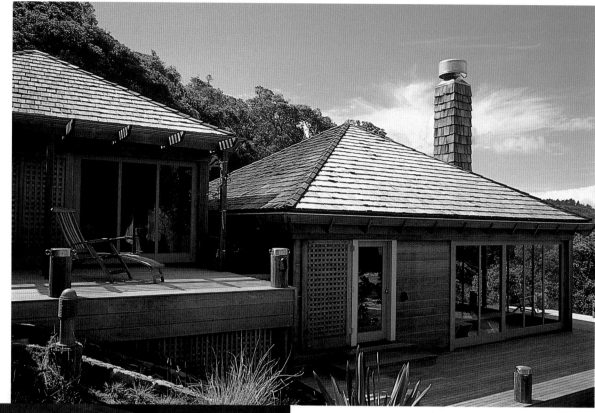

Wood-framed structures are ideal for use in earthquake zones. Residence at Coromandel, NZ (Architects: J. Schulze and F. Poursoltan; Photograph: J. Schulze)

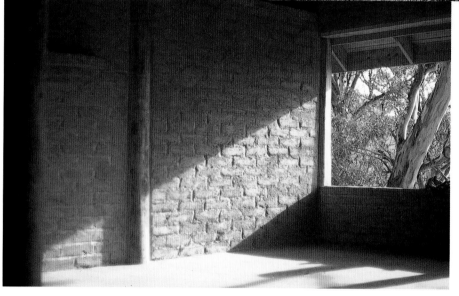

Wood-framed, earth-brick infill and earth floor building under construction at Thredbo, NSW, Aust. (Architect: N. Mortensen; Photograph: N. Mortensen)

symptoms such as rashes, respiratory problems, seizures, hair loss, blackouts, eye irritation and muscle cramps; high arsenic levels were found in the air and in hair samples of those exposed (Croft, et al 1984).

There is a relatively benign wood treatment for preventing pest and fungus attack, ammoniated copper quartenary (ACQ). Unfortunately, plantation pine treated with ACQ is not yet available in Australia for use in pole houses. It is, to date, only available for traditional building construction and landscaping. If you wish to build a pole house, careful termite-resistant detailing is essential (see Chapter 10).

◉ Wood-frame, earth-brick construction ◉

The hybrid wood-frame, earth-brick house represents the ideal biologically appropriate construction method. It creates a house that simultaneously breathes yet stores heat for energy efficiency, as the hygroscopic nature of wood is combined with the high thermal mass qualities of earth-bricks. It is a good construction method for earthquake or cyclone zones. It is also a flexible method, in that the roof can first be constructed on posts so that the earth-brick walls can be worked on beneath the roof. The wood-frame, earth-brick house can be constructed with reusable materials, creating a low-impact, ecologically acceptable building.

◉ Straw bale walls ◉

Basically a waste material, straw has a high cellulose content and is identical to wood in composition. A highly effective and environmentally sound use for straw can be found in the simple, low cost practice of straw bale construction. It is a technique that was developed on the treeless plains of Nebraska in the late 1800s and is carried on today in the United States, Canada, Britain, Europe, China, Russia, Mexico and South America.

A wall can be made by stacking bales of straw in a brick-like manner then staking them with steel spikes. Chicken mesh is stitched on with wires passing through the bales from either side. Each side of the wall is then given three coats of cement and lime-modified adobe stucco. The resulting wall is 50 centimetres (19 inches) thick and can be used as either a load-bearing wall or an infill panel. Cellulose material from sources such as oats, rye, barley, wheat, rice or even baled waste paper and cardboard free of printing ink is suitable.

The bales hold enough air to provide impressive thermal insulation but not enough to support combustion, so they have both a high thermal insulation value and a high resistance to fire. They are also very resistant to vermin because the cellulose material is so closely packed together that there is less space for vermin than in an ordinary framed or sheeted wall construction. The layers of adobe stucco provide a tight seal to prevent the ingress of even relatively small insects. Termites can be excluded by installing larger than normal ant-caps and termite mesh 'socks' on the structural poles. Straw bale construction is susceptible to moisture damage, but the three adobe stucco coats (one of which should be waterproofed), the elevation of the structure and the overhangs and verandahs give a good weather-resistant finish overall.

⊚ Wood-framed walls ⊚

Wood-frame construction, while not having the thermal mass to store heat energy, does have the benefit of reacting quickly to climatic change, hence cooling more rapidly than brick or earth-brick on summer nights. Insulation is necessary within the frame to control heat transfer. If your primary aim is to create a passive-solar design, utilising high thermal mass materials, wood will not be of value to you. In such circumstances, it would be better to use earth-bricks to construct your walls. Wood-framed walls are, however, the most acceptable type of wall from the viewpoint of health, provided they have pervious linings and insulation.

ENGINEERED TIMBER BEAMS

Many of the large supporting beams used in house construction are chosen because they have only a small number of knots — but this is usually a good indication that the timber was extracted from an old-growth forest. Timber-engineered beams avoid the necessity of using old-growth timber. They are produced by assembling a number of smaller timber sections into composite beams that achieve the same result. There is one drawback to using such beams: they rely upon steel components, which have the potential to alter the electroclimate of a building for the worse. The timber veneer laminated beam is usually manufactured from layers of plantation pine veneer, using patented joining technology. Although the glues are formaldehyde-based, tests indicate extremely low levels of outgassing of this chemical, which is a Group 2A carcinogen.

PLYWOOD

An assembly of glued layers of wood veneer, plywood is principally used for interior and exterior wall panelling, door sheeting and formwork to retain concrete when it is poured. One of the major sources of plywood for veneer is the rainforests of Indonesia. Try to ensure that your plywood is made from plantation timber only.

There are many categories of plywood manufactured: structural, marine, exterior, interior, overlaid formwork and laminated veneer lumber (LVL). It ranges in thickness from 3 centimetres (⅛ inch) to 4.5 centimetres (1¾ inch). It is bonded with either phenol-formaldehyde, melamine urea formaldehyde or urea formaldehyde resin, in each case less than 8 per cent of

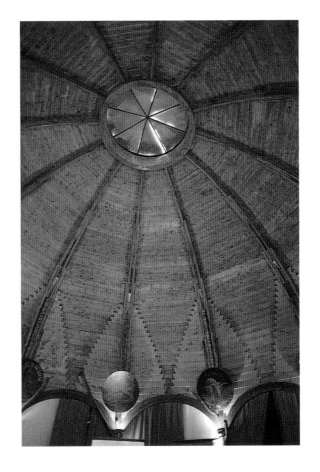

This earth-sheltered environment studies centre in Hungary shows a magnificent use of wood (Architect: I. Makovez; Photograph: D. Pearson)

the total mass of the plywood. During manufacture, the resin used to bond the veneer is cured and becomes inert. The emissions of chemicals from plywood products are well below the level recommended by the World Health Organisation. However, workers using plywood are exposed to pine dust which may cause allergic dermatitis and asthma. Inhalation of pine dust over a long period can increase the risk of nasal and paranasal sinus cancers. Wear a mask and wear protective clothing when working with plywood.

Plywood may be a reasonable solution when you have a large area to cover, but remember that it lacks permeability and is not an optimum 'breathing' material. If you feel the need to confirm the manufacturer's claims as to the levels of formaldehyde in the plywood, it is possible to purchase a sampling pump with tubes (see Resources List) to do your own independent test. Alternatively, you could take readings several months after the completion of another project where the same type of plywood has been used. The ideal reading is 0.01 parts per million (ppm), and no higher than 0.05 ppm (Plywood Association of Australia 1984).

HARDBOARD

Hardboard is made from wood fibres which have been rebonded under heat and pressure. It is usually paint-coated on all surfaces. The paint used is a pigmented primer, usually containing less than 1 per cent titanium dioxide. There is a further 4 per cent maximum of paraffin wax and the major proportion consists of wood fibre (CSR Ltd 1993). In Australasia,

Table 9.3: Plasterboard ancillary products containing synthetic chemicals

PRODUCT	USE	SYNTHETIC CHEMICALS	NATURAL PRODUCTS
Plasterboard (gypsum plaster core and paper liner)	Interior walls and ceilings		Gypsum, liner paper, starch, paper pulp
Fire-resistant plasterboard	Fire-resistant linings	Fibreglass filaments	Natural gypsum, vermiculite, clay, starch
Finish coat	Top coating or finishing plasterboard joints	PVA adhesive	Calcium carbonate, talc, mica, clay
Vinyl-lined plasterboard	Interior ceilings	PVC laminate, PVA adhesive	Natural gypsum, starch, paper pulp
Water-resistant plasterboard	Interior water-resistant walls and ceilings	Paraffin wax	Natural gypsum, starch, paper pulp
Reinforced plasterboard	Interior water-resistant walls and ceilings	Paraffin wax and fibreglass filaments	Natural gypsum, starch, paper pulp
Waterproofing compound	Waterproofing plasterboard	Synthetic rubber	Bitumen emulsion, water
Moisture and fire-resistant plasterboard	Water-resistant lining board to fire-resistant systems	Fibreglass filaments	Natural gypsum, vermiculite, clay, starch and paraffin wax
Priming and sealing coat to plasterboard	On aerated concrete blocks and panels prior to adhesive and plasterboard	PVA adhesive	Cellulose, water
Adhesive	Fixing plasterboard to metal and timber studs	Acrylic copolymer emulsion, PVA emulsion, plasticiser, preservative, anti-foam	Water, pigment
Adhesive alternative	Fixing plasterboard to metal and timber studs	PVA resin, toluene	Calcium carbonate, water, clay
Jointing top coat	Top coat to joints in plasterboard	PVA adhesive	Calcium carbonate, water, talc, mica, clay
Hardwall plaster	Trowel-on smooth finish to walls	Cellulose ether, calcium sulphate hemihydrate (calcined calcium sulphate dihydrate or gypsum)	Calcium carbonate, keratin retarder, hydrated lime
Cornice cement	Adhesive to fix cornice to plasterboard	PV alcohol	Calcined gypsum, calcium carbonate, mica
Base coat	Bedding coat for flush-jointing plasterboard	PV alcohol	Calcined gypsum, calcium carbonate, mica, talc
Join finish plaster	Finish top coat to cornice cement	PVA adhesive (clay can be omitted and starch added)	Calcium carbonate, water, (bentonite used for a white result) talc, mica, clay (perlite sometimes added)
Interior wall plaster	Finishing plaster coat to masonry wall	Cellulose ether, detergent	Calcined gypsum, calcium carbonate hydrated lime, clay, talc, perlite, keratin
Interior texture compound	For coating plasterboard, brick and concrete		Calcium carbonate, talc, mica, starch, cellulose
Adhesive	For fixing plasterboard and cornices to masonry	PV alcohol	Calcined gypsum, hydrated lime (calcium oxide)
Patching compound	Patching for holes in masonry, wood, plaster, plasterboard, fibre cement	PV alcohol	Calcined gypsum, hydrated lime (calcium oxide)
Plaster	Wall plastering, stopping, casting and spraying	PV alcohol	Calcined gypsum, gypsum, keratin retarder
Reinforced plasterboard	Rigid plasterboard for wider batten spacing	Silicone continuous filament glass fibres	Gypsum starch
Accelerator	To accelerate setting of plaster and as a stabiliser		Gypsum starch, calcined gypsum
Additive	To waterproof plasterboard in manufacture	Paraffin wax, potassium hydroxide (styrene maleic hydroxide can also be added with petroleum resin)	Water

the wood fibre usually comes from mixed Eucalyptus species. Hardboard is available as plain or rusticated weatherboards and planks. Some hardboard contains a polyvinylchloride spline in the back.

Workers using hardboard and all other timber-based boards may increase their risk of sinus cancers if they fail to follow the manufacturers' safety instructions. There are certain general precautions which should always be taken when using these types of boards: wear long sleeved shirts, long trousers and socks to avoid contact with sawdust; work in a well-ventilated space; vacuum your work area frequently; and wear a mask to avoid inhaling sawdust.

Essentially, hardboard is a reasonably permeable material and has a place in the healthy, naturally breathing house. Try to obtain it without the pigmented primer finish so you can apply a diffusive finish yourself.

PLASTERBOARD

Biological building materials such as plasterboard are very acceptable for use in the healthy building, providing that any accompanying products that contain chemicals are checked for their level of outgassing. It is composed of a gypsum plaster core, encased in a paper lining. It is manufactured by grinding gypsum and heating it to a very high temperature so that calcium sulphate hemihydrate is formed. As the gypsum reforms after heating, crystals interlock, increase in strength, and bind with the paper. In most circumstances it is free of radioactive emissions, but radiation can occur if the gypsum has been manufactured with calcium sulphate dehydrate produced from a byproduct of nuclear power generation. Hence in Europe, the United States, the United Kingdom and perhaps parts of Asia, it would be wise to test the product with a geiger counter before installation. We tested natural gypsum and found that it was not radioactive. However, plasterboard made with talc or mica was shown to emit $radon_{222}$ and gamma radiation 10 per cent above background levels.

There are a range of ancillary plasterboard products, some of which are free of synthetic chemicals and have very little, if any, glass filament. Consequently, they have a low level of ionised radiation, making them ideal for use in the healthy building. It is recommended that you use alternative, non-chemical means of fixing and finishing plasterboard. Provided pervious coatings are used, a plasterboard wall will breathe satisfactorily.

MOULDED-GLASS, REINFORCED-CEMENT BOARD

Moulded-glass, reinforced-cement panels are mainly used for wall cladding. They comprise Portland cement (up to 60 per cent), silica (up to 30 per cent) and glass filaments (up to 10 per cent) (James Hardie & Co Pty Ltd 1994a). If an excessive amount of dust is created by workers using these boards, eye irritation can result, and if the dust is inhaled, it can lead to upper respiratory tract irritation. The glass filaments can also cause skin irritation. From the point of view of the occupant though, the presence of these materials is benign and its level of permeability is acceptable, providing pervious finishes are applied.

FIBRE CEMENT BOARD

Fibre cement building boards are used as external and internal cladding as well as for roofing and flooring. (Fibre cement is also used for irrigation, storm water and sewage pipes, electrical conduits and various types of columns.) It comprises calcium silicate (hydrate), silica and cellulose, the proportions depending on the intended use of the material. These boards are basically benign in their impact on human health and are relatively permeable. They provide a reasonable material for the healthy building, providing pervious surface finishes are used. (James Hardie and Co Pty Ltd 1994b)

JOINERY

Cupboards

If you have the misfortune of suffering from allergic reactions to chemical emissions, building boards containing formaldehyde will be unsuitable for use in constructing cupboards. We do not recommend the use of pressed particle boards and medium-density and high-density fibreboards. Their outgassing can only be controlled by sealing with paint, varnish or other decorative finishes which do not breathe adequately. The glues used in cupboard construction can also create outgassing problems. Of all the synthetic glues, polyvinylacetate (PVA), water soluble glue is the least offensive. There are several PVA wood glues that are claimed to be non-toxic after the initial outgassing occurs prior to setting. These glues are only water resistant and cannot be exposed continuously to water. Cross-linked PVA emulsions, in the form of hot-melt glues, are completely unacceptable as they outgas formaldehyde at 0.1 parts per million.

Rather than choosing modern techniques, it is preferable to follow the old-fashioned methods of timber cupboard construction, developed before the invention of synthetic glues.

Some people are allergic not only to the chemicals used in building boards, but also to the resins and oils in natural timber. In this case, cupboards can be designed to utilise stainless steel, fibre-cement sheets, brickwork and polished granite. Depending on the cost of local stone, it is also an option to create open shelving using thin stone slabs in the walls. Glass shelving could replace timber, but its entropy debt is high. (A material with a high entropic debt is manufactured by a process that requires an excessive amount of energy and results in considerable waste heat being released into the Earth's atmosphere.)

The ideal type of cupboard (or of any furniture) is the antique, as the chemicals have outgassed long ago and are now inert. Second hand cupboards are the best choice if you are willing to live with the old finish or to sand it back and reseal with a non-toxic finish — you will have to make sure that no lead-based paints were used on the furniture if this is your intention.

If you are going to construct your own cupboards from scratch, opt for properly jointed timber-framed cupboards and doors with, say, 9 millimetre (⅜ inch) thick infill panels. In the early days, cupboard doors often had glass infills. If the old panelled or pioneer-cottage style is unsuitable for your purposes, you could follow the construction methods prevalent in the immediate post-World War 2 period. This involved having reasonably rough, unjointed frames (often secured at the corners with strips of corrugated metal called wriggle nails) sheeted with hardboard. The edges were finished with a higher quality strip. If you consider that plywood is acceptable, you can use this method, substituting superior quality plywood for hardboard.

◎ Bench tops ◎

Marble and granite are suitable materials for bench tops, as when the slab is polished on top and sealed with a natural seal on the underside, exposure to radiation from the mineral content of the stone is minimised. If we were to choose the most allergy-free bench top, it would be stainless steel (as would the cupboards), provided all protective sealants were completely removed from the stainless steel before delivery. For the Gaian, the principal issues in this case are that stainless steel has a very high entropic debt and that because of its high conductivity it has the potential to distort the natural electric field, sustaining its own electrostatic field. Its appearance is also very sterile. From the *feng shui* point of view, the use of so much metal in the kitchen is unacceptable because the Fire element (the cooking process) threatens the Metal element (the large number of metal appliances found in the kitchen).

◎ Doors and windows ◎

The best doors and windows for a Gaian healthy house can be found at second-hand yards or demolition sites. All timbers need to be checked to make sure they have not been subjected to chemical treatment in order to give them an aged appearance. If you decide to use second-hand materials, ensure that they are on site before the wall framing or bricklaying commences. Choose doors with no movement in the joints and with reasonably preserved surfaces. Scratch the paint and rub the undercoat with a lead test stick, which is a short, cigarette shaped paper implement saturated with a yellow chemical that turns pink in the presence of lead. If the test indicates the presence of lead be sure you are happy with the surface finish, because when you strip back such a door or window you risk disturbing the harmful lead-based coatings.

Opposite page, top: Earth-built Anthroposophical school at Jarna, Sweden (Architects: Prisma Architects; Photograph: D. Pearson)

Opposite page, bottom: Permaculture Institute of Europe, Steyerberg, Germany (Architect: Prof. D. Kennedy; Photograph: D. Kennedy)

Below: Low toxicity family room, Mill Valley, California USA. Gypsum board with natural paint and all natural timbers and finishes (Architect: C. Venolia)

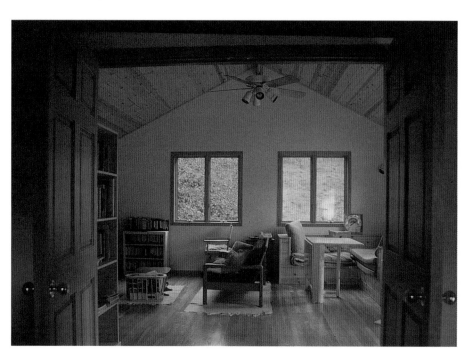

NEW DOORS AND WINDOWS

With new doors the simplest hollow-core construction can be undertaken using a similar method to that described earlier for cupboard doors. If you are not using second-hand windows choose a window type that will maximise ventilation. The old-fashioned double sash window, which consists of two vertically sliding sashes (a sash is a frame containing a pane of glass), is not a good choice as it requires too much detailed construction if the old counterweight system is used, or results in a high entropic debt if spring-balance hardware is used. Further, double sash windows only achieve 50 per cent of free opening for ventilation.

When sashes are vertically hinged (like French doors), they are called casement sashes. If casement sashes are designed to open outwards, they present no waterproofing problems, but if such sashes are unintentionally left open and unsecured, the glass could be broken in the wind. Outward-opening sashes also obstruct access if space outside is limited, and they are difficult to screen against insects.

For maximum energy conservation and ventilation use friction-type casement stays that hold the sash open and allow it to be turned inside for cleaning.

Flyscreens for outward-opening windows must be mounted inside the house, so to gain access to the window the whole screen must be hinged, which may interfere with the curtains and internal spaces.

In regard to inward-opening casement windows, it is very difficult to make wind and watertight the gap between the bottom of the sashes and the top of the sill. We do not recommend the installation of sliding doors and windows because they also provide only 50 per cent of the total area for ventilation. In addition they involve mechanisms and materials of high entropic debt.

A major source of heat leakage is the window. A bare, traditional window is a 'black hole' that creates almost perfect conditions for heat transfer. Insulating windows with double glazing or using window shutters at night, during heat waves and cold spells prevents the building from gaining or losing heat at inappropriate times. Curtains with thermal linings can help, but remember that they create dust and outgassing problems. Probably the best system for privacy and sun control is a double glazed window system containing movable metal sun-control louvres within the glazing cavity. These give totally dustproof and flexible privacy and sunlight control.

Glazing

ULTRAVIOLET RADIATION

Except for glass that has been especially manufactured to allow ultraviolet light to penetrate, all glazing excludes most ultraviolet radiation. Countries that experience long, cold winters need ultraviolet radiation to enter the interiors of their homes. Low iron-content glass is 90 per cent transparent to ultraviolet radiation, but it is very expensive. Professor L. Schneider, the head of the Baubiologie™ Institute in Germany, recommends that quartz glass be used in countries where days are short, particularly for windows in sanatoriums. In countries with plentiful sunshine, ultraviolet radiation should be minimised inside the home because of the risk of skin cancer, so normal glass is best.

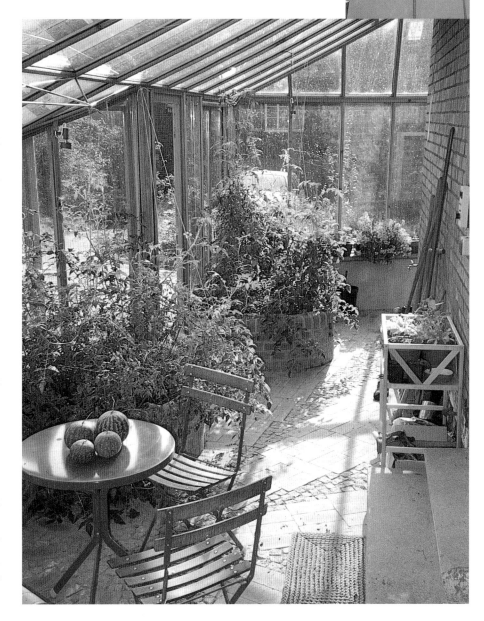

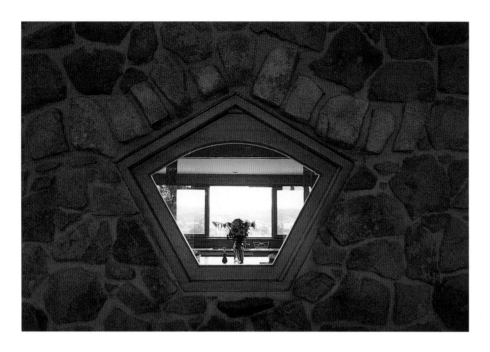

The pentagonal shape of this window reflects the plan shape of the whole house, Armidale, NSW, Aust. (Architect: M. Baxter; Photograph: M. Baxter)

Physical safety should be a prime consideration when choosing glass. Children aged up to 4 years old have the highest number of injuries involving glass — 71 per cent of these injuries occur in the living or sleeping area of the house (Ozanne-Smith 1993). Choose your glazing with the thickness and strength of the glass in mind. It is preferable to use toughened or laminated glass for low windows and door panels, especially near stairs and landings. Special care should be taken with glazing from floor level up to 1 metre (3 feet 3 inches) high. One solution is to install an intermediate rail at around 1 metre (3 feet 3 inches) from the floor, with safety glass below and ordinary glass above.

METALWORK, HEATING AND PLUMBING

The key to making decisions about all conductive materials normally used in the building process is to be aware of what happens when they interfere with natural electrical and magnetic fields. The Earth's electrostatic field is normally positive, directed from the positively charged ionosphere, towards the negatively charged Earth. Steel-framed houses and those with metal roofs disrupt the flow of cosmic radiation entering the house, usually resulting in a neutral electrostatic field. When plastics are added to the interior, the field becomes measurably negative, and a negative electrostatic field can create and exacerbate fatigue, irritability and apathy.

When geomagnetic anomalies or geo-pathogenic zones are bridged by structural concrete containing steel reinforcement, the adverse health effects will be carried throughout the building, as long as there is steel in contact with steel. The metal in reinforced concrete, steel frames and metal plumbing functions as a conductor of microwave, television and radio frequencies. The metal randomly distributes these frequencies over the whole area in which such systems and elements are used. Similarly, electrical wiring carrying alternating current can create unhealthy ELF fields throughout the building.

The situation is best avoided by dispensing with reinforced concrete. Fibreglass and ceramic reinforcement are suitable, but are expensive compared to steel. The use of glass-reinforced plastic rods, as an alternative to steel reinforcement, is being researched by the Institute of Polymer Technology and Materials Engineering in the United Kingdom. In New Zealand, a product is being developed that utilises a material stronger than steel, produced by pulling a continuous filament of special glass through a polyester resin bath and then through a heated die. The material is highly resistant to corrosion from salts, acids and alkalis over a wide temperature range. It is ideal for prestressing in concrete and, in the future, may provide an alternative to steel reinforcing. Biocement, a combination of crushed limestone aggregate, sand and cement, is being developed by the scientist Doctor Palm. In Japan, glass/polypropylene reinforcement is being developed and in Australia, short fibreglass filaments are already being used in certain types of reinforced concrete.

As these projects are all in developmental stages, or are very expensive, steel remains the most common reinforcement for structural concrete. Reinforced concrete is best considered as a 'trade-off' material, its practical value (its high thermal mass) being offset by the electroclimate problems it can create. If you cannot avoid using reinforced concrete, metal frames or metal plumbing, they should be discontinuous and earthed using a copper rod permanently connected to the conductor, and taken down to relatively constant soil-moisture conditions. In both clay and free-draining soils, the optimum depth is around 1.2 metres (4½ feet), but in free-draining soils, the hole for the conductor should be widened and filled with dry clay and charcoal which expands and binds with the surrounding soil when watered.

METAL PIPE LAYOUT

The distortion of pulsed electromagnetic fields can be avoided by laying the plumbing pipelines around the outside of a building, with short pipelines leading off the main pipeline into the building. Alternatively, the main pipeline can lead to a point in the building roughly equidistant from all the taps and other fittings; short pipelines can then run to each fitting from that central point.

Keeping pipes well outside the building not only seems likely to avoid electromagnetic field distortion but also makes maintenance access easier. All metal piping should be kept away from the electrical wiring and earthed, as for steel reinforcement. The GMF interference caused by metal reinforcement and plumbing cannot be completely corrected by mechanical means. Only total avoidance of such systems can eradicate the potential health problems.

STEEL-FRAME BUILDINGS

The problems associated with reinforced concrete are even greater for structural steel framing. Your sleeping quarters should be located away from any steel, including metal door and window frames. The medical scientist Doctor von Pohl (1978) is very critical of steel girders and steel frames in homes, and reinforced concrete-frame buildings in general. He associates this building type with nervous restlessness, headaches, uneasy sleep, sleepwalking and lack of sleep.

STEEL HEATING SYSTEMS

Heating units and steam or hot water reticulation units made of steel are to be avoided as they create problems with the indoor electroclimate of a house. Should you decide on an electric hot water storage unit, it is important to locate it no closer than 15 metres (49 feet) from a bed, lounge room or any other room where you stay for long periods. Solar collectors on the roof should be given the same buffer space.

In Europe, masonry or clay ovens are often used for both cooking and heating. They do not create problems for the indoor electroclimate so their installation could be considered in a healthy house. In general, radiant heating devices are preferable as convective heating of air creates electrostatic charges.

GALVANISED IRON AND COPPER PIPES

The installation of hot and cold water reticulation systems present the serious Gaian home owner with some difficult issues to resolve. Apart from stainless steel, which is very expensive, there are no materials for carrying water that are not inherently problematic for the healthy building. When copper tubes and galvanised iron pipes are used for water reticulation in conjunction with brass fittings, a moderate degree of electrolysis occurs due to differences between the metals. This may occur when a galvanised pipe is used at a brass T-fitting and copper tubing is connected to the same fitting. The result of the electrolytic process is that oxides of copper and zinc enter the water, and hence the bodies of the people who use the water.

One solution to this problem is to avoid zinc and copper altogether, the other is to install a filter system. Such a system should not concentrate only on purifying the drinking water, as the skin is the largest organ of the human body and can assimilate metals in the shower or bath. A very large filter system is necessary to treat all the water used in the house. It should also filter out chlorine. Rainwater collected in tanks is not a viable solution, as tanks are usually made from galvanised iron, causing the same metallic pollution problem. Concrete tanks should also be avoided, as the extent of radon emissions from concrete aggregates has not been investigated properly.

A European clay oven (Architect: D. Kennedy; Photograph: D. Kennedy)

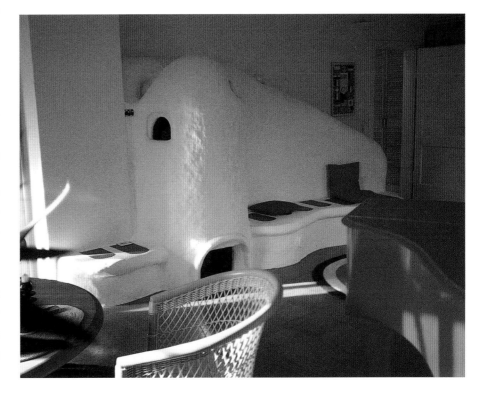

PLASTIC TUBING

In terms of plastic tubing for water supplies, PVC is the most widely used, even though it is made from 'vinylchloride monomer which is highly toxic and a known carcinogen' (Kabos 1986). Over time, plastic water pipes also release pseudo-oestrogens into the water. Pseudo-oestrogens have been implicated in decreasing sperm counts and increasing feminisation of male animals (including humans) throughout the world.

Polypropylene piping is probably the best of the plastic tubings in terms of quality and cleanliness. Polybutylene piping is also a reasonable compromise material.

SOLAR DOMESTIC HOT WATER

Solar hot water systems can deliver water at temperatures of up to 50 degrees Celsius (122 degrees Fahrenheit). When installed as part of an independent power system, solar heating can be coupled with a wet-back fuel stove (one which has a built-in water heating unit) as well as primary heating sources like gas. Low temperature solar collectors are the type most commonly installed. They use the infrared radiation of the sun to provide hot water for washing and bathing.

Solar hot water systems can either be connected to the mains pressure or create their own head of pressure from an elevated storage tank. Their black, heat-absorbing surfaces are in constant contact with the water being heated. Solar radiation passes through transparent covering sheets and is absorbed by the black plate. The infrared radiation from the heated plate cannot reradiate through the transparent cover to the outside air. Hence the temperature of the plate rises and the heat is absorbed by the circulating fluid. The back of the plate is insulated to prevent loss of heat. The collector should face north (in the southern hemisphere) or south (in the northern hemisphere).

In a closed solar collector system, the fluid flows in tubes or ducts that are securely fixed to the heating surface. The bottom of the hot water tank must be above the collector, as it operates on the principle that water rises when heated, just as air does. The warmer water rises, while the relatively cooler water at the bottom of the tank flows down to the collector for reheating. The fluid 'thermosiphons' around the system without having to be pumped. In countries with cold winters, the system may have to contain antifreeze or be drained each night. This system is usually used to supply domestic hot water to a conventional hot water cylinder.

To avoid locating the water tank above the collector, and hence sometimes intruding above the roof line, a pump can be located in the circuit allowing the tank and collector to be located independently of each other.

FLOOR COVERINGS

A floor surface should be durable, neutral in odour, an efficient thermal insulator, skid-proof when wet, of low conductivity and unable to carry an electrostatic charge. Very few floor finishes fulfil these criteria and can be considered completely benign to human health.

CARPET

All synthetic and blended synthetic/wool carpets are unsuitable for a healthy home, as they create and hold electrostatic fields, and outgas chemicals. If woollen carpets were pure, they would be acceptable, but they are treated to repel insects and to make it easy for stains to be removed. The chemicals used in these treatments outgas into the air. Underlay, whether synthetic or latex, and the joining strips and glues, also outgas. Rubber is the most acceptable underlay, though it does contain chlorine. We know of a family who had pure wool carpet installed on rubber underlay, believing that their decision would be reasonably safe. However, they were not informed that the synthetic glue used to bond the carpet to the backing material was toxic and had an objectionable odour. The smell was so intense that the newly carpeted rooms could not be used as bedrooms for 12 months because outgassing caused asthma in several family members.

Carpet becomes a major breeding ground for the house dust mite unless treated with a chemical compound, which outgasses. If you are living in rented premises and are unable to remove the carpet, you have to make a decision about whether to live with the dust mite or endure the outgassing of chemicals from the expensive, three-monthly treatment to kill the pest.

Even though flock, jute and jute/hair underfelt is available as a safe underlay, there is no carpet that can be considered 100 per cent safe.

SHEET AND TILE FLOOR COVERINGS

Of all the sheeting and tiles available, only linoleum is both composed of organic materials and easy to clean with plain soap and water. When common, highly contagious microbes were placed on samples of Marmoleum, a specific brand of linoleum, it was found to have an anti-microbial effect (Hartog and Pouw 1994).

NATURAL FINISH WOOD FLOORING

Wooden floors are preferable in a healthy house, so long as the wood has not been treated with toxic finishes. The most frequently used synthetic sealants outgas toxic chemicals and flake off. The only way to restore the surface to a safe and healthy state is to sand back to raw wood and begin again with a suitable non-toxic finish. Remember that 'low allergy' does not mean 'allergy free' and some sensitive people may react to the oils and resins in such products, even though they are natural. Discuss this issue with the supplier prior to purchase — highly sensitive individuals may be able to test the product simply by sniffing and waiting to see if there is a reaction.

CERAMIC AND STONE TILES

Kiln-baked ceramic tiles provide an ideal healthy house floor surface provided only natural sealants are applied to them. The best base for such a floor is concrete, provided that you have avoided the use of steel reinforcement, as discussed earlier in this chapter. If you have a wooden sub-floor, the major problem posed by a ceramic tile floor is the difference in expansion and contraction between the ceramic tiles' cement mortar bed and the wooden floor structure supporting it. This differential movement is solved by ensuring that the materials are not in direct contact, for instance by having a layer of bituminous building paper between them.

A poorly constructed wooden floor system may not be able to bear the weight of a ceramic tile covering. On the ground floor, the floor joists need to be checked to ensure that they are resting properly on bearers or wall plates; timber wedges may need to be driven under any components that are not firmly supported. In suspended floors, you must check that the deeper floor joists are not springy. If they are, they will need reinforcing to take the extra load from the new materials.

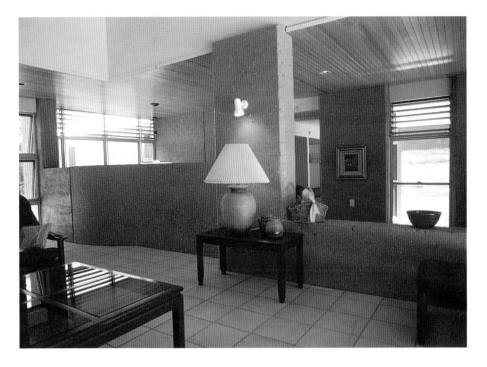

Tiled floor in rammed-earth residence in northern NSW, Aust. (Architect: D. Oliver, Greenway Architects; Photograph: D. Oliver)

Breakages occur frequently on ceramic tile floors, but the danger can be minimised by using washable cotton throw-rugs in the areas where breakages are most likely. Backing products are available to stop mats slipping, but unfortunately they all outgas.

PAINTING

The solvents and chemicals outgassed by paint finishes create air pollution problems. The most common house paints are either water-based, or have mineral turps as their base. Sensitive people can easily react to the fumes from either of these types of paint. Internationally, there has been a call to develop standards for testing emissions and to set maximum limits. In Europe, manufacturers of coatings have to 'decrease volatile organic compound (VOC) emissions by 70 per cent during manufacture and use' (Brown 1994). This may mean that paints must be reformulated, or produced with new polymers or new production systems.

Some water-based latex paints contain mercury-based chemicals which inhibit mould and mildew formation. Over a long period, exposure to mercury causes a cumulative effect in brain and other tissue. Symptoms include gingivitis and neurological disturbances such as tremor and personality changes. For their members' protection, the Operative Painters and Decorators Union of Australia points out (in the

Painters Hazard Handbook, by Noni Holmes) that the following types of cancer are linked to painting and decorating: lung, bladder, oesophagus, stomach, leukaemia, lymphatic system, mouth, larynx, skin, prostate, mesothelia, gall bladder, bile duct, pancreas and testes. An American study in 1988 concluded that: 'studies based on painters consistently demonstrated a significant increase of risk of cancer of all sites combined'. The World Health Organisation also conducted studies on the carcinogenic effects of occupational exposure to paint products. Both studies failed to identify the specific substances in paint that cause health problems — as paints and coatings are cocktails of chemicals, there are many potential causal agents.

Table 9.4: Known carcinogens and their likely sources*

KNOWN CARCINOGENS	LIKELY SOURCES	POTENTIAL HAZARD
Antimony oxide	Some pigments, fire-protection coatings	Possible cancer
Asbestos	Surface preparation, formerly used in texture finishes	Lung cancer
Benzene	Contaminant in some thinners and organic solvents, formerly used as thinner and organic solvent	Cancer of reproductive system; 'painters' syndrome'
Benzidine-based dyes	Art dyes	Probable cancer
Cadmium	Pigments	Possible cancer; kidney damage
Carbon tetrachloride	Contaminant in some chlorinated rubber coatings	Possible cancer; liver and kidney damage
Chromates	Primers, pigments	Cancer; allergic-contact dermatitis
Coal-tar pitch	Coal-tar epoxies	Cancer; occupational skin disease
3,3,-Dichlorobenzidine	Pigments	Possible cancer; allergic contact dermatitis
Epichlorohydrin	Contaminant in some epoxy resins	Probable cancer
Formaldehyde	Phenol-formaldehyde resins, urea-formaldehyde resins	Cancer; allergic-contact dermatitis; occupational asthma
Lead	Primers, driers and some pigments	Hazardous to reproduction; peripheral nerve damage; possible cancer; lead poisoning; mental retardation in infants
Methylene chloride	Paint strippers	Occupational cancer; 'painters' syndrome; kidney and liver damage
Nickel compounds	Pigments	Cancer; allergic-contact dermatitis
2-Nitropropane	Used as organic solvent until 1981	Possible cancer; 'painters' syndrome'
Silica (crystalline)	Sandblasting dust, some pigment	Probable cancer; occupational lung disease
Styrene oxide	Breakdown product of styrene	Probable cancer; 'painters' syndrome'; liver and kidney damage
Tetrachloroethylene	Organic solvent, for degreasing	Possible cancer; 'painters' syndrome'
Toluene Diisocyanate	Some polyurethanes	Possible cancer; asthma; hazardous to reproduction

* after Holmes (1990)

◉ Painters' syndrome ◉

Most painters are familiar with the short-term effects of exposure to organic solvents: dizziness, headache, nausea, tiredness, or a feeling of being 'wired' or 'high'. These effects usually disappear when exposure stops. Long-term exposure, however, can result in permanent damage. The organic solvents in paint enter the body as vapours, some being absorbed through the skin, others being breathed in through the lungs.

Studies conducted in Sweden and Denmark have shown that long-term exposure to paint products results in symptoms such as memory difficulties, reduction in intellectual capacity, tiredness and changes in personality. In Holland, studies found that construction workers were more likely to be on a psychiatric pension if painting had been part of their work. In England, the results of painters in mental ability tests were worse than for any other type of worker tested. In studies carried out in the United States, painters have reported increased forgetfulness, feelings of weakness, increased mood swings, depression and confusion. All these symptoms comprise what is termed 'painters' syndrome'.

If you must use a synthetic chemical product, make sure you know as much as possible about the product. In Australia, you can write to the manufacturer and ask for a Material Safety Data Sheet (MSDS). Similar publications may be available in other countries. The MSDS will tell you what chemicals are contained in a product. You can then check the effects of those chemicals and decide whether you think it is safe to use the product.

Bear in mind that the outgassing periods of paint chemicals have not yet been fully researched. Remember also that the generic name of a product should not be confused with the chemical name. For example, some paints are said to contain 'glycol ether', yet there are several different types of glycol ether which all have different effects on human health. Ethylene glycol, for instance, may cause 'painters' syndrome' while 2-ethoxyethanol (another glycol ether) may cause the testicles to atrophy. Give each product careful consideration as the descriptions of chemical ingredients in the products may be deliberately unclear and may avoid using the correct chemical names.

Solvent-based versus water-based paint

Despite the fact that compared to solvent-based paints, the rate of VOC emission from water-based paint is low, adverse reactions have been recorded in relation to water-based paint. A Swedish study of 239 occupants of dwellings freshly painted with water-based paint recorded a significantly high number of complaints of airway irritation, eye irritation, breathlessness during rest, and of waking up during the night due to tightness in the chest (Wieslander, et al 1993). Earlier studies by the same group of scientists showed that the biocides found in water-based paints resulted in skin sensitisation.

Healthy surface treatment of wood

The simplest, and usually the best, approach to wood is to leave it untreated. Materials should be allowed to express their own characters. There are circumstances, though, where it is necessary to treat wooden surfaces. Certain rooms may look monotonous without accents of colour. You may need to minimise the amount of dust that collects on a rough or porous wood surface, or you may need to seal a wood floor from dirt or moisture. Natural wax finishes on wood can also help eliminate electrostatic charges.

If you are going to treat your wood, use natural paints made from plant and earth derivatives. Any paint, varnish, lacquer, stain or wax should smell pleasant or neutral. It should be permeable, allowing the wood to breathe and dry out, equalising the interior air humidity. A floor finish should not encourage electrostatic charges to build up, as may happen during dry weather when people walk over a wood floor coated with a hard plastic-based finish containing epoxy resins or polyurethane. Paints, binding agents and solvents should not emit hazardous or obnoxious smelling fumes. Non-gloss surface finishes are preferable, as they maximise noise absorption and keep reflection and glare to a minimum. Floors should only be treated with non-slip finishes. You should take care that the materials you choose do not pollute either the person applying them, those who will live in their atmosphere, or the water and air of the outdoor environment when brushes and rollers are washed. Shellac, for instance, can be quite harmful in terms of the solvents it contains and the chemicals it outgasses, even though it is a natural product derived from a resin secreted by insects.

CHEMICAL FAMILY	CHEMICAL NAME	POTENTIAL HAZARD
Alcohols	Amyl alcohol, ethanol, benzyl alcohol, methylated spirits	'Painters' syndrome'
Aliphatic hydrocarbons	Kerosene, n-heptane	'Painters' syndrome'
Aromatic hydrocarbons	Styrene, xylene (or xylol), trimethyl benzene (also known as mesitylene or 1,3,5-Trimethylbenzene)	Cancer; 'painters' syndrome'; liver and kidney damage
Chlorinated solvents	1,1,-trichloroethane (methyl chloroform, methyl trichloromethane), methylene chloride (also known as dichloromethan, methane dichloride or methylene bichloride)	Cancer; 'painters' syndrome'; liver and kidney damage
Esters	Amyl acetate, iso-butyl isobutyrate, benzyl acetate, iso-propyl acetate, 2-methoxy-1-propyl acetate	'Painters' syndrome'
Glycols	Ethylene glycol, propylene glycol	'Painters' syndrome'
Glycol ethers	2-ethoxyethanol, 2-butoxyethanol, propylene glycol, monoethyl ether, diethylene glycol	'Painters' syndrome'; hazardous to reproduction
Ketones and aldehydes	Acetone, methyl iso-butyl ketone, cyclohexanone	'Painters' syndrome'; peripheral nerve damage
	Methyl methacrylate (monomer)	Asthma; dermatitis; peripheral nerve damage; hazardous to reproduction
	Diethylene triamine	Asthma; dermatitis
	Triethylene tetramine	Asthma; dermatitis

* after Holmes (1990)

Table 9.5: Organic solvents in paints and coatings*

Sodium carbonate solution has been used on Alpine log houses for centuries. A 3 per cent carbonate solution is washed or scrubbed onto the wood every 2 or 3 years. This prevents the wood from greying with age and protects it from fungal and insect infestation. A similar strength solution made from wood ash is even more effective. Ash is placed in a cloth bag, boiled in water for 30–60 minutes, allowed to cool, recooked and allowed to ferment. This produces a weather-resistant finish, the colour of which is dependent upon the type of bark added during the boiling process.

Treatment of brick and plaster

Whitewash is a safe surface treatment for plaster, and it also kills bacteria. You can make your own whitewash at home for use on plaster walls and ceilings by adding water gradually to quick lime. The solution will begin to boil; add water until the boiling stops. Allow the solution to reduce to a 'sludge' with a creamy consistency. Store this sludge, just covered with water, in a plastic-lined container for at least a year before use. Earth or plant colours can be added for pigment (maximum 10 per cent by volume) and linseed oil (raw or boiled) can be added as a binder. Alternatively skim milk can be added as a binder to the slaked lime. Casein powder (or white cheese) as well as natural glues can also be added. By adding a binder of a mixture of beef fat, waxes and resins to the whitewash the durability is even further improved although diffusibility decreases. Such a mix is suitable for exterior walls.

If you do not wish to whitewash your exterior walls, potash waterglass (a mixture of sodium or potassium silicate and water) and silicate paints in general are weather resistant while still being relatively permeable. When such paints are used on wood, they function as a fire-protection measure as well as making it fungus and insect resistant. The mix for potash paint is one part potash water and one part borax applied in a 10 per cent solution (diluted with water). A weather-proof outer skin can be achieved on plaster or brick by using white cement (the type used as grouting between tiles) to which an equal amount of calcium hydroxide has been added. This gives a reasonably diffuse finish that breathes well.

On interior plaster or brick walls, water-saturated chalk with added glue and colour pigments can be used. The glues should not contain animal extracts, but plant derivatives instead. Cellulose glues are excellent because they do not support the growth of moulds, but as they remain water soluble they cannot come in contact with moisture.

Pigmented, elutriated clay (the result of washing the clay with water and retaining the larger particles) treated with fat or fish oil after drying has been used as a surface finish in Asia and Europe for thousands of years. The result is good in humid conditions for both interior and exterior surfaces.

Cellulose-based wallpapers can be useful for lime-plaster walls, provided they have been manu-factured in the same way as ordinary unbleached paper and do not contain sealers or chemical binders. They should be fixed with cellulose adhesives (do not use fungicides), and should not be sealed with varnishes or oil-based materials.

◉ Natural paints ◉

There can be no doubt that conventional synthetic paint creates problems. As one natural paint company's brochure says:

> the paint you've probably been using contains
> fungicides, pesticides, preservatives, foam-control
> agents, acrylic resins, isocyanides and formaldehyde
> which evaporate over time into the air you breathe
> every day and night. Water-based paints are nothing
> but chemicals dispersed in water. (Livos Australia)

Natural paints, on the other hand, are derived from plants and trees, and natural resins and waxes that are far less likely to cause allergies. In natural paints, herbal extracts perform the same function as the synthetic pesticides and herbicides found in conventional paints. Natural paints for both interior and exterior surfaces are based upon solvents which do not contain chemicals like benzene, toluene or xylene, and the colours are produced using natural pigments.

From a practical point of view, the main stumbling block to painting with natural products is that, unlike the use of conventional products, the process requires a little more understanding and input than simply stirring a paint pot and slapping a brush to the wall. If tradespeople are used for the application of natural products, prices tend to be slightly higher than standard, but this is not universal.

ELECTRICAL INSTALLATIONS

The configuration of the electrical system of your house is vital to your health, so it should be installed by a bio-electrician. An electrician with an understanding of the wider biological implications of electrical installation will be able to consult with you about the concepts and advice in this section so you can ensure that your building is free from rogue electromagnetic fields which may damage the occupants' health.

Hardly a building exists in which some rooms are not electrically contaminated, but whether you are building from scratch or renovating an existing house, there are steps you can take to minimise the build-up of electromagnetic fields inside your home. Most of these basic procedures can be applied equally to the 50 Hertz (240–250 volt) system used throughout much of the world and the 60 Hertz (110 volt) system used in North America.

In most conventionally wired homes, even when appliances plugged into the system are turned off such a strong pulsed field is produced that it is wise, when sleeping or relaxing, to be 2 metres (6½ feet) from any appliance and 3 metres (10 feet) from a television set. The intensity and spatial distribution of the field produced by an appliance is proportional to its amperage (current intensity) and depends on the type of wiring and appliance being used. Above all, avoid appliances with built-in transformers, such as clock-radios. You should only use battery-powered appliances in your bedroom; those with earthed metal casings are also acceptable.

Not only are microwave ovens an unacceptable means of preparing food, they also contribute to rogue electromagnetic fields. Cataracts, alterations in hormone levels and digestive problems are associated with their presence (Schneider 1988). In a typical kitchen, electromagnetic pollution is everywhere, particularly if induction hotplates are used with elements that emanate electromagnetic fields. These fields can be measured with a magnetometer. The ELF count on the magnetometer should not be more than 100 gamma (100 nanoTesla or 1 milliGauss) in the home environment.

Rooms containing clothes driers, washing machines, irons and sewing machines connected to multiple power outlets present a high degree of electromagnetic field contamination. In addition, the metallic surfaces of these appliances sustain an electrostatic charge in dry conditions. Bathrooms are sometimes over-equipped with power and light outlets. Living, dining, rumpus and work rooms are characteristically over-supplied with electrical outlets. The bedroom, where one third of life is spent, is very open to the potential damage of rogue electromagnetic fields. Electric radios, clocks, blankets and water beds containing transformers are unacceptable in the healthy bedroom. Offices, shops and work places create similar pathological electroclimates.

Exterior walls constructed of earth or other materials that have a high mineral and moisture content do not create many problems with electromagnetic fields because of their high electrical conductivity. Dry interior walls are another matter, as they create strong electrical fields whether the power is flowing through the electrical wiring or not.

◉ Problem wiring configurations ◉

Very high electromagnetic fields can be produced when a current-carrying wire has been located separately from its earth wire. When separated, the wires no longer cancel out each other's magnetic fields, and these become rogue electromagnetic fields. A current-carrying wire and its accompanying neutral wire must always remain together. It is generally only in older houses that the wires are separated; the change can usually be made at the switch box by an electrician. Where two-way switching has been employed, opposite wires run along different paths and electromagnetism builds up because the neutral wire does not follow the same path as the energised wire.

In Europe, electricity is grounded only at substations, which means that the current makes huge rings or loops through whole blocks of buildings, creating the potential for rogue magnetic fields to form. In the United States, there are multiple earthings all along the path of the current, resulting in several rings or loops which again create stray electromagnetic fields.

◉ The earthing system ◉

Metallic water pipes, or metal and steel in walls, floors and ceilings, cable television lines, coaxial cables and telephone lines create indirect induction rings or loops which conduct electromagnetism unless the earthing for each system has been carefully designed. In the past, metallic water pipes have commonly been used as an earthing device for a building's electricity supply, but this does not create a healthy electroclimate and should not be done.

A house's electrical system is grounded to earth by connecting the neutral wire (coming from the switchboard) to metallic objects and appliances such as stoves and hot water systems that are themselves electrically earthed to ground electrodes. When an appliance is used, it draws current, and unless the same amount of current is drawn off to balance it on another circuit in the building, the difference between the amount of power being used by one circuit compared to the other will cause a current to flow in the neutral wire.

If you are constructing a new house, and hence a new wiring layout, you should only earth the system to ground conductors, not to metal plumbing tubing. This will eliminate almost all ground currents. Existing electrical installations should be retrofitted so that they are grounded to earth conductors.

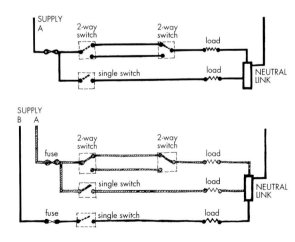

Figure 9.5: An extra load on two-way wiring can imbalance the system and raise ELF electromagnetism to an unsafe level at each two-way switch

The Electric Power Research Institute runs a major research facility at Lenox, Massachusetts at which a small residential neighbourhood has been modelled. It includes overhead power lines, distribution transformers, and basic houses with typical wiring and earthing arrangements. Research undertaken at the facility concluded that:

• Peaks in residential magnetic fields are caused by residual currents in the vertical wiring that leads from the electrical supply to the house's switchboard, and by currents in the earthing system within the ground.

• The use of power in one house tends to generate ground currents in adjoining houses.

• If the usual method of earthing to metallic water piping is avoided and earthing rods are used instead, ground currents are practically eliminated.

Wiring precautions

The biological impacts arising from exposure to the non-ionising radiation of rogue electromagnetic or stray electrostatic fields can be avoided if the following precautions are taken when the electrical service, fixtures and fittings are being installed:

• Avoid overuse of electrical appliances and resist the temptation to install excessive numbers of power and light outlets. One or two power outlets near doors is all that is needed. Do not use equipment with built-in transformers.

• Only use materials that create a benign electroclimate.

• The earth of your electrical installation should be as far as possible from the point where the house is connected to the power supply.

• The mains supply is best located underground and the meter box should be placed well away from bedrooms and work areas.

• Avoid all two-way, switched wiring rings or loops and minimise the number of power outlets in the house.

• Switches, power outlets and junction boxes should be made of metal and connected to a protective cover or sheathing on the wiring, or a metal conduit or wire mesh covering.

• The shielding or mesh on wiring should end inside the earthed metal meter box.

• Wiring should not be ringed or looped; radial layouts are preferable.

• Wiring should be well shielded by a wire-mesh covering or (where permissible by local authorities) galvanised metal tube. Both types of metal shielding have to be earthed with conductive wire. You can shield electrical fields by using aluminium foil around the wiring, and earthing the foil. The earthed aluminium foil can be attached inside the wall with glue but this may create a condensation problem. Only perforated metal foil should be used.

• Rogue electromagnetic fields can also be reduced by twisting the wires of the cable. In some countries cable can be purchased pre-twisted. If the wires are twisted at a complete 360 degree pitch, magnetic fields are reduced by 80 per cent. This reduces electromagnetic fields only if the junctions are made of metal, are connected to the protective conductor, and are themselves shielded with a metal tube or wire mesh. In Australia, however, domestic wiring is flat, thermoplastic sheathed (TPS). The mains should be located underground and the wiring should come up (through metal ducting) to the centre of the floor like a trunk branching off to each outlet.

• Install earth-leakage breakers and a safety switch as protection against electrocution.

• Use battery-operated equipment, for example, radios and clocks, especially in bedrooms. Eliminate circuitry as much as possible.

• Only use computer terminals that are shielded against electrostatic and electromagnetic fields.

• All appliances must be earthed.

• Poor insulation can cause fields strong enough to be felt as a tingle or slight shock, especially in metal lamps and ceiling pendants. Exposure to these fields results in itching, insomnia, nervousness, circulation disorders, heart problems, headaches, immune system breakdown, kidney disease and rheumatism. Television sets, stoves, radios and clocks with built-in transformers, as well as computers, can cause the same health problems if they are located close to people. All such equipment is much safer if the body is made of metal rather than plastic. The power supply cord needs to be encased in aluminium foil sheathing or metal pipe, both of which are grounded. The metal casing of equipment with two-wire cables may feature a small screw, usually on the base, to take an earth wire. Use a small field-tester to determine if equipment is carrying current when switched off.

• If you are renting premises and cannot alter the wiring or fittings, some other precautions can be taken. Wiring can be inactivated by turning off unused circuits overnight at the switchboard, particularly those to bedrooms. A better alternative is to install a demand switch at the switchboard, which automatically neutralises all wiring under its control once the last appliance or light is turned off. (Deepfreezes, refrigerators and smoke-detectors operate independently of this switch.) A cheaper option is a control switch within the building which allows you to cut off circuits to sleeping areas.

Choosing electrical equipment

Before purchasing electrical equipment, check it with a portable magnetometer (see Resources List). This is an essential purchase if you are serious about correcting an unhealthy electroclimate. Ideally, when the piece of electrical equipment is connected to the mains power supply, the meter should read no more than 100 gamma (100 nanoTeslas or 1 milliGauss). Take your measurement from the distance you will be at when exposed to the appliance. For example, the magnetometer should be about a centimetre (¼ inch) away when testing a hairdryer, but about 50 centimetres (20 inches) away when testing a computer monitor.

In most existing houses you will probably find that a reading of 100–200 gamma (100–200 nanoTeslas or 1–2 milliGauss) or more prevails due to the stray magnetic fields created by conventional wiring. You may find hot spots where the readings are much higher. You should generally aim to keep the level below 100 gamma (100 nanoTeslas or 1 milliGauss). In bedrooms you should aim to keep the levels down to 10 gamma (10 nanoTeslas or 0.1 milliGauss). Your decision to purchase an electrical appliance should be made according to whether or not it pushes the reading over the limit.

Artificial lighting

The unique spectrum of ultraviolet light to which the human body has become attuned and which we need to maintain our health is not present in artificial lighting. However, the use of artificial light is unavoidable — our task is to make sure that the artificial lighting we choose is suitable for the safe and healthy house.

Fluorescent lights are to be avoided, not only for the disruption they cause to the electromagnetic field inside the home, but also because of their link with an increased incidence of melanoma, squamous cell carcinoma and possibly cataracts. Working under fluorescent lights for 8 hours is equivalent to receiving 5 minutes of exposure to the midday sun; the effect is cumulative. This means that in a year of working under fluorescent lights, you would have been exposed to the equivalent of about 18 hours of midday sunlight. One study has shown that continuous exposure to fluorescent light made mice, rabbits and rats more aggressive and irritable, to the extent that they ate their young (Ott 1982). A separate study of children showed a 32 per cent drop in hyperactivity when fluorescent lighting was removed from their schools (Johnson 1981). If you are forced to use fluorescent lighting, for example at work, insist on full-spectrum tubes.

Although quartz halogen lighting now includes glass filters to screen out ultraviolet radiation, because it requires transformers, the associated electro-magnetic field precludes their use in a healthy house. The best type of artificial lighting is that from incandescent bulbs.

Alternative energy sources

No reasonably priced wind or solar generating system can cope with a household that watches colour television while running electric lights, a refrigerator, cooking appliances, a dishwasher, and a radiator or air conditioner simultaneously. However, when wind and solar generating systems are combined, such loadings are possible as long as a sensible selection has been made of appliances and other types of fuel are used where appropriate, for example gas cooking and refrigeration. Ultimately, the rising price of grid electricity will make alternative electricity generation an economical alternative.

An electricity generating system based on wind energy may cost thousands of dollars, and the electrical supply halts during calm periods. The same type of problem occurs with photovoltaic (solar) systems during cloudy periods. This problem can be overcome by installing a bank of deep-cycle batteries to store surplus power during windy (or sunny) periods; energy can be fed back into the system when needed. This is only a partial solution, as it poses some problems as well.

• The amount of storage capacity available to you will be dictated by economics.

• All electrical equipment in the house has to be converted to run on a 12, 30 or 110 volt supply, depending on the storage battery. (A licensed electrician should be contracted to wire this part of the system.)

• Batteries store only enough energy for lighting and a limited number of appliances for 2 or 3 days.

• The batteries must be stored outside on several square metres (several square yards) of well-ventilated storage racks.

You can achieve the maximum benefit of an alternative energy system with minimum cost by sharing the system in a communal arrangement. Several families can share the cost of the initial installation and the subsequent benefits. This is particularly relevant to the installation of a methane digester waste system. The system turns farm animal, household and treated human waste into methane gas which can be used for cooking, heating and perhaps even lighting. Exotic alternatives such as the separation of water into hydrogen and oxygen by electrolysis have tremendous potential but belong to the future.

SOLAR-GENERATED ELECTRICITY

Photovoltaic cells utilise some of the electromagnetic radiation generated by the sun. Photons from the sun hit the photovoltaic cell and cause electrons to be ejected from the atoms of the material in the cell. The light causes other substances in the cell to accept those electrons. The electrons flow through a conductor, generating electricity. The photovoltaic cell has no moving mechanical parts, so nothing wears out and no fuel is used, making it the ultimate energy generator.

Solar panels are comprised of many of these photovoltaic cells. The direct current (DC) generated by the cells is changed by an inverter into alternating current (AC). Solar panels are used extensively, particularly in remote areas, as they are easy and fast to install and require little prior preparation on-site. Although the energy efficiency of most reasonably priced systems is currently only 10 to 15 per cent, the technology is improving all the time. (The more highly priced solar energy systems have energy efficiency levels around 30 per cent.)

An experienced solar designer or a fully qualified dealer or distributor of solar energy equipment should be consulted when you are installing a solar energy system. He or she will ensure that your system is correctly located and mounted, that the photovoltaic modules are properly oriented and that you have the correct wiring, circuitry, regulators, batteries and fuses.

When economically feasible, solar panels should be designed to track the movement of the sun throughout the day, as this increases the overall efficiency of the system, particularly in winter. As a compromise, you could install a mounting system that can be moved manually several times throughout the year. Table 9.6 is to be read in conjunction with local observations of any shadowing produced by obstructions surrounding your site. The information in the table assumes a wide expanse of open, flat, unobstructed land and does not take into consideration the regional issue of

Table 9.6: Calculating the number of daylight hours a site receives

LATITUDE OF SITE	SUMMER DAYLIGHT HOURS	WINTER DAYLIGHT HOURS
10 deg	12.71	11.54
15 deg	13.02	11.24
20 deg	13.34	10.92
25 deg	13.70	10.58
30 deg	14.08	10.21
35 deg	14.52	9.80
40 deg	15.02	9.33
45 deg	15.62	8.76

Table 9.6

Table 9.7: Tilting a photovoltaic module to improve efficiency*

LATITUDE OF SITE	RECOMMENDED ANGLE OF TILT
0–15 deg	15 deg
15–25 deg	Angle of latitude
25–30 deg	Angle of latitude + 5 deg
30–35 deg	Angle of latitude + 10 deg
35–40 deg	Angle of latitude + 15 deg
40+ deg	Angle of latitude + 20 deg

* adapted from Pedals 1992

Table 9.7

Table 9.8: The advantage of using a tracking device (calculated for a cloudless day)

HOURS OF SUNLIGHT	PERCENTAGE GAIN
4	5
5	7
6	11
7	15
8	21
9	28
10	36
11	47
12	57
13	70
14	83
15	96

Table 9.8

cloudiness (Pedals 1992). If you are not using a mechanical solar tracker, face your photovoltaic modules at right angles to the midday sun and at an angle of tilt from the horizontal approximately equal to the latitude of your site. The photovoltaic modules can be oriented up to 15 degrees away from magnetic north (in the southern hemisphere) or south (in the northern hemisphere) without radically affecting efficiency, but it is preferable to orient them to solar north or south wherever possible.

WIND AND WATER POWER

The conversion of wind power to electricity is more economical than the direct conversion of solar energy. It has proven an effective source of power over the centuries — some ancient windmills are still in use today. In the modern era, the heating of water and interior spaces by wind energy requires relatively sophisticated, and expensive, wind generators.

The energy in wind power is dependent on the wind's speed, hence site selection should take into consideration the speed of prevailing winds as well as their frequency. The ideal site for wind power generation faces a sea or desert from which the wind blows consistently. Both seas and deserts present little frictional resistance and hence impede air flow the least. Rounded hill tops are better than open flat ground because aerodynamic funnelling results from their topography.

Wind is of two principal types, planetary and local. Planetary winds are vast masses of moving air, constant in direction and varying with high and low pressure systems as well as with the seasons. Local winds, such as mountain and valley winds, are the result of local temperature differences. The best sites are subject to both types of winds.

To estimate how much wind energy a site can potentially produce, first obtain the 10 year average data from your nearest meteorological station. With an anemometer (see Resources List) take wind speed measurements every day for one month and compare the average for that month with the average provided by the meteorological station for the same month. Divide your figure by the meteorological station's figure — the result will be a fraction. You can then multiply each month's figures from the meteorological station by this fraction to predict the average amount of wind energy your site will receive in a year.

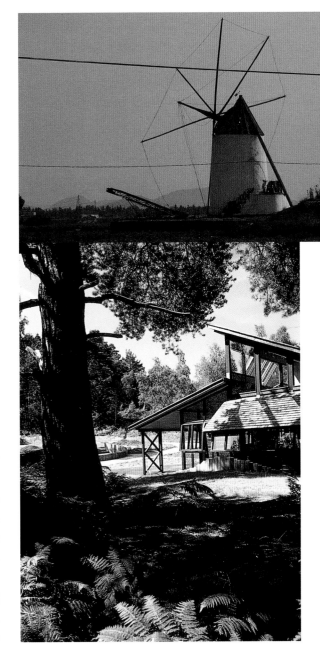

Above: Windmill still in use today near Ivinghoe Beacon, UK

Left: An award-winning school building designed for a cold, damp climate. Woodlea Primary School, Hampshire, UK (Architect: N. Churcher; Photograph: N. Churcher)

Micro hydro is a form of energy generation which utilises a continuous flow of water from a creek or river. The micro hydro unit is usually located away from the building so some power loss must be allowed for. Such a system can supply all the energy needs of a household using only a quarter of the energy of a wind-powered generator.

THERMAL INSULATION

Thermal insulation serves to reduce the amount of heat flowing through the envelope of a building. It slows down the passage of heat from the exterior to the interior in summer, and vice versa in winter. To some extent the building envelope itself insulates against climatic extremes and ideally, it should not need insulating. However, unless you are planning to build an earth-sheltered building, there will be times when climatic conditions are too extreme and the building envelope will be thermally inadequate.

There are two types of insulation, bulk and reflective. Bulk insulation works by means of small pockets or trapped bubbles of air or other gases. These pockets retard the flow of heat inside the material. If made from organic materials such as coconut fibre or cellulose, bulk insulation will allow the building envelope to take part in the air-exchange process.

Reflective insulation, such as aluminium foil laminates, reduce the transfer of heat by reflecting radiant heat away from the material on the heated side. This type of insulation is not acceptable in the healthy building because it lacks diffusivity, does not encourage the building envelope to exchange air with the exterior environment and does not help to absorb interior gaseous pollution.

A variety of heat transmission ratings are used throughout the world. In Australia, an R-value describes an insulation material's resistance to heat transmission. The higher a material's R-value, the more effective it is. In temperate climates, the aim is to have a roof with insulation that performs at R1.5–2. An uninsulated tiled roof has an R value of 0.3. The ratings for hygroscopic insulation are: cellulose fibre R2.6, seagrass R2–2.7 and wool R2.5. The ratings for less hygroscopic, and hence less acceptable, insulation are: glass-fibre batts R2.0, rockwool R2.5 and double-sided, aluminium foil-sarking R1–1.4 (NSW State News Building Industry Connection 1994a).

A house insulated to keep heat out in the summer but not designed with other passive-solar features, such as shaded windows, eventually heats up after a few hours. When night-time cooling begins after a hot summer day, the inside heat may be slow to escape, especially if it is a poorly designed brick or concrete building. While night-time ventilation helps in the cooling process, buildings need to be designed according to passive-solar principles to make full use of the daily heat cycle.

An architect can advise you on what type of insulation gives the best control of heat flow, but it is for you to decide which type is the most acceptable from a Gaian viewpoint. Try to find an architect trained in environmental issues. The insulation you use should reduce heat transmission efficiently yet be diffusive enough to help the walls, floors and ceilings breathe. It should be able to absorb and neutralise chemicals and odours and help balance the moisture content of the air in the room; it should not encourage condensation to form. You should consider the material's impact on human health, including its impact in fire conditions. Ideally, insulation material should be produced without a high energy demand and should have a minimal impact upon the environment during its manufacture and installation. For example, because a relatively small amount of energy is used in the manufacture of cellulose insulation, it 'pays back' the energy debt incurred in its production and installation within 3 weeks, while polyurethane makes up for its debt only after 9–23 months have passed.

Insulation materials can contain harmful chemicals, for example, glass and rockwool mineral fibres contain phenol-formaldehyde resin. Foam insulation also contains harmful chemicals. During its manufacture certain ingredients do not fully polymerise (convert into large molecules like the bulk of the insulation). Over the years, these free molecules, along with softeners and fireproofing chemicals, are released into the indoor air. Many of these chemicals, such as formaldehyde, isocyanate and styrol, are carcinogenic. The potentially harmful health effects of insulation, along with the amount of energy used in mining and/or manufacturing it are all part of the environmental impact issue for you to consider.

Insulation materials derived from natural sources, such as recycled paper, timber shavings and sawdust, are produced with low entropic debts and come from renewable resources. Unfortunately, these materials are not available everywhere, and can be costly. John Ruskin, the 19th century author and architect, once said: 'there is hardly anything in the world that some men cannot make a little worse and sell a little cheaper, and the people who consider price only are this man's lawful prey'. Insulation is one of those things. However, the rising costs of maintaining health and environmental quality are something we all have to share. For years now architects and engineers have considered the thermal conductivity of insulation as the main issue when evaluating insulation in terms of economics. We are now inhabiting their buildings and dealing with the problems caused by their approach.

In selecting the right insulation material, we should consider a range of issues, not just the thermal conductivity of the insulation itself. The whole house should make a contribution to the process of insulation. The type of insulation we choose should depend upon how well the house has been designed for passive-solar heat storage and cold storage, the type of heating used inside the building, the orientation of the building to the sunlight, the type of windows and ventilation. The amount of heat from incoming solar radiation stored in the thermal mass of exterior walls is another factor, as walls are a type of insulation in themselves. Thermal mass storage in the walls reduces the heat energy that could be lost and helps to reduce the need to heat in winter (and vice versa in summer).

Walls that allow diffusion between the air inside and outside a building carry heat energy; air and water molecules flowing through the outside surface of the wall leave their heat energy in the cells of the wall material in winter. Incoming particles then absorb the heat energy in their passage through to the building's interior. Heavier building materials have a higher heat storage capacity than lighter materials. Generally speaking, synthetic building materials have less heat storage capacity than natural ones.

Table 9.9 is intended as a guide, about which your architect, engineer or builder will be able to give you further advice. A score of six or more indicates an appropriate material from the viewpoint of Gaian building biology and ecology philosophy.

Cellulose insulation materials

Cellulose is a good insulation choice, but as it is more easily ignited than other materials, it is dependent upon fireproofing agents. As we search for natural materials with a low entropy debt we find that the usual fireproofing chemicals cannot be classified as acceptable to Gaian principles.

A harmless fireproofing and fungus treatment for waste product insulation materials such as paper, wood shavings, woodchips, bark, straw, coconut fibre, reed and sawdust can be made by mixing one part of borax (boric acid) with one part of waterglass (sodium silicate), then to one part of the borax and waterglass mixture adding nine parts of water. Calcium and

Table 9.9: Comparison of insulation materials:

+2= very advantageous to use

+1= advantageous

0=neutral

-1=disadvantageous

-2= very disadvantageous

Insulating Material	Insulation Value	Toxicity	Waste Disposal	Diffusivity	Hygro-scopicity	Draught-proofing	Fire-resistance	Cost	Overall Score
Natural									
Straw and clay mix	-1	0	0	+2	+2	+2	+2	+2	+9
Woodwool	+1	0	+2	+2	+2	0	-1	+2	+8
Sawdust or shavings with bark	+1	0	+2	+2	+2	0	-1	+2	+8
Strawboard	+1	0	+2	+2	+2	+1	-1	-1	+6
Cellulose (recycled paper)	+2	-1	0	+2	+2	0	-1	+2	+6
Cork (Baked)	+2	0	+2	+2	+2	+1	-1	-2	+5
Coconut fibre	+2	0	+2	+2	+2	+1	-1	-2	+5
Foam glass	+2	0	+1	0	0	+1	+2	-1	+5
Foamed lime or cellulose	+1	0	0	+1	+1	+2	+2	-1	+5
Clay bead ('Liapor')	-1	0	0	+2	+1	0	+2	+2	+4
Vermiculite or Perlite	+1	-1	0	+2	0	+1	+2	-2	+2
Synthetic									
Mineral wool (glass, rock fibre)	+2	-2	-2	-2	-2	+1	0	+1	-6
Polystyrol	+2	-2	-2	-2	-2	0	-2	+2	-8
Urea formaldehyde	+2	-2	-2	-2	-2	0	-2	+1	-9
Polyurethane	+2	-2	-2	-2	-2	0	-2	-1	-11

adapted from Kanuka-Fuchs 1991

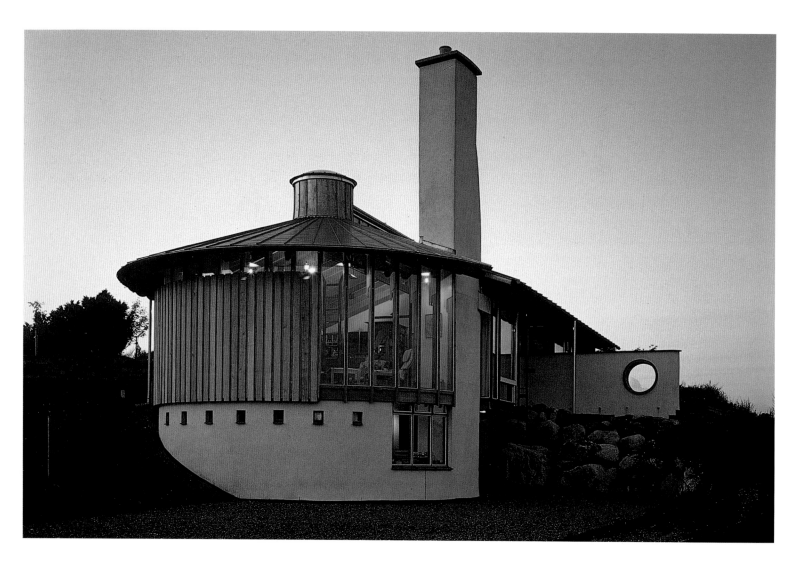

'Clach Mohr', in the Scottish highlands, has a slate-finished roof (Architect: R. Langmuir, Edward Cullinan and Associates; Photograph: R. Langmuir)

magnesium sulphate can also be added to cellulose insulation materials to promote fire resistance and control fungus. All of these treatments are benign, almost as safe to ingest as common house salt. During a fire, mineral salts emit only carbon dioxide and steam, and no combustible gases.

Wool insulation

Wool appears to have all the right characteristics to qualify it as an environmentally safe product, but we must not forget that the wool batt insulation available for purchase has been treated with chemicals to control moths and larvae, beetles, mites, fungi and rodents. These chemicals can cause skin and eye irritation during manufacture, and the jury is still out on the potential for outgassing in a hot roof. The presence of these chemicals in wool insulation is also a serious fire safety issue. Because wool has a very high ignition point (400 degrees Celsius, or 752 degrees Fahrenheit), fires are unlikely to commence in wool insulation, but if a fire starts elsewhere and the

insulation is burnt, noxious gases, including carbon monoxide and hydrogen cyanide, will be emitted.

Overall, wool insulation should only be considered as a compromise to avoid the use of insulation made from synthetic mineral fibres. A wool layer 11 centimetres thick (4¼ inches) can have an R rating of 2.5, similar to that of synthetic mineral fibre insulation.

Quality control is essential, as wool insulation often uses the cheapest grades of wool available. Reclaimed wool fibre should always be checked for the presence of other fibres and pieces of hide. Wool insulation already contains 10–15 per cent water, and will absorb additional water into its fibres to up to 35 per cent of its volume. Should roof leaks occur, wool insulation has a good resistance to rotting but it can be damaged by prolonged wetting. There is currently no data on whether moisture from condensation or roof leaks could induce the growth of the fungus *Scopulariopsis brevicaulis*, which has the potential to produce deadly arsene.

⊚ Insulation with under 0.1 per cent formaldehyde resin ⊚

BONDED MINERAL WOOL

Bonded mineral wool is also known as rockwool, slagwool and mineral-fibre insulation-wool. It is used for thermal and acoustic insulation and fire protection. It is 95 per cent rock and blast furnace slag, less than 5 per cent heat-cured, urea-modified phenol-formaldehyde resin, and less than 2 per cent refined mineral oil. Rockwool dust can cause skin rashes and eye, nose, throat and lung irritation. Its use cannot be recommended in a healthy building.

BONDED GLASSWOOL OR FIBREGLASS INSULATION

Bonded glasswool is also referred to as glass fibre, glasswool, fibreglass insulation (or batts), insulation batts, insulation wool and glasswool insulation. Used for thermal and acoustic insulation, it is made up of borosilicate glass, heat-cured phenol-formaldehyde resin and a solvent-refined mineral-oil. The health effects of exposure to this material are the same as for bonded mineral wool.

POLYESTER INSULATION

Polyester insulation is a bonded, long-chain synthetic-polymer material, hence outgassing of chemicals is a major issue. It is also used for duct wrapping and lining, wadding for furniture and to filter air. Although its air-exchange capacity is reasonable, the material itself is not diffusive and permeable, so it is unsatisfactory.

ROOFING

In a healthy house the roof must breathe, allowing air to be exchanged between the inside and outside of the building. Impervious roof membranes are not acceptable. Steel sheet roofing is also out, as it encourages the formation of rogue electromagnetic fields, disturbing the natural path of cosmic, microwave and terrestrial radiation into the building. Aluminium roofing is non-magnetic so will not create rogue magnetic fields but, as it conducts electricity, it can create problems with DC fields and distort natural radiation. You should opt either for pervious materials such as terracotta roof tiles or impervious ones such as slate tiles that have adequate air gaps around them. Earth-covered and sod-roofs are acceptable, provided there is a drainage layer (beneath an inert membrane) connected to the atmosphere.

CORRUGATED FIBRE-CEMENT ROOFING

Fibre-cement (not asbestos cement) is an acceptable roofing material but it requires a long-wearing coating for weather resistance. Cement-based water paints are appropriate, provided they do not contain solvents and toxic chemicals.

SPLIT AND SAWN TIMBER-SHINGLE ROOFING

The wooden shingle, split or sawn from durable timber (hardwood in Australia, oak in the United Kingdom and cedar in the United States) has been used for human shelter for thousands of years. The shingles overlap, three layers thick, and the resultant roof is not only the most hygroscopic type but also has excellent insulation qualities. A shingle roof has excellent wind resistance, so is ideal for sites exposed to cyclones and tornadoes. In general, shingles should not be used in forest or bushfire prone areas.

Below: The flexibility of wood shingle roofing is beautifully illustrated by the clever detailing in this house in New Zealand (Architect: R. Kanuka-Fuchs; Photograph: R. Kanuka-Fuchs)

Bottom: An Australian hardwood shingle roof (Photograph: P. Kelly, The Shingle Roofing Co.)

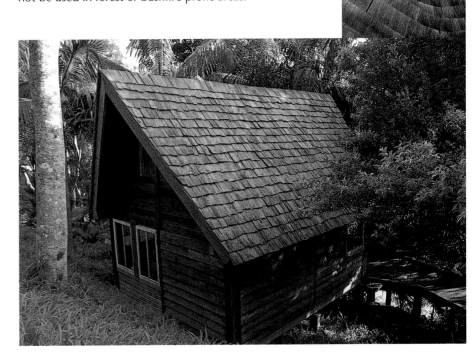

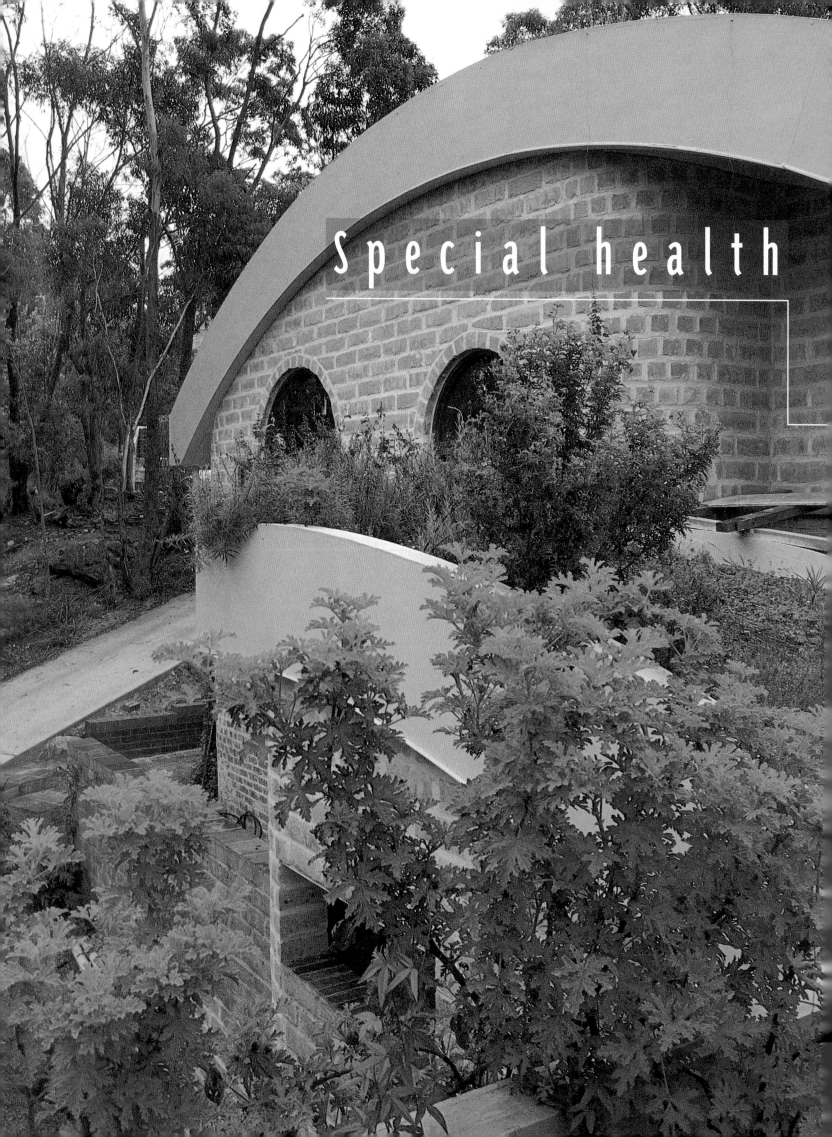

Special health

and safety issues

to create a truly healthy building, you need to consider a number of specific health and safety issues which require special building construction techniques. In this chapter we outline procedures to exclude termites, radon and noise from your building, reduce accident 'black spots', and make your building resistant to bushfires and earthquakes.

You cannot predict every event that may threaten your house, but there are a number of preventative measures you can incorporate into your design to gain maximum protection from household accidents and natural disasters.

TERMITES

The organochlorines used in pest control are known to accumulate in the fat cells of humans and have been shown to produce cancer in animals. The United States Environmental Protection Authority has banned chlordane, heptachlor, aldrin and dieldrin. In Australia, manufacturers were slow to respond and dangerous organochlorines remained in the marketplace long after they should have been removed. The effects of the recommended substitute for organochlorines, chlorpyrifos (an organophosphate that lasts some 5–8 years in the ground), have never been fully tested but chlorpyrifos is known to cross the blood–brain barrier and act as a 'slow' poison (Short 1994). But how do we protect against termite attack without flooding the ground beneath us with poison or spraying toxic chemicals onto the underside of our flooring?

⚬ Protection from termite attack ⚬

It is absolutely essential that all buildings containing timber are designed and built to exclude the local species of termites. You must first find out which species live in your region. There are well over 300 known species of termites in Australia, not all of which cause problems to buildings.

Termites can generally be identified by the type of nests they build. Subterranean termites build above-ground mud tunnels that can be traced back to their nest. They usually locate their nests beneath buildings or in the bole of a tree or tree stump. They may also construct small nests, scattered beneath concrete floor slabs, paving slabs or verandahs resting on the ground. Subterranean species can build tunnels reaching to the upper storeys of high buildings. Their tunnels can be 60 or more metres (197 feet) long, providing the termites have continuous access to moisture and soil. The most widespread and destructive termite, *Coptotermes acinaciformis*, is a tunnel-builder. They may also build nests above ground and a mature colony can contain some one million insects. Termites are capable of penetrating a range of building materials, including most types of brick mortar, some adobe earth blocks and even lower-strength concrete.

To find out the species in your area, obtain several intact specimens and send them for identification to the closest entomology department (Australian readers can contact the Commonwealth Scientific and Industrial Research Organisation's Division of Entomology — see Resources List for details).

⚬ Chemical methods of termite control ⚬

Since the 1950s, dangerous organochlorines (mainly cyclodeines) were used for termite control. Though thousands of tonnes of chemicals have entered and continue to enter our soils, termite infestations are steadily increasing. The cyclodeines still on sale in Australia, for example, are chlordane, a potential neurotoxin (sold either as Chlordane™ or 800EC™) and heptachlor, which causes long-term genetic damage (sold as Heptachlor™, 400EC™ or HC80™). While Aldrin (Aldrex 60™) and Dieldrin (Dieldrex 30™) are no longer manufactured, they remain active in the soil for 20–30 years.

The only registered alternative to the cyclodeines in Australia is chlorpyrifos (sold as Dursban™ or Deter™). Chlorpyrifos is a synthetic pyrethroid and probably the least hazardous of the organophosphates. Although it has not yet been associated with cancer in animals, 'it is toxic to both vertebrate and invertebrate animals' (Short 1994). Symptoms from pyrethroid pesticide exposure include abnormal facial sensations, fatigue, nausea, dizziness, headache and loss of appetite.

Apart from chlorpyrifos, the only other chemical that can be used as a barrier to termites is arsenic trioxide. It can only be used on termites that construct tunnels. It is a useful alternative, provided the chemical does not come into contact with humans or animals. If the arsenic-treated termite tunnels are broken, a person or animal could be poisoned by contacting the toxic compound. It is a slow-acting cumulative stomach poison but it needs to build up in the gut to cause serious illness, however it is extremely carcinogenic (Verkerk 1990). Only licensed, experienced operators who understand termite biology and building construction should be employed.

Cyfluthrin was used in Australia by the Commonwealth Scientific and Industrial Research Organisation (CSIRO) in their first synthetic pyrethroid trial in 1987. Research into its efficacy is ongoing as well as into alpha cypermethrin, esvenvalerate, bifenthrin and deltamethrin (Verkerk 1990).

A termite control procedure has been developed in Hawaii involving an underground pipeline system installed in the ground beneath the concrete floor slab. Termiticide is released through slits in the pipe so that it penetrates the ground. Another version uses injection tubing built into the slab.

All chemical pretreatment procedures have to reach 5 centimetres (2 inches) into the soil, hence they cannot be used where buildings have been constructed on rock. If the soil is overwet, or if it happens to rain after the injection or spraying of termiticides, the poisons can enter the ground water system and reach creeks, rivers and coasts where they cause extensive environmental damage.

A team led by Melbourne-based entomologist Doctor John French of the CSIRO is working on a toxic bait system using an organochlorine (Mirex™) under restricted and controlled conditions in conjunction with an agar and sawdust mixture. The baits are highly toxic and must be removed when the termites have been exterminated. Before they die, the termites carry small doses of the chemical into the soil.

The CSIRO has obtained promising results from research into biological control of termites. One strategy is to inhibit the production of chitin, which is essential to the development of the insects' exoskeletons. Other research has been based on encouraging fungus and roundworms to enter the bodies of termites.

Several companies have had success with products that do not include any of the scheduled poisons, but rather the botanical insecticides of pyrethrin, eucalyptus, tea-tree, lavender and citronella. However, the public's perception of safety may be misplaced in the case of pyrethrin, as it can cause serious eye damage (Short 1994).

Termite box-traps (in conjunction with arsenic trioxide and boron or sulfluramid) can be used to control identified termite colonies.

◉ Physical barriers ◉

The problem with all chemical termite control systems is that they will eventually impact on the natural environment and on human ecology. Termites are part of the natural environment's wood–cellulose cycle. In urban areas, people removing all their timber debris could replace the actions of termites, but in the natural environment, termites serve a definite purpose, so total extermination is not an option. The best Gaian approach is to use physical barriers or safe chemical repellents.

Physical barriers place impediments in the path of termites which force them to come out into visible locations as they try to enter the building's structure. Integral to the success of a physical barrier system is clear visibility, access and regular inspection. If you have chosen to construct an earth-brick home, and you live in a termite area, it should be elevated above the ground for ease of inspection.

BASALT GRAVEL BEDS

This method involves the laying of a thick bed of gravel beneath a concrete slab floor. It was originally developed for use in Hawaii, where only one species of termite is found, *Coptathermes formosanus*, the Formosan termite. The crushed basalt is so hard that the termites cannot penetrate it, so small that they

cannot fit through the gaps between the grains, yet large enough that they are unable to remove it. The situation in some tropical regions of Africa, South America, Australia and the Pacific Islands (north of the Tropic of Capricorn and south of the Tropic of Cancer) is more complex than that in Hawaii because several different species of termites may coexist, and a different size of gravel is needed to stop each species. In such regions, a multiple-layer barrier must be used, where more than one type of gravel is laid to stop each termite species.

WOVEN STAINLESS STEEL MESH

Stainless steel mesh will control even the smallest species of termite, such as *Heterotermes vagus*. Stainless steel mesh is suitable for peat and heavy humus soils and coastal environments. It does not suffer any significant corrosion, including galvanic corrosion.

Quality control is probably the most difficult aspect of using the mesh protection technique. It is of paramount importance that there are no breaks or holes in the mesh barrier, so most careful professionals will insist on continuous site supervision to make sure that wear and tear in vulnerable areas is attended to.

The stainless steel mesh method can be used in all types of buildings with concrete floors, including double brick and brick veneer walls that have been erected on concrete strip footings. The mesh is installed after the plumbing and footings are finished but if ducts, pipes or other components have to pass through a concrete floor slab, a collar of mesh can be stretched around the component and fastened with a stainless steel hose clamp. The termites are prevented from entering the building via the cavity walls or footings.

The mesh provides extra security for the damp-proof or waterproof membrane which is subsequently laid on top of the mesh. The mesh stops termites from penetrating the membrane at a later date, when access to the membrane is no longer possible. It also eradicates the problem of construction workers accidentally punching holes in the membrane, by providing a buffer between the membrane and the ground.

The reinforced concrete slab floor must be free of cracks for the mesh to be effective. If the engineering specifications and quality control procedures implemented in your construction are able to guarantee that cracking in the concrete slab will be absolutely minimal (no cracks wider than 0.5 millimetre (1/50 inch), the area beneath main floor slabs need not be equipped with anti-termite mesh. There will, however, be some risk that termites may penetrate the waterproof membrane. Assuming that quality control standards are high, the mesh will prevent termite entry above the floor level of a building.

WOODEN FLOOR CONSTRUCTION

The installation of anti-termite mesh in buildings with wooden floors aims to protect all wood in the superstructure of the building. There must be no wood present in the substructure below the termite barrier. More common than mesh is galvanised metal anti-termite capping located on top of brick piers and isolating the floor timbers above. The main purpose of galvanised metal anti-termite capping is to force the termites to build their tunnels where they can be easily detected. Stainless steel mesh is flexible and is therefore a much more effective barrier than the capping, as the termites find it difficult to build their stiff mud tunnels on it.

From an aesthetic viewpoint, some people object to the mesh being visible from the building exterior. Though the supplier of the mesh in Australia has advised that it is acceptable to set the stainless steel up to 2 centimetres (¾ inch) inside the exterior face of the joint, this is not in the best interests of good termite proofing. Insist that the mesh be visible so you can see any termite tunnels attempting to bridge the barrier.

Other preventative procedures

GAPS BETWEEN TIMBER

When timber does not have clear space around it for air to circulate, fungal infestations like dry rot and wet rot can set in, encouraging termites. Wet rot occurs in wood in contact with moisture from the ground, or from poor plumbing or weatherproofing, while dry rot occurs when air circulation is inhibited and results in cracked and dry wood. Fungal infestation can be avoided by creating air gaps between timber in the building structure and the other parts of the structure that can be accessed by termites. It is easy to ensure this when constructing a new building, but the feasibility of creating such gaps in an existing building must be investigated by an architect.

There should be a gap of at least 2.5 centimetres (1 inch) between structural wood (particularly its end grain) and other structural parts of a building. A gap of at least 5 centimetres (2 inches), but preferably 7.5 centimetres (3 inches), is necessary between the earth and any piece of wood near the ground (verandah or pergola posts for instance). Fence palings need to be placed 7.5 centimetres (3 inches) above the ground, and precast concrete or galvanised steel fence posts installed. If wooden posts are used, a sock of anti-termite mesh should be wrapped around the end of the post in the ground, rising 10 centimetres (4 inches) above the ground on all sides and the bottom of the post should sit on a bed of crushed rock to keep the endgrain away from the soil.

LIGHT AND VENTILATION IN THE SUB-FLOOR

Lack of ventilation in any part of the building, especially the crawl space underneath the building, can encourage dry rot, which in turn encourages termites. You should have a generous, even excessive, number of ventilators built into the foundation walls. There are products available made specifically for foundation ventilation. They are larger in size than the standard 'air bricks' and are equipped with galvanised mesh, to protect against rodents.

Should you discover a termite infestation but you do not wish to exterminate it, apply incandescent or halogen lights, which create their own heat, and fan-forced ventilation for several weeks to dry out the termite tunnels. The light and the increasing dryness of the soil will encourage the colony to move. This is an accepted method amongst some natural pest controllers, but it is a repellent only, and you will have to continuously monitor the termites to make sure you are not driving them into other areas of the house. Installing continuously running sub-floor lighting is a possible preventative method, provided the lighting is powered by photovoltaic panels.

INSTALLING INGROUND BARRIERS TO EXISTING BUILDINGS

An existing building can be protected from termites by encircling it with a termite-proof shield constructed from stainless steel mesh or galvanised steel sheet (or roofing). The joints between the sheets of metal must be completely sealed to avoid termite entry. As this is very difficult and costly to achieve in sheet steel, you could install a gravel barrier in a trench. It is important to check the type of termites capable of living on your site, as the depth to which you must build the shield will depend on this — some species of termites have been known to extend their workings down to some 3 metres (10 feet).

For up-to-date information about construction methods designed to protect buildings from termites, refer to your local building authority and Environmental Protection Agency. (Australian readers should contact the Standards Association of Australia.)

RADON

Radiation is all around us, it can come from the sun and from space, from an x-ray or even a luminous watch dial. Exposure to radiation continues throughout life. In our houses, particularly if they are inadequately ventilated, exposure can be continuous, night and day. Radioactive radiation has a cumulative effect, so there is no harmless level of exposure. Low-level exposure for long periods is significantly more dangerous than a brief period at a high level. Leukaemia, a radiation cancer, is one example of the long-term (20–30 years) effects of radiation; birth defects, genetic mutation and infant mortality are among the more immediate effects.

In 1990, Bristol University scientists reported that internationally, the incidence of myeloid (bone marrow) leukaemia, kidney cancer, melanoma and certain childhood cancers all show a significant correlation with radon exposure in the home.

Radon$_{222}$ is formed during the radioactive breakdown of uranium in the earth. During this process, the radon produces a number of daughter products. These radioactive ions attach themselves to dust and other particles in the air. Radon is considered a serious source of noxious pollution in some regions of the world. In Sweden, for example, the amount of ionised radiation recorded inside buildings due to radon was found by the Council for Building Research to be 10 times greater than that found in the air after the Chernobyl nuclear disaster (Holdsworth and Sealey 1992). In a United States survey of 11,600 homes across 10 states, 21 per cent were found to have radon levels above the recommended level (Pierce 1987). In fact, radon is so common in the United States that it is blamed for 5000 deaths in non-smokers every year. In Britain 'between 50,000 and 90,000 homes may have levels that exceed the government's "action level"' (New Scientist, 22 September 1988), which is four times the level set for exposure of employees at nuclear power stations.

The amount of radon in the soil and air of a site is gauged either with a dosimeter or a track-etch detector (see Resources List). The metric measurements used are Becquerels per cubic metre (Bq/m^3) and, in the United States, picoCurie per litre in cgs (centimetre, gram and second units).

If the radon level is 20–203 Becquerels per cubic metre 0.5–5.5 picoCurie per litre), action should be taken within one year. At 100–750 Becquerels per cubic metre (3–20 picoCurie per litre) it should be taken within a month, and over 7500 Becquerels per cubic metre (203 picoCurie per litre), within a few weeks.

Does simple ventilation help in ridding the house of radon? Based upon the results of a university study undertaken in the mid–1980s, the government of New South Wales, Australia, recommended that opening the windows is enough to prevent radon-related health problems (Ferrari, et al 1988). However, when we conducted a study in conjunction with the Queensland Institute of Technology we found that the air exchange rate bore no relationship to the amount of radon present in the home (Baggs and Wong 1987). These findings have also been borne out by a study conducted by international expert, Doctor Anthony Nero Jr in 1986.

What our study and Nero's found was that simply leaving windows ajar is not sufficient to prevent radon build-up, but that large air movements have the desired effect. Because only a large volume of air flowing through the building washes the house out completely, it is necessary to open all windows and doors as wide as possible at least twice a day, particularly in breezy weather. Better still, seal all cavities and cracks in the house with non-toxic sealants. The most effective method of ridding a timber-floor house of radon is to install solar-driven fans in the sub-floor of the house to continually evacuate the air containing radon.

Smokers should be asked to smoke outside, because many studies have established that smoking amongst miners exposed to radon increases their risk of dying from lung cancer by up to 15 times, thus adding 15,000 lung cancer deaths to the annual toll (New Scientist, 22 September 1988).

◎ Detailing to exclude radon ◎

Ionised radiation can be artificially concentrated in a building's interior because the wrong type of building materials have been chosen, or the methods of construction do not adequately exclude the radon gas rising from the soil.

The Swedes are presently using special wells (reservoirs) to control radon. It is a particularly successful method where gravel forms the underlying strata to a building. The Swedish example uses a well that is 4 metres (13 feet) deep and 800 millimetres (2 feet 7 inches) in diameter in the vicinity of 15 four-bedroom houses with basements. Such an installation will drain radon from 1 hectare (2.5 acres) of land. This control treatment reduces radon concentration by 96–98 per cent in all buildings. If installed in a single residence, a smaller pipe would have to be used. Also the depth should be governed by readings taken in bore holes around the site (when used with buildings without basements, the depth would be much less). Ideally such a device should use photovoltaics for the necessary mechanical fan. The designers of the radon well strongly recommend continuous monitoring of radon daughter products in conjunction with a professional consultant to supervise the method and the results (Clarensjo and Kumlin 1984). According to the Institute of Building Research at Gavle in Sweden, the radon well costs approximately the same amount as a good quality washing machine. It generates no noise, takes up no space within the building and can be run by photo-voltaic cells.

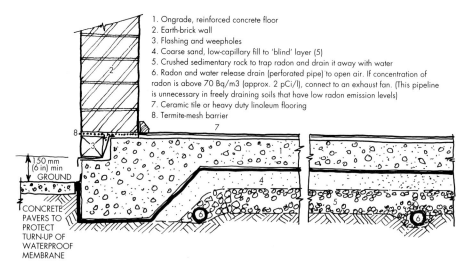

1. Ongrade, reinforced concrete floor
2. Earth-brick wall
3. Flashing and weepholes
4. Coarse sand, low-capillary fill to 'blind' layer (5)
5. Crushed sedimentary rock to trap radon and drain it away with water
6. Radon and water release drain (perforated pipe) to open air. If concentration of radon is above 70 Bq/m3 (approx. 2 pCi/l), connect to an exhaust fan. (This pipeline is unnecessary in freely draining soils that have low radon emission levels)
7. Ceramic tile or heavy duty linoleum flooring
8. Termite-mesh barrier

150 mm (6 in) min GROUND

CONCRETE PAVERS TO PROTECT TURN-UP OF WATERPROOF MEMBRANE

Figure 10.1

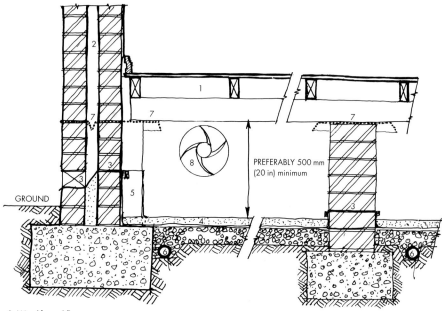

PREFERABLY 500 mm (20 in) minimum

GROUND

1. Wood-framed floor
2. Cavity type, double-skin brick wall
3. Flashing, weepholes and damp-proof course
4. Coarse sand, low-capillary fill to protect layer (5)
5. Radon barrier, polyethylene membrane (only if absolutely essential)
6. Radon and water release drain (perforated pipe) to open air. If concentration of radon is above 70 Bq/m3 (approx. 2 pCi/l), connect to an exhaust fan. (This pipeline is unnecessary in freely draining soils that have low radon emission levels)
7. Termite-mesh barrier

Figure 10.2

HOUSE
GROUND

RADON RESERVOIR LOCATED HIGH ABOVE WATER TABLE

4 m (13 ft) deep in Swedish examples with basements but depth depends on radon measurements taken in preliminary test bores

WATER TABLE

1. Pipe perforated at bottom. In the Swedish cases this was 4 m deep and 0.8 m diameter to vent radon for 15 x 4 bedroom houses. Scaled down for a single house, this could be 0.2 m (8 in) diameter pipe, 1 m (3 ft 3 in) deep in most soils. In soils with a coarse gravel content radon can travel though 4 m (13 ft) of such soil before decaying into its daughter products, hence the depth of the pipe would increase to 4 m (13 ft) (Pearce 1987)
2. Exhaust fan to create pressure gradient
3. Sealed cover in concrete frame
4. Ventilation pipe carried above roof
5. Industrial grade polythene cover permanently fixed to pipe
6. Crushed sandstone or similar sedimentary rock to form suction well to concentrate radon withdrawal from surrounding area

Figure 10.3

◉ Radiation from building materials ◉

If you are using compressed earth-bricks, rammed earth construction or adobe blocks, check all the materials for radon outgassing before proceeding with the construction. If radon is present and no alternative sources are available, seal all exposed, interior faces with a non-toxic, breathing sealer. Outgassing of radon from concrete, brick, earth and gypsum can be controlled by sealing the surface with a non-allergenic paint or seal, but this is a poor substitute.

In addition to radon there are a number of other sources of ionising radiation in building materials that contribute to indoor pollution. The careful selection of materials is the most fundamental step in avoiding high indoor radiation levels.

Radioactivity in a building material is caused by the presence of radioactive materials such as potassium (k_{40}), thorium (th_{232}) and radium (ra_{226}). When added together the radionucleic contents of each of these ingredients in a building material should not, as a general rule, exceed half a Becquerel per kilogram (6 picoCurie per pound) of the material. See Table 10.1.

NOISE

Sometimes a fine view or a site's proximity to schools may be such an important factor in the final decision to buy the site that you accept a prevailing noise problem as a trade-off. Noise exposure can cause anxiety and even illness, but there are a range of strategies that can turn a noisy site into a quiet home environment.

MATERIAL	RADIOACTIVITY
PREFERRED MATERIALS	
Lime	0.12 Bq/kg (1.47 pC/lb)
Aggregates	0.27 Bq/kg (3.31 pC/lb)
Basalt and lava rock	0.33 Bq/kg (4.04 pC/lb)
Composite (reconstituted) stone	0.38 Bq/kg (4.65 pC/lb)
Sandstone and limestone	0.46 Bq/kg (5.63 pC/lb)
LESS ACCEPTABLE MATERIALS	
Kiln-burnt bricks	0.55 Bq/kg (6.76 pC/lb)
Glazed wall tiles	0.56 Bq/kg (6.86 pC/lb)
Granite and slate rocks	0.94 Bq/kg (11.51 pC/lb)
Pumice and tuff rocks	0.90 Bq/kg (11.02 pC/lb)
Slag 'grit' and blocks	1.03 Bq/kg (12.61 pC/lb)
Pumice and slag aggregate	1.20 Bq/kg (14.70 pC/lb)
Synthetic plaster	1.37 Bq/kg (16.78 pC/lb)

* Schneider (1988)

Table 10.1

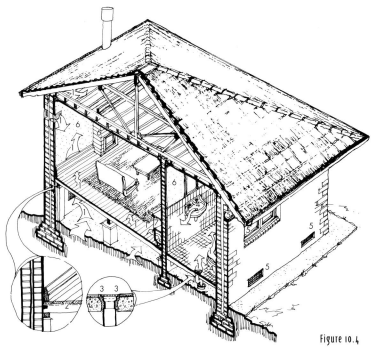

Figure 10.4

1. Radon gas emitted from the soil becomes concentrated in the crawl space under the sub-floor and enters the building's interior through cavities in brick walls, ventilators, the roof space, cracks in ceilings and cornices, cracks between skirtings and walls, and through the floorboards.
2. Seal off all cracks with heavy PVC tape or with a caulking compound. Line the underside of the floor joists with fibre-cement or Greenboard and tape the joints.
3. In the bathroom, radon enters via cracks in a concrete floor, between the floor and the walls, and around floor pipes. Seal all cracks with waterproof caulking.
4. Radon is also present in the water we use. Because radon gas rises out of the water and enters the air of a room, leave plugs in place in kitchen sinks, laundry tubs, basins and baths (this saves water if you have dripping taps) and use a snug-fitting toilet seat and leave the lid down. (Not only does this stop radon emission but also stops germs being spread by the aerosol effect of flushing the toilet.) A dry floor waste (one that does not receive water from a basin, bath or shower) is preferable to a water-sealed one if authorities permit its use.
5. Add ventilation by installing casement or awning windows, as 100 per cent of their area can be opened for ventilation. Install large ventilators in the sub-floor crawl space and extraction fans in bathrooms, toilets and kitchens, and even under the house if your budget can stretch to it.
6. Do not forget that many materials that come from the earth (gypsum plaster, clay and earth bricks, concrete and stone) can release radon gas and should be sealed with a natural sealer or paint.
7. Seal off any unusual vents between the sub-floor crawl space and the interior. For example, some kitchen cupboards ventilate to the sub-floor to have a draft of air passing through a vegetable storage cupboard. Seal these vents off.

Figure 10.4: Reducing radon levels in an existing house

Sound is measured in decibels (dBA). The murmur of water and soft conversation is around 30–40dBA; a normal conversation is 40–50dBA; a conversation at 1 metre (3 feet 3 inches) apart, and the sound of a distant train, is 50–60dBA. The optimum sound level in a house is ideally 25dBA in bedrooms and 32–35dBA in living rooms (see Table 2.1 in Chapter 2). At 35dBA, 32 per cent of people wake up; at 45dBA, 42 per cent wake up; and at 60dBA, 80 per cent. When a material reduces the amount of noise on a site, it is said to attenuate the noise.

◉ Controlling noise ◉

BRICK WALLS

A brick wall 23 centimetres (9 inches) thick and 2 metres (6 feet 6 inches) high, built around the boundary of the site, will reduce noise by 6dBA. If it is 2.5 metres (8 feet 2 inches) high, the noise will be reduced by 8dBA, and if 3 metres (10 feet) high, by 10dBA.

Table 10.1: Radioactivity of building materials (by weight)*

WINDOWS

A 5–20dBA attenuation of sound can be achieved by closing windows. From the point of view of reducing noise, it would be better that windows face away from the source of noise, but for health reasons it is often more important that the windows be reduced in size (to lessen the noise impact) rather than be removed from that side of the building. If feasible, in areas with high noise levels, it is wise to open only the windows that do not face the source of noise; windows facing the noise could remain permanently shut and sealed if alternative and adequate ventilation exists in the room.

A closed window glazed with a single pane of 3 millimetre (⅛ inch) thick glass will attenuate noise by 20dBA. If weather stripping (metal, wood or rubber placed on windows or doors to exclude draughts) is installed on a window glazed with 4 millimetre (⅛ inch) thick glass, up to 23dBA attenuation is possible. Attenuation of 27dBA can be achieved if 6 millimetre (¼ inch) thick glass is used, and 30dBA if it is 112 millimetres (½ inch) thick.

Double glazing achieves the best noise reduction results. For example, a window with two closed weather-stripped sashes of 4 millimetre (⅛ inch) thick glass will attenuate noise by up to 30dBA. Using 6 millimetre (¼ inch) thick panes of glass, the attenuation rises to 35dBA. When one pane of the double glazed window is 6 millimetres (¼ inch) thick and the other is 12 millimetres (½ inch) thick, up to 40dBA noise attenuation can be achieved. The recommended minimum air space between the two panes is 5 centimetres (2 inches), but by increasing the space up to 20 centimetres (8 inches), a further drop in noise of 3dBA occurs. Such a reduction is equivalent to halving the amount of traffic in the street outside. The gap between the panes needs to be indirectly ventilated, by small holes in the sashes allowing air to enter the cavity and move out again, to reduce the likelihood of condensation forming, and should be equipped with sound-absorbing material. In windows sound-absorbing material usually consists of perforated acoustic metal with insulating wool behind the metal, and is located on the sashes in the cavity between the panes of glass to absorb sound that could reverberate in the cavity.

WALL VENTILATORS

It is better to study the air circulation of the room and devise ways to encourage ventilation by convection rather than by wall ventilators. Any wall ventilators that face noise sources need to have built-in baffles.

INSULATION

As well as considering the thermal qualities of an insulation material, you should also look at its capacity to keep out sound.

WALL INSULATION: Simply by constructing double brick cavity walls, you will achieve a noise attenuation of 44dBA. For example, a brick veneer external wall with a cavity separating it from a timber-stud wall that has gypsum board attached to the inside face of the studs will reduce noise by 40dBA. A timber-stud wall 100 millimetres (4 inches) thick, lined on the outside with weatherboard and on the inside with 10 millimetre

Figure 10.5:

(a) Acoustic weakness at eave of a brick veneer house

(b) Use of vibration-damping cork to isolate a house from low-frequency vibration noise in the ground

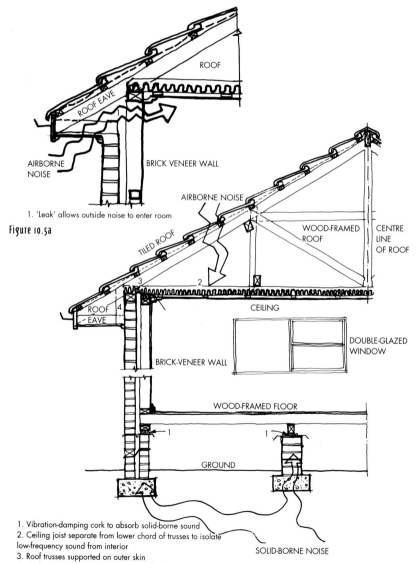

1. 'Leak' allows outside noise to enter room

Figure 10.5a

1. Vibration-damping cork to absorb solid-borne sound
2. Ceiling joist separate from lower chord of trusses to isolate low-frequency sound from interior
3. Roof trusses supported on outer skin
4. Brick outer-wall skin carried up to roof closes 'leak' shown in previous figure

Figure 10.5b

(½ inch) gypsum board, results in a 26dBA drop in noise. Adding 100 millimetre (4 inch) thick insulation between the timber studs of this type of wall, or to a brick veneer wall, achieves a further 5dBA drop in noise level. It is important that there are no gaps in the mortar joints and no windows or doors with attenuation values less than the wall in which they occur.

CEILINGS: A normal, tiled, pitched roof with a 9 millimetre (⅜ inch) thick plasterboard ceiling reduces noise by 27dBA. The noise level is reduced even further when insulation is added to the roof. Cellulose insulation 120 millimetres (4¾ inches) thick, with a density of 46 kilograms per cubic metre (3 pounds per cubic foot), gives an attenuation of 8dBA in a pitched roof and 9dBA in a flat roof. Fibreglass insulation 50 millimetres (2 inches) thick gives 4dBA attenuation in a pitched roof and 5dBA in a flat roof. Fibreglass insulation 100 millimetres (4 inches) thick gives 5dBA attenuation in a pitched roof and 6dBA in a flat roof. There are no figures yet available on the capacity of wool insulation to attenuate noise.

The use of the right ceiling insulation and roof construction methods can achieve as much noise reduction as a correctly constructed double-glazed window.

EXTREME CASES

If you live on a site unpleasantly close to a major source of noise such as an airport, highway or train line, consider a totally different approach than that outlined above. The earth-sheltered house attenuates noise far better than any of the usual types of buildings.

LOW FREQUENCY (SOLID-BORNE) NOISE

One of the most persistent noise problems is the transfer of low frequency noise into a building from outside. These low frequency, solid-borne noises are similar in effect to the sounds tapped out at one end of a long steel pipe handrail which can be heard by putting your ear to the pipe further down. Noise, like that from heavy vehicles, trains (particularly in underground systems) and from engine testing at airport hangars, can be transferred through sandy soil or rock in the ground into the floor of the house. These noises can be controlled using vibration damping technology — a commonly used household material is vibration-damping cork, known as VDC, used in the foundation walls.

HOME SAFETY

In Australia, 72 per cent of all accidents are home-related. An average of 5000 children need medical attention each day at a doctor's surgery or hospital; 200 of these enter hospital, and one or two die (Child Accident Prevention Foundation of Australia 1992). How can we design to minimise the chance of accidents in the home? Just as there are traffic accident black spots in every city, our homes also have certain areas where the risk of accidents is higher. In a typical home, these accident black spots are the bathroom and toilet, the swimming pool, any slippery floor, the kitchen and the laundry.

Falls are a major source of home accidents; in Germany they account for 80 per cent of all home accidents (Schneider 1988). In general, surface falls, caused by slipping on rugs and runners, tripping over single steps and uneven surfaces, and inadequate lighting, are mostly experienced by elderly people. Falls from heights mostly happen to the young.

The main cause of mortality in children under one year old is suffocation due to Sudden Infant Death Syndrome (SIDS, or cot death), soft pillows, faulty and negligent use of restraints, plastic bags and other plastic sheeting. (Plastic can carry an electrostatic charge and adhere to the face.) Burns are a serious safety issue and are more likely to occur when hot saucepans, kettles and teapots are accessible to children. Younger children can be badly burnt when the home water heater is on a high setting. Poisoning is responsible for an increasing number of accidents. Pools are a major source of drowning, while falls in bathtubs with smooth bottoms (lubricated by bubble-bath, soap or shampoo) are also responsible for a number of drownings.

Although the absence of stairs, electricity and swimming pools would make homes safer for children than they currently are, children would still remain ignorant of other dangers, so parental guidance is basic to the safety of children. We need to expand our idea of a child safety zone from the safety of the womb, cot, change table and bedroom, to the whole house, the garden, the street block and eventually, at around five years of age, the whole neighbourhood. These zones are continuously being explored by children, and adults need to anticipate likely causes of accidents.

Crawling, walking or climbing into potential danger is common childhood behaviour, but many designers think only about the needs of adults, forgetting the necessity to minimise childhood accidents. There are many instances of poor design: high chairs and walking frames that tip over easily, stairs without safe handrails, floor surfaces that are slippery when wet or if walked on wearing only socks, strollers that fold too easily, plastic bags without breathing holes, the list goes on and on. While adult supervision overrides all other factors, safe design should accommodate young children. Their growing urges to explore their environment, with their limited control of body movement, need to be catered for by household design. The needs of elderly people, whose mobility may be restricted, should also be considered.

◎ Child safety ◎

The best way to ensure that your house is safe for children as well as adults is to use the following checklist.

KITCHEN

Plan your kitchen so that foot traffic is not encouraged within the triangle of space contained by the sink, refrigerator and stove. Ensure that kitchen windows allow supervision of outside and inside play areas. Use a movable barrier to halt crawling children, or install a stable door, the bottom of which can be closed to restrain children while the top remains open for ventilation and communication. Limit the number of doors leading outside to one.

Ensure that the heating elements of the stove are out of reach. Gas stoves with self-lighting burners and child-proof knobs should be used. Saucepan handles should always be turned away from the edge of the stove, out of arm's reach, and other hot items like teapots placed well away from the reach of children. Install a 15 centimetre (6 inch) high stove-top guard made of light aluminium, hinged to fold away and of the same size as the stove top; this needs to be solid metal to serve as both fence and splash guard. Wall ovens should be mounted at eye level. Do not place curtains or cupboards above or near the stove. Install smoke detectors and fire extinguishers for electrical and oil fires.

The hot water temperature should not exceed 55 degrees Celsius (131 degrees Fahrenheit). Hot and cold taps should be clearly marked and fitted with a selective temperature control valve. The hot tap should be covered with a child-proof knob if children are likely to play at the sink. Install power points away from water and close to where electrical equipment will be used. Avoid dangling electrical leads.

Kitchen drawers should not be able to be removed by a child. They should be located away from the stove and be equipped with safety knobs on all doors. Overhead cupboards should be low enough to be accessed without the need of a step ladder. Install at least one child-proof cupboard in which to store injurious products or kitchen ware. Eliminate sharp edges and corners on all kitchen surfaces. A non-slip floor is essential in the kitchen.

BATHROOM

Mark hot and cold taps clearly and control hot water temperature to 50 degrees Celsius (122 degrees Fahrenheit). Make sure that the temperature does not fall below 50 degrees Celsius (122 degrees Fahrenheit) or you will increase the risk of Legionnaires' Disease developing. (See the Resources List for equipment to control water temperature.) Place child-proof knobs over all the hot taps. Hot water pipes should be insulated and concealed.

Use a non-slip floor surface and always place a rubber mat in the shower recess to avoid slipping. Pick up the bath mat after you have finished, to avoid mould growing beneath it (mould is a major source of allergies). The bath should have a non-slip bottom and the shower taps should be accessible from the shower recess doorway, not located near the shower rose.

Eliminate sharp corners and edges, like projecting soap holders. Avoid overhanging hand basins, as children tend to swing from them. Towel rails should be strong and well secured, and one should be located near the bath. Shower screens should be made of laminated glass. Design the bathroom so that there is no climbing access near windows. Use safety door locks and knobs on bathroom cupboards and install a child-proof medicine cabinet.

Power points should be equipped with safety switches and located in a dry zone, away from the bath, shower or toilet. Avoid extendable cords that allow electrical equipment to be carried to wet areas.

LAUNDRY OR UTILITY ROOM

Use a stable door or a movable barrier. The ironing board should be firmly secured and have adequate space around it. A non-slip floor is essential. Wherever a sewing machine is in use, a floor surface that shows up pins easily should be laid. Install a child-proof cupboard at a high level for detergents and other harmful substances.

Install your clothes washing machine so that a hot water connection is permanently available, as very hot water is required to eradicate dust mites from bed linen. Power points should be equipped with safety switches and be located in a dry zone, clear of all tubs, taps and the washing machine. Avoid extendable cords that allow electrical equipment to be carried to wet areas. All taps should be out of children's reach.

LIVING ROOM

Ensure that you can supervise activities in the living room from the kitchen. Design the room so that there is a clear space for recreation which does not receive cross-traffic. Do not locate seating areas near glass panels. You should provide toy storage space at a low level, accessible to children, and higher level storage for adults. All wall storage and bookshelves need to be securely fixed to the wall or stable enough that they will not topple over should a child climb up on the shelves. Eliminate sharp corners and edges where possible.

There should be safety screens and guards around all heating units. All power points should be equipped with safety plugs. Security screens should preferably be attached inside and open inwards, rather than being fixed permanently on the outside, making escape impossible in the event of a fire. You should not engage dead-locks or security door locks at night — if you must, make sure that the keys are placed on a hook beside the door for easy escape in the event of fire. Train children how to escape should such a situation occur.

CHILDREN'S BEDROOMS

Children's bedrooms need to be easily supervised, so the door should have an unbreakable glass panel in it. Windows should only open 10 centimetres (4 inches) wide. In glassed areas up to 1 metre (3 feet 3 inches) from the floor, use safety glass only. Locate beds away from windows and avoid the use of furniture or toys that can be used to provide access to windows.

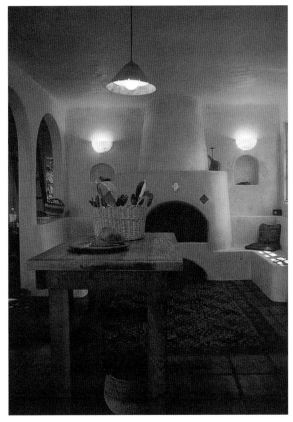

Avoid double bunks in order to prevent serious falls, or at least ensure that children under the age of nine do not use the top bunk. Eliminate sharp corners and edges. A soft floor surface that minimises impact should be used (not carpet, because of dust mites). Provide plenty of accessible toy storage space. If you have toys handed down to you from your parents or grandparents, check to make sure they contain no lead. Keep toys that contain small parts away from toddlers. Choose toys such as sit-in rockers and rocking horses carefully, as some can squash children's toes or fingers. If you have an exercise bike, place a strap tightly around the wheel so that children cannot damage their fingers. Trampolines and plastic-sheet water-slides can be prime accident sites and must be well supervised at all times.

Do not use walking or bouncing frames and make sure that high chairs and cots are stable and well constructed. The vertical slats or dowels on cots should be close together so that an infant's head cannot pass through and become jammed. Choose a stroller that does not fold up too easily, as otherwise it may fold with the infant inside. Do not load the stroller with so many parcels that it may tip over. If you have a cot that rocks, make sure the locking device is engaged when the rocker is not in use.

Do not use rotating ceiling fans, as they present a challenge to growing children to rope onto them and use them for play. If you have rotating ceiling fans, cover them with a guard. Avoid using blinds and curtains with cords.

HIGH-LEVEL BALCONIES AND STAIRS

In general, a split level house is safer than a two storey. Balcony railings should be designed as child-proof barriers, preferably 1.35 metres (4½ feet) high, but at least 1.2 metres (4 feet) high. Avoid designing balconies with glass — if you use glass, up to 1 metre (3 feet 3 inches) from the floor, you should install laminated safety glass. Doors should not open onto landings. There should be good, shadow-free lighting on stairs. Light switches should have bold or luminescent markings on them for easy access in the dark. Any glass at or near the foot of the stairs should be laminated safety glass (not wired or toughened glass, as these cannot be considered tough enough to withstand major impacts with hard materials).

The treads on stairs should be non-slip, the intermediate landings should be at least three treads wide, and the stairs should be easy to clean. Handrails should be placed no less than 86.5 centimetres (2 feet 10 inches) above the line joining the treads of the stairs. There should be an additional top rail at 1 metre (3 feet 3 inches) high. Each stair should be no higher than 14–15 centimetres (5½–6 inches). The balusters (which fill in the space between the handrail and the stairs) must be vertical, as horizontal balusters can be climbed on — balusters should be no further apart than 7 centimetres (2¾ inches) — and risers should be closed in, not left open.

All stairs and landings need a handrail each side with balusters (as above) to the open side of the stair, including basement, attic and spiral stairs. Any accessible roof areas should have a safety barrier of some type. Landings onto which doors open should be as long as the door is wide.

HEATING SYSTEMS AND FIRE PREVENTION

Do not use electric floor heaters or kerosene heaters. Make sure that all fixed heaters are well secured. Fit spark arresters (bronze wire mesh cages to intercept red-hot embers) to fireplace flues and chimneys. Fuel stove flues and chimneys should be well insulated.

All exhaust fans from the kitchen should be ducted to the outside air, as fat and dust build-up is a fire hazard. Smoke detectors should be installed at least in the kitchen, bedrooms and laundry. Fire extinguishers and fire blankets should be located at appropriate places in the house, including the garage.

When designing the house, ensure that the family can evacuate quickly, bypassing areas with flammable furnishings. Provide two separate escape routes for every floor. Discuss the escape routes with the family. Avoid using materials or surface finishes that give off toxic fumes when they burn.

FRONT GARDEN AND ENTRANCES

Separate the areas of the garden used by children from the areas used by vehicles. Avoid providing access from the rear garden into the garage and thence to the front garden. Install child-proof catches to all outside gates and doors. Locate the front door lock at least 1.5 metres (5 feet) above floor level. Do not have doors opening onto the driveway. Design your front garden so that it includes 'go' and 'no-go' areas for children. All ponds and fountains must be safety-fenced, or situated so that children cannot gain access. Place a light at the front and rear entrances to the house. Make sure that there is no climbing access up to roofs and other high places. Avoid using power leads in the garden by installing waterproof power outlets for garden areas. Choose outdoor play equipment and the type of ground surface beneath it with safety in mind.

GARAGE

Your garage should be built far enough away from the house so that vehicle fumes cannot enter the building. If you have an electronically operated garage door, you should also provide a lockable second exit should the door malfunction. Place vents at floor level so that carbon monoxide from car exhaust fumes does not build up.

Choose a floor surface that does not become slippery when wet, and allow for a fall of at least 1:100 (1 centimetre in 100 centimetres, 1 inch in 100 inches, and so on) to an outside drain.

If the garage is to double as a workshop, place duckboards near the workbench so that your feet are not in contact with the concrete floor. Provide lockable cupboards for storage of dangerous materials. Do not store hazardous substances like petrol or pool chlorine in the garage. Do not store toys or play equipment in the garage, or allow children to have access to the garage without supervision. Dispose of toxic materials in the approved way. Group your power points together in one place and install them thoughtfully so that you do not need to use double adapters or extension cords.

Provide a child-proof safety fence, preferably 1.5 metres (5 feet) high, or at least 1.3 metres (4½ feet) high. The fence should be of a type approved by your local authority and must be equipped with a child-proof gate that opens out, away from the fence. Make sure that trees do not grow over the swimming pool enclosure. Use paving that is non-slippery when wet.

Remove all non-pool equipment from inside the swimming area and make sure that all garden furniture is well away from the pool fence and too heavy for a child to move. Store chlorine, other pool and gardening chemicals and gardening tools in a locked storage shed away from the house.

The suction outlets of certain types of pool filters must be equipped with covers in order to deter children from sitting in them. The overflow skim tank (which collects leaves and debris as the water passes through a strainer or leaf basket before it is sucked to the main filter) often has a vacuum cover that can be removed by children. Make sure your suction outlet is larger than a child's buttocks, lest a child sit on the tank and the suction pull them onto the rim of the tank, creating conditions for a very nasty accident (children have been disembowelled this way).

FIRE

◎ Wood heaters ◎

Wood contains a high percentage of water, so a lot of heat energy is required in the initial stage of a fire to dry out the wood before combustion can actually begin. Once the wood has dried out and has started to burn properly, gases are driven out of it, most of which burn. The flames of a fire are these ignited gases. Certain gases will only burn in the temperature range of 100–700 degrees Celsius (212–1292 degrees Fahrenheit). Open fires and some wood heaters do not reach this temperature range, so not all of the

gases are burnt off. Some are released as vapour that condenses on the walls of the flue, causing creosote to form; the remainder enter the air as pollution. Once the gases have been removed from the wood, oxygen in the surrounding air feeds the burning wood, which starts to glow red.

In the most efficient wood heater, complete combustion takes place, which means that all the hydrogen, carbon and oxygen atoms of the wood have been transformed into water and carbon dioxide at the temperature of the air in the room. Under these conditions there is no pollution, odour or smoke. The burner of an efficient heater or stove is designed to encourage the thorough mixing of air and combustion gases, as this will ensure that the wood burns completely. When selecting a heater or stove, look for one with a burner that creates a turbulent condition and hence encourages the complete mixture of air and combustion gases. It is preferable to find a burner that recycles combustion air so the air is used more than once.

Heaters should be airtight because if a heater's combustion chamber utilises the air of a room to mix with the wood gases for the combustion process, major problems can occur. The first and most obvious problem is that the room air on which the occupants depend becomes depleted of oxygen. This happens in the old-fashioned open fire, and even some of the modern heaters and stoves have air intakes that draw on room air. The second problem is that a proportion of the warmed room air will be consumed by the combustion process, wasting valuable energy. Lastly, if all the products of combustion do not pass up the flue, an open combustion system will allow these products to pollute the room. These gases can be highly noxious. The best airtight heaters have an independent ducted supply of outside air and offer efficient, controlled combustion and heat output.

◎ Accidental fires ◎

During a building fire, heavy gases form as a result of combustion. To dispose of these gases, provide high outlets for hot smoke exhaust and adequate cross ventilation at floor level. Install non-ionising smoke alarms in key locations of the house, and check the batteries annually. In the event of a fire, exit quickly to safety in the outside air. In the first minute or so of the fire, you should crawl from the room as there will be more oxygen at floor level, but after that time, you should stand upright because heavy toxic gases will begin to pool at floor level.

PYROLYSIS, THE HIDDEN HAZARD OF ACCIDENTAL FIRES

Pyrolysis is the decomposition of substances due to heat. A multitude of substances are used in modern buildings which, when burnt, change their chemical composition and emit toxic gases. When a fire occurs, more people die from inhaling smoke and toxic gases than because of the flames.

NATURAL MATERIALS: Even non-toxic, environmentally benign materials can become dangerous in a fire. When these materials combust, they give off gases heavier than air which begin to pool at floor level within minutes. Natural materials like wool, cotton and silk are composed of oxygen, carbon and hydrogen atoms, the structure of which is reformed upon heating, resulting in the creation of new molecules. Carbon and oxygen produce carbon monoxide or carbon dioxide, both highly dangerous gases in unventilated conditions. Nitrogen and oxygen molecules produce oxides of nitrogen, which have an immediate toxic effect on the body. Although not considered a significant fire risk, pure wool and wool-based products emit carbon monoxide, carbon dioxide, copious noxious fumes and acrid smoke when they combust. When wool products smoulder, they also give off dangerous gases like ammonia, hydrogen cyanide, hydrogen sulphide and methane.

COMBUSTION PRODUCTS: Fossil fuels, and wood and plant materials that are often used for space heating and cooking mostly emit carbon monoxide and oxides of nitrogen. Gas cooking appliances and unflued gas and kerosene space heaters also yield combustion products that cause serious indoor pollution.

SYNTHETIC MATERIALS: All synthetic textiles, such as polyester and nylon, emit carbon monoxide, hydrogen chloride and hydrogen cyanide during combustion. Plastics generally emit carbon monoxide, hydrogen chloride, hydrogen cyanide and phosgene (a poisonous gas used in chemical warfare and the manufacture of pesticides and polyurethane). Lightweight foam insulation is impregnated with toxic solvents for fire-protection, and when ignited it creates highly toxic gases, including carbon monoxide. When polystyrene foam burns it develops 'candles' that emit flares equivalent in effect to napalm.

HEAVIER-THAN-AIR COMBUSTION GASES: The synthetic and organic chemicals with which we are surrounded turn our environment into a lethal gaseous inferno within several minutes of ignition. Some of the toxic, heavier-than-air gases produced during a fire are listed below.

• Ether is sometimes used as a refrigerant. It is toxic, colourless, nonflammable and smells like sulphur.

• Sulphur dioxide can also be used as a refrigerant. It is colourless, sulphurous in smell, nonflammable and toxic.

• Hydrogen chloride is a pungent, poisonous gas that irritates the nose and respiratory tract and is dangerous to the eyes.

• Liquefied petroleum gas (LPG) is made up of propane or butane, or a mixture of both. It is often used for heating, cooking and refrigeration in areas where normal electrical and natural gas supplies are unavailable. The gas itself is highly flammable and suffocating if it is released uncombusted. If used for cooking or refrigeration it must be stored in special cylinders outside the building.

• Carbon monoxide is a highly toxic gas which is produced by many substances when they combust; it is also found in car exhaust fumes, so can accumulate inside the house if the garage is adjoining.

• The dangerous gas hydrogen cyanide can be released when seemingly inert chemicals like the glue in cupboards or the foam in cushions combust.

House construction to withstand bush and forest fire

Recommendations on detailing for bush and forest fire resistance can usually be found in local fire regulations and guidelines. Your building should be designed and constructed to resist the wind forces nominated by your regional authority as appropriate to the site so that it can resist the winds accompanying a bushfire.

No fire-retardant treatment applied to building materials will make your house completely fireproof. These treatments tend to leach or flake off over time when exposed to the weather. They also outgas chemicals, although when they are used in the open air, this is not a serious problem. While fire-retardant treatments may afford some protection, there is no substitute for sensible, fire-aware design and precautions.

The ideas outlined here relate to our experiences in Australasia. For methods of detailing your building to prevent bush or forest fire, ask your local fire authority and refer to the building standard relevant to your region. (Australian readers should contact the Standards Association of Australia, and British readers the British Standards Association.)

PLAN SHAPE

As a general rule, the closer a building plan is to an elliptical or circular shape, the less it is likely to accumulate burning debris during a bushfire. This also applies to projections of roofs and pergolas. For most situations the simple square or rectangular plan is best. In the overall building plan it is not wise to use porches deeply recessed back from the main building line or recesses that create nooks and crannies where litter and burning debris can collect. Care should be taken that any additions or alterations to the building conform to these overall guidelines.

From the point of view of minimising the effects of bush or forest fire, garages and carports are better sited beneath the main roof of the house. However, according to the principles of healthy house design, the house and garage must be separated. The best compromise in bushfire-prone areas is to make sure that the garage is separated from the main building by at least a 3 metre (10 feet) gap. This will avoid wind-eddying and debris accumulation.

ROOFS

Simple roof shapes, without dormer windows, roof valleys, roof lights and vents, are the most fireproof. The pitch of the roof should be continuous and should not be altered at verandahs and porches. If it is unavoidable for the pitch of the roof to change, the change should be gradual. Gutters should be enclosed to avoid the build-up of debris.

A major danger in the face of a bushfire is that the house can sustain serious window and roof damage due to flying debris. Some say that low-profile buildings fare better in a bushfire than normal buildings, but there is no evidence to prove this.

In bushfire-prone areas, timber shingles should not be used unless special care is taken to install roof sprinklers and use timber species with low flammability. The underside of roof rafters in open-eave construction should be lined with non-combustible material, though this is not necessary in closed (boxed) eaves.

FLOOR CONSTRUCTION

Floor systems appropriate for use in bushfire-prone areas to provide protection from burning debris have differing qualities with respect to healthy house construction. Consult your local fire authority for construction types that comply with their regulations and guidelines.

In bushfire-prone areas it is appropriate to have an on-grade reinforced concrete floor slab or a suspended concrete or timber floor on concrete or brick columns (timber should be treated to your local authority's standards). A suspended concrete or timber floor not more than 60 centimetres (24 inches) above the ground is also suitable, but the flooring, bearers, beams and floor joists need to be treated with chemical fire retardant. The gap around the perimeter of the building, between the ground and the floor, needs to be covered with a non-combustible infill panel no less than 30 centimetres (12 inches) above the final ground level. If fibre cement is used in this panel infill it should be at least 6 millimetres (¼ inch) thick, the joints should be sealed and covered, and all plants should be kept well clear of the walls.

WALLS

If an exterior wall, or its cladding, is made of combustible material (such as wooden weatherboards or clapboards), it will need to be protected from the accumulation of wind-blown fire debris for at least 30 centimetres (12 inches) above the ground level by a non-combustible material such as fibre-cement or galvanised sheet metal. It is not recommended that timber be given a fire-retardant treatment as all these treatments outgas (with the exception of borax, which is not a permanent treatment).

DOORS AND WINDOWS

Windows can be made resistant to wind-blown debris and sparks by installing corrosion-resistant metallic mesh, the holes in which are no bigger than 2 millimetres (¹⁄₁₂ inch). These screens should be designed so that they can be in place when the windows are open. Ventilation openings and weepholes in the exterior walls need to be protected with the same type of mesh.

Exterior doors need self-closing weatherstrips at the bottom of the door. These weatherstrips are designed to move down firmly onto the threshold as the door closes.

WINDOW FRAMES, GLAZING AND SHUTTERS

The least combustible types of window frames and shutters are aluminium and steel, although both can become distorted in shape when exposed to extreme heat. Fire-resistant hardwood is a most suitable material; most other types of timber are also suitable, particularly if they have been coated with a fire-retardant treatment. Timber shutters may ignite when exposed to intense radiant heat. Louvred shutters are unsuitable unless they are constructed of fire-resistant timber, backed by a layer of spark-arresting metal mesh. Avoid PVC frames as they, and all other plastics, will melt.

METAL FIRE SHUTTERS

Metal fire shutters on windows and doors must be close-fitting and have no gaps at the edges. Automatic fire shutters should have an emergency release mechanism fitted in case the electricity fails during a fire and prevents the occupants from escaping. Metal shade screens (of heavier material than wire screens) in front of the windows on the outside and toughened wired glass in the windows themselves all need to be considered as second lines of defence to the use of shutters.

VERANDAHS AND DECKS

To prevent a fire passing through a verandah or deck, the following materials are acceptable: solid timber decking (including tongued and grooved), waterproof plywood or compressed fibre-cement at least 5 millimetres (⅕ inch) thick. Particle board is not a suitable material as it outgasses.

If the deck is no more than 60 centimetres (2 feet) above ground level, the joints between the boards have to be sealed or covered as fire debris trapped beneath the floor is inaccessible and flames will pass through any gaps and set fire to the wall above. The gaps between flooring timbers in an open deck construction should be at least 8 millimetres (³⁄₁₀

inch) wide. The vertical space for access under the deck should not be sealed off, to allow fire-fighter access.

WATER AND GAS PIPES

If pipes carrying gas or water are exposed on the outside of the building, they should be made of metal. For fireproofing purposes, any non-metal pipes should be buried to a depth of 30 centimetres (12 inches).

EARTHQUAKE

When designing a building in an earthquake-prone region, the aim should be to try and ensure the safety of the occupants during and after the earthquake and minimise damage to the structure. Designing for earthquake impact is a complex issue, which may involve factors such as earthquake-generated landslides or soil liquefaction, but the most common earthquake risk to our buildings and personal safety is the effect of lateral ground motion.

Most earthquakes occur along the boundaries of the major tectonic plates (the large, moving plates that make up the Earth's crust) but can also occur far from a plate edge. They generally occur when two plates converge and grind together, or shift past each other. When the strain caused by the tectonic plates exceeds the strength of the rock, sudden fracturing, or faulting, occurs. Ground vibrations result, which are recorded as seismic waves. The magnitude of an earthquake is expressed in terms of the Richter scale, a logarithmic scale in which an increase of one unit denotes a tenfold increase in the earthquake's intensity. Thus, an earthquake that is 8 on the Richter scale is 10 times more intense than that at 7, 100 times greater than that at 6, 1000 times greater than that at 5, and so on.

PLAN SHAPES

In general, square plan shapes will have far greater resistance to structural damage compared to rectangular shapes. Wings and projections extending out from the central core of a building increase the risk. Discontinuities in the building's frame, such as skylights, windows and doors, and any irregular shapes, are all points of high stress which weaken the structure.

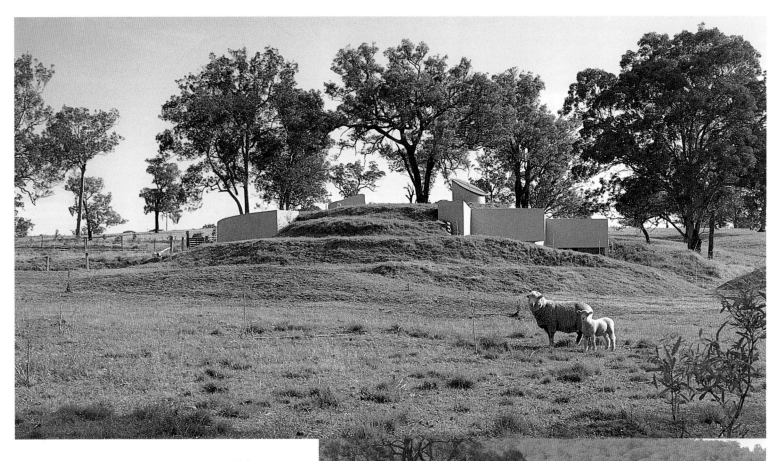

EARTH-SHELTERED BUILDINGS

The most earthquake-stable building type is the earth-sheltered building. In earthquakes most loss of life is caused by collapsing buildings. During an earthquake, massive horizontal forces pass through the ground, as though it is a carpet being shaken. A building sitting on top of such a horizontal wave is flicked by the force, but an earth-sheltered building moves with the earth *en masse*, minimising the twisting and whipping effect of the earthquake. If there is sufficient flexibility in the jointing of the water, gas and electricity service pipes, the building will move with the earthquake, without its structure breaking.

ABOVE-GROUND BUILDINGS

In Australia, a relatively stable continent, the Standards Association has developed codes to control the design of buildings for wind loadings and for earthquakes. Under many circumstances compliance with the standards for wind loading will cover earthquakes but this depends on whether there has been a history of earthquakes in the area where you wish to build, and risk needs to be assessed against economic considerations. If there has been such a record the process of designing to withstand earthquakes will increase your building costs and you will need to consult an engineer to optimise the necessary design considerations and to control costs. In other countries, earthquake codes need to be consulted by your engineer for your regional conditions.

This earth-sheltered house in the Hunter Valley, Aust., withstood the 1989 Newcastle earthquake (5.5 on the Richter scale) without even suffering cracks in interior paint applied shortly before (Architects: ECA Space Design Pty Ltd)

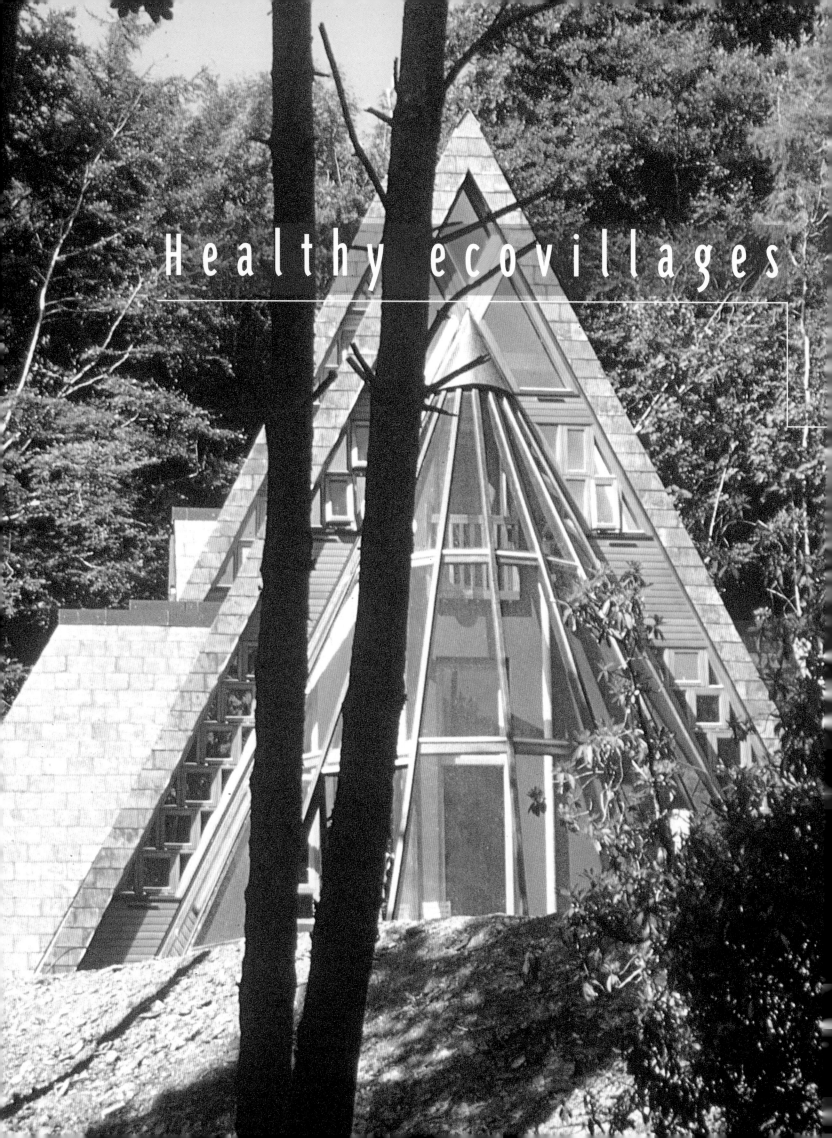

Healthy ecovillages

and ecotowns

althought the ideas in this book have been directed to helping you design and build a healthy home it is possible to apply them to whole groups of houses, communes, retirement villages and so on. The ecovillages and ecotowns in this chapter may stimulate ideas should you become involved in the planning and development of group housing.

Gaian ecovillages represent our best chance to solve the problems of city living, giving us the opportunity to achieve the highest possible levels of ecological sustainability, autonomy and harmony with the environment.

Those who grew up in a village-size community surrounded and interpenetrated by open space in which they were able to run wild, watch the growth of towns and cities with dismay. Where are our grandchildren to experience the unlimited sand hills many of us knew as children and which have disappeared into the concrete around us? Where will they find tadpoles and frogs, or disappear for hours in safety? Has this time passed? Perhaps with the right type of investors and a common philosophy, people may again be able to find a way to live with and within nature.

In the past, various religious and philosophical sects have attempted to forge new ways of communal living with nature, but the 'glue' that held such communities together often became 'unstuck', usually because of intolerance. However, in the last decade, a number of secular alternatives have been proposed, some of which are being implemented. These ecovillages reflect the Gaian principles of ecological sustainability, harmony with the natural environment and near autonomy.

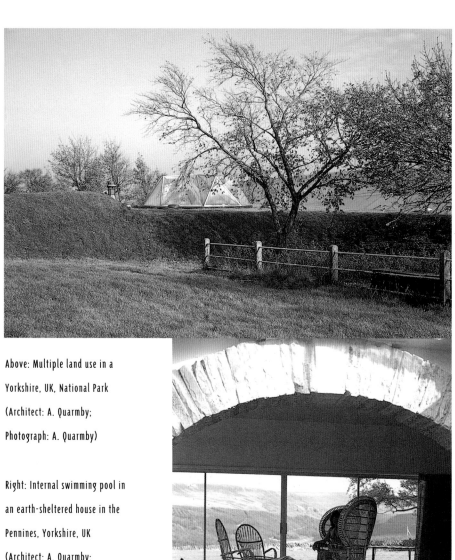

Above: Multiple land use in a Yorkshire, UK, National Park (Architect: A. Quarmby; Photograph: A. Quarmby)

Right: Internal swimming pool in an earth-sheltered house in the Pennines, Yorkshire, UK (Architect: A. Quarmby; Photograph: A. Quarmby)

Page 194: The Eco-house in Bandon, Cork, UK, faithfully follows ecological building principles (Architect: P. Leech, Gaia Associates; Photograph: P. Leech)

It is an encouraging sign that in Australia a code of residential development (AMCORD) has been established, providing guidelines for the development of residential areas, with street layouts designed for optimum solar access, solar energy use, noise control, bushfire resistance and water conservation. While the formation of such a code is a step in the right direction, a greater effort is needed to reach the goal of an ecologically sustainable way of life.

Described in this chapter are a number of examples of ecovillages and ecotowns 24 hectares (60 acres) or more in size. The construction of several of these has already begun, while others are in the planning stage, awaiting the establishment of an ethical source of funding. All are of interest in terms of the physical, emotional, mental and spiritual health they will facilitate for future generations.

Throughout the world, particularly in Scandinavia, many smaller eco community projects are either underway or in the planning stage. The Danish Environmental Protection Agency is developing a handbook of environmentally sound design and will conduct trials of the methods contained in it. Their aim is for people and nature to be burdened as little as possible throughout life. In Bamberton in British Columbia, Canada, a cohousing project has been planned which will house up to 12,000 people who will be able to participate in planning the development. The proposal embodies 'biodiversity policy, conservation zones, vegetation protection zones, share community facilities, organic agriculture, water and energy conservation' (*Eco-Communities* 1994).

Financing and management of ecovillages is a major consideration, as they need to be as self-sustaining as possible. A management plan is also needed for areas of open space so that they remain wild communal parks, maintained at the same standard as the national parks in Australia, for instance. (In the United States and the United Kingdom multiple-use national parks that combine two or more land uses, including limited residential in some cases, are commonplace.)

Before the end of this millennium there will be more people living in cities than in rural areas (Hinsley 1995). The problems of urban living need to be solved. This can only be achieved if there are firm democratic systems in place to encourage debate and the eventual development of sustainable projects. Sustainability, in this sense, must encompass ecological, economic, political and cultural sustainability.

The latest developments in information technology are not necessarily liberating. Without democratic involvement they can become discriminatory and elitist. Citizens' groups need to be fully informed — only then can they play a major role in urban development. When citizens' groups are highly informed and have direct access to professional consultants, they can achieve a lot, such as the successful replanning of inner city districts in London, including the development of the Kings Cross railway land and the implementation of the Greenwich waterfront projects in the United Kingdom.

While urban design cannot solve all of the problems that plague cities, such as pollution, crime, unemployment and poverty, the work of urban designers and architects can be interlocked with that of sociologists and citizens groups, so that the problems of city living are considered in the overall brief. This principle underlies all of the following projects.

◉ Ecovillage proposal, New South Wales, Australia ◉

This ecovillage will be situated on 180 hectares (446 acres) of land with gently undulating terrain and a number of watercourses feeding to a main creek. The principal concern of this development is that it should have minimal environmental impact, be virtually autonomous and be ecologically sustainable in the long term.

It is designed to have a high proportion of indigenous vegetation to balance human-generated carbon dioxide. Trees that grow well in the area without introduced water or nutrients will be selected. All effluent and storm water from the village will be three-stage treated (including reed-bed filtration) and final nutrient removal will make it available for all uses. Water will be totally and independently supplied to the township from within its boundaries by collection in a catchment and by recharging, oxygenating and reusing the ground water. Inside the ecovillage, residents will be able to commute by electric vehicles or by riding on the bicycle paths. The maximum walk to public transport will be 500 metres (547 yards).

Groups of home owners will take responsibility for their section of common to raise organically grown fruit and produce. The orchard areas will be under the overall maintenance plan. Energy will be produced within the village from solar collectors and photovoltaic cells; excess electricity will be sold to the regional grid. Building materials will be chosen that have a low entropic debt, require minimum maintenance and have a long useful life. Buildings will therefore last longer, counteracting the higher initial cost of the autonomous energy systems.

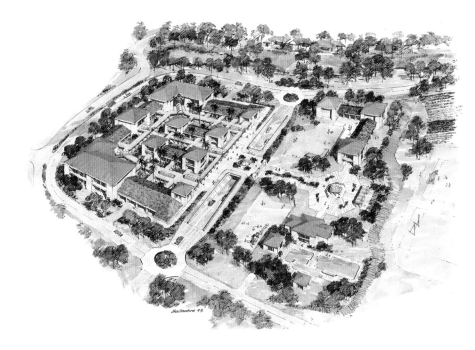

All buildings will be designed to create a biologically healthy environment for the occupants and will make minimum demands on the ecology of the country or the village itself. Overall design and planning will be based on bioenergy principles. Harmonic dimensions, colours and textures will be used to promote emotional, physical, mental and spiritual health. The space of the development property will be optimised by having a judicious mix of closer density housing than is currently evident in urban developments. This increased housing density will be balanced by comfortable private outdoor space and easily accessible open spaces, which will have multiple uses, such as market and crop gardens, water management and urban reafforestation, in addition to recreation.

Social interaction and community integration is an important aspect of this ecovillage. There will be neighbourhood activity centres, business facilities for those who work at home, and facilities for the sharing of resources and information by the whole village. The village will provide opportunities for residential ownership and business investment. All planning, design and development within the village will be accountable by auditing, public exhibition and public debate. Decisions will be based on sociological data gathered from occupants and potential occupants of the village.

Ecovillage civic precinct with marketplace, district school, neighbourhood centre, village square, underground carpark (abandoned brick quarry), commons (including orchards and 'wild' natural areas), turf roofs, walkways, courtyard and mixed-use areas, NSW, Aust. (Architects/Engineers and Urban Designers: The PEOPL Group)

Ethical investment trusts will be responsible for the management and security of all areas, including communal orchards and wild open space.

The ecovillage project will address the high standards of environmental sustainability and social accountability within the planning and design process. As a result it is expected that the correspondingly high standards that have been established for ethical investment will also be matched. This high standard is important not only for achieving an ethical goal but it also may be beneficial to encourage the participation of Ethical Investment Managed Trusts for cost-efficient financing of a staged development or part of the total project. Ethical Investment Managed Trusts may be sought to target the key results of purchasing advantages for sales promotion and the opportunity for reduced purchase-costs by future home buyers.
(The PEOPL Group 1994)

◎ Ecocity proposal, New South Wales, Australia ◎

Surrounded by national parks, state forests, conservation and organic agricultural zones and with 8 kilometres (5 miles) of Pacific Ocean beachfront, the ecocity will be a collection of ecovillages within easy bicycle reach of one another and a Central Business District (CBD). The ecocity will accommodate a large population and there will be room for expansion that causes minimal ecological damage to the beautiful natural environment. There will be a vast area of useable open space in the CBD because the majority of buildings will be earth-integrated, incorporating linked roof gardens.

The buildings will be designed to create allergy-free, healthy environments. The materials used will be as free of chemicals as is practical. Only natural materials will be used in furnishings, finishes and fittings. In the industrial parks and some of the residential areas, there will be continuous open space over the top of the buildings. Light and sunshine will enter buildings through atria or large diameter photonic conduits which are similar in effect to the fibre optic cables that carry telecommunications signals. Incandescent lighting systems will cut in when the sun is not shining.

The streets will not be crammed with polluting vehicles, but will have a predominance of pedestrian malls. Pollution-free public buses and private amphibious electric vehicles will be able to access the malls via underground traffic conduits and an environmentally clean street-canal system.

City blocks will contain commercial or residential buildings of five storeys, with some storeys underground. Commercial space will open on to wide sunlit courtyards landscaped with pools, waterfalls and vegetation. There will be roof-top parklands both at mall level and at five storeys above the pedestrian malls. They could be linked by 'people-movers' such as escalators, moving footways and a canal system with electric amphibious buses and private cars.

All services and facilities will be nonpolluting. Electricity will be generated from a low-head, offstream hydro-dam and will be augmented by solar, wind and other proven alternative energy systems. Energy will be sold to the national grid in off-peak periods. In order to avoid the use of air conditioning, the whole city will have a ventilation system based on computer-controlled, environmental sensor-directed air scoops and a stack-effect ventilation system which vents at high level outlets in the mountain range behind the city. When humidity is excessive, the ventilation air stream will be directed through chambers within the earth for snap cooling. Condensate can be collected and recycled.

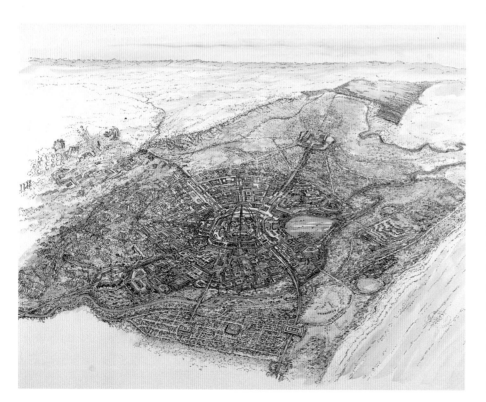

Ecocity proposal, NSW, Aust.
(Architects/Engineers and Urban Designers: The PEOPL Group)

The CBD would not be a typical business district, but an island space where social gathering and entertainment would be of pre-eminent importance. Enjoyment and relaxation will be brought into the work environment. There will be disabled access to all spaces and vehicles, and the network of roof gardens will be easily accessible.

Connected by ramps to the canals and parking areas, there will be a major underground tunnel system with concrete roads which will offer faster transit conditions for private vehicles than prevail on the canals. At the next level down from the private transit tunnel there will be a public transit system. Below that, a transportation network will handle all deliveries of goods. Beneath that again, conduits will carry all services (electricity, gas and water) and waste processing systems as well as accommodating the city's ventilation ducts, cooling and dehumidifying chambers and localised pollution treatment. These tunnels and conduits will be constructed of bioconcrete with reinforcing mesh made from glass/polypropylene to avoid the distortion of electromagnetic fields and to allow incoming deep space and terrestrial radiation to enter without distortion.

It is proposed that the ecocity will be supported by an ethical method of funding based on community ownership of all commons and public land. Citizens will make an initial investment for their residence and an amphibious electric vehicle. As the city proceeds the citizens will share in the increasing value of the estate. City construction and maintenance will be the responsibility of city council members who will be chosen on the basis of their professional skills. The council will be answerable to a Board of Trustees which will also audit all financial transactions.

◎ Halifax Ecopolis Project, South Australia ◎

The Halifax Ecopolis Project will be connected to the infrastructure of the City of Adelaide, South Australia. It is not designed as a stand-alone village but as a 'piece of eco-city'. As an Ecology Centre is planned, the project could become an educational, ecotourism destination. The design proposes a community of 800–1000 people with pedestrian streets, squares and courtyards, and energy-efficient buildings three to five

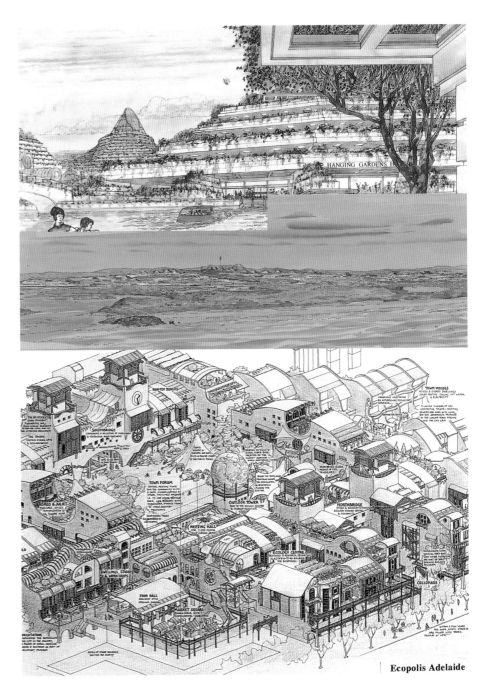

Ecopolis Adelaide

storeys high with lookout towers rising above them. The construction will be of stabilised earth, concrete and timber. The aim is to create spaces which respond to the needs and creativity of the inhabitants and the demands of healthy environmental performance and ecological responsibility. Integral to the functioning of the passive-solar cooling and heating of the buildings is the presence of vegetation, including Permaculture and a corridor of native species.

The residences will be designed based upon the Danish model of cohousing, where each household has their own dwelling comprised of bedrooms, bathroom, living and dining areas and a small kitchen. The dwellings will be clustered around a

Top and centre: Proposal for an ecocity on the New South Wales coast. (Urban designers: The P.E.O.P.L. Group)
Below: The Halifax Ecocity project, Adelaide, South Australia. (Urban designers: Urban Ecology Australia and Ecopolis Pty Ltd)

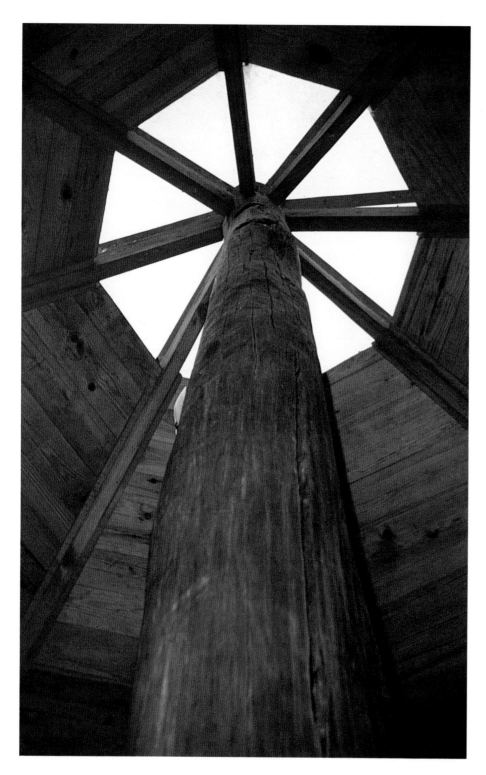

urban sprawl. Its creators hope to optimise energy performance, contribute to the economy, provide health and security, encourage the formation of a community and promote social equity. It has been designed to respect history, enrich the cultural landscape and contribute to the repair, replenishment and improvement of the biosphere.

The Multi Function Polis (MFP), Adelaide, South Australia

South Australia's long-dormant and much maligned Multi Function Polis (MFP) is planned for a site on Adelaide's swamplands. The new MFP Australia board and chief executive expect the project to take 20 years to complete. It is said that it will eventually be an innovative, globally focused and environmentally friendly home for more than 30,000 people.

Crystal Waters ecovillage, Queensland, Australia

On a 258 hectare (640 acre) site about one hour from the Sunshine Coast in Queensland, Crystal Waters ecovillage will house a population of 250–300 people. Houses will be grouped in clusters, oriented to the sun. A charter of commonly accepted ethical principles require residents to care for the Earth and for other people, and to make their own surplus available to the community.

The Tui community, Golden Bay, New Zealand

Reinhard Kanuka-Fuchs, director of the Building Biology and Ecology Institute of New Zealand, has designed and built his own house to be part of an ecologically sustainable, healthy development on 57 hectares (140 acres) of coastal land. A Charitable Land Trust owns and administers the property, and those who build on it are its caretakers. They are:

. . . committed by Trust objectives to enhance [its] environmental, social, educational, cultural and spiritual qualities . . . An environmental-impact plan outlines various problems and solutions involved in the maintenance of the ecological balance, fire safety, land stability and aesthetic appeal of the site . . . Building biology and bio-harmonic design have been considered for the planning and implementation of this project. (Kanuka-Fuchs 1994)

Natural light is integrated with the structure of this excellent example of harmonic architecture, which is to be part of the Tui community ecovillage, Golden Bay, NZ (Architect: R. Kanuka-Fuchs; Photograph: R. Kanuka-Fuchs)

common house which consists of the laundry, workshops, soundproof rooms for music or children's play, and the kitchen and dining room where dinner is shared regularly.

The ecopolis seeks to create patterns of human settlement in which built forms and natural processes are functionally integrated, satisfying human needs as part of the dynamic ecological balance of living systems. The ecopolis development aims to restore degraded land, fit in with the bioregion and halt

Ecovillage, Fiji

A project similar to the Tui community has been planned for an island in Fiji. Centred around ethical investment, its aim is to be a haven for health, relaxation and learning, and to contribute to the local economy. The project will be developed according to the principles of ecological site-planning, Permaculture, *feng shui* and geoenergetics. It will incorporate environmental architecture, making use of biologically benign and natural materials. All buildings will be designed to promote a healthy environment and to integrate sensitively into the cultural setting.

Davis Ecovillage, California, United States

The development of the city of Davis, California, began in the early 1970s in response to energy shortages. Integral to the planning of the city was the use of solar energy and bicycle transport. Two hundred houses were established on 24 hectares (60 acres) of market garden land, in accordance with a 'village homes' concept that the home owner should be involved in the urban planning process. Homes are sited in groups of eight, all facing north/south. The land surrounding the houses, the Common, is controlled by the residents, who use it for growing vegetables, holding social activities and as a children's playground. Greenbelts are allocated for the use of the entire community, as bicycle ways, small orchards and mini-parks. A fifth of the land is used for fruit trees and vines, and just over a tenth for communal gardens and personal garden plots. Residents pay 40 per cent less for their energy than the remainder of Davis City (Hopkins 1992).

Celebration, Florida, United States

When Walt Disney died in 1966 he was in the midst of planning what he called the Experimental Prototype Community of Tomorrow, a high-tech town featuring monorails, moving pavements, centralised computer control and roadways enclosed in a climate-control dome. Several decades on, The Walt Disney Company has resurrected the idea in the form of the town of Celebration, Florida. While the town will be equipped

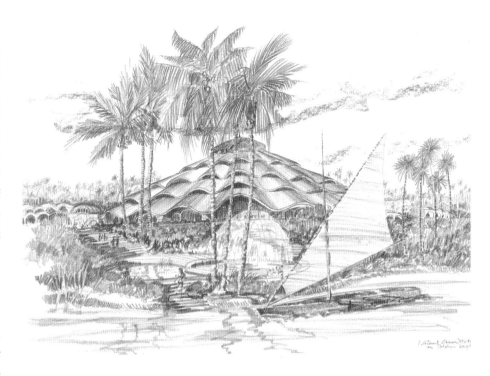

with technology well beyond what could have been imagined in the 1960s, the planners of Celebration have diverged from Walt Disney's futuristic vision, concentrating instead on people's desire to belong to a community.

Walkways, cycle paths and parks will dominate the town which will take up 2025 hectares (5000 acres) and be surrounded by 1863 hectares (4600 acres) of wilderness area. The downtown area will be small and built around a lake. All water, gas, sewerage and electricity services will utilise the latest technology and be designed with environmental principles in mind. Telephone services will be supplied via fibre optic cable. For the local children traditional classrooms will be a thing of the past. The school buildings will contain large 'hearth' areas with comfortable reading chairs and window seats overlooking wetlands. Every student will have access to computers linked to the town's information system and the Internet. The town will be serviced by a hospital that has been designed not just as a place for the sick, but as a facility for providing information and fostering a healthy lifestyle.

It is planned that Celebration will eventually contain around 8000 homes and have a population of about 20,000 people.

Thatch-roofed communal centre and hotel for the Fijian ecovillage (Architects/Engineers and Urban Designers: The PEOPL Group)

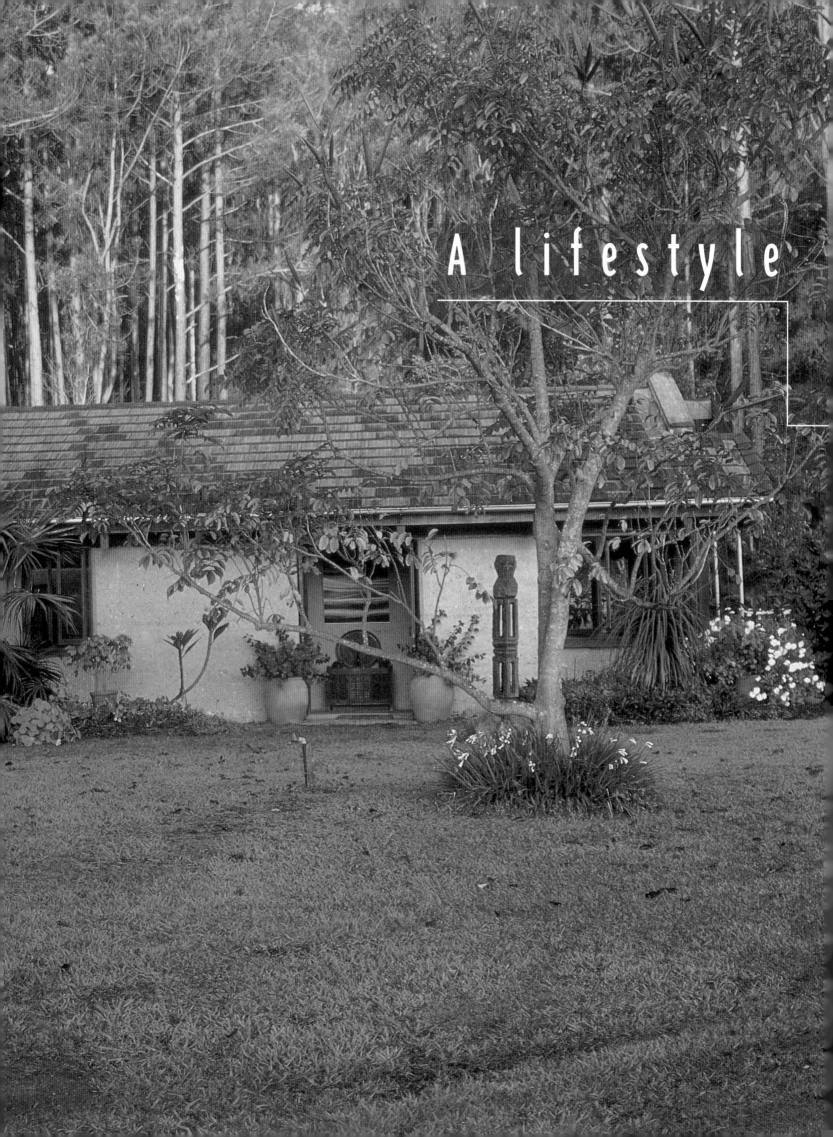

A lifestyle

that respects gaia

deforestation, soil degradation and air, water and heat pollution are degrading the Earth's natural solar-drive chain, which begins when plants turn sunlight and carbon dioxide into carbohydrates through the process of photosynthesis. The stored energy of the carbohydrates is released when combined with oxygen during the plants' respiration. Animals, including humans, in turn consume the plants and respire. During both photosynthesis and respiration, heat is released, to be absorbed by the planet and the atmosphere. This heat, which is the ultimate pollutant, has been entering the planet's 'heat sink' for billions of years.

I use the term Gaia not to propose a human feminine goddess, but to encompass the idea that the entire living pelt of our planet, its thin green rind of life, is actually one single life-form with senses, intelligence and the power to act. (Pedler 1979)

ENTROPIC DEBT

The Second Law of Thermodynamics states that all processes eventually tend towards disorder or chaos, known as entropy. Entropy is the heat released when a pen moves across paper, the heat released by the friction generated when you rub your hands together, the heat in the flaming sweep of a comet falling through the atmosphere. This heat loss was first termed entropy in 1850 by the German physicist, Arthur Eddington, who considered it the supreme law of nature. Entropy exists in all systems.

As a system functions, it loses heat to the atmosphere and its entropic debt increases. When a great deal of energy has been invested in the manufacture of something, it can be said to have a high entropic debt. It incurs that debt because energy has been used to reorganise its particles to form a special shape, for example, when bauxite is transformed into aluminium, which is in turn transformed into a window frame. If we recycled the window frame by melting it down, the resulting aluminium ingot would have a low entropic debt, but if we made the ingot into an automobile part we would again increase its entropic debt. A raw material, such as bauxite, can be said to have *high entropy*, as its molecules are still in their original chaotic state. Once energy has been expended on the bauxite, the resulting aluminium can be said to have *low entropy*, because the molecules have been ordered into a particular form, and a *high entropic debt* because of the waste heat generated in its processing.

In its lifetime, a plant or animal produces minimal waste heat because when it dies it re-enters the solar-drive chain by decaying into soil nutrients, which then sustain new plant growth. Humans, on the other hand, are great creators of waste heat because they use science and technology to order physical matter, creating objects such as buildings and machinery. Every item that human beings have ever made, whether from artificial or synthetic materials, has added to the total heat stored by the planet. Since the industrial age began, the rate of creation of waste heat has increased exponentially. Only 28 per cent of the fuel used by a power plant is turned into electricity, the remaining 72 per cent is converted into waste heat. These generating plants should be called 'waste heat generators' as they produce more heat and chaos than electricity.

Since the lifeweb of Gaia began, humankind is the only species to have altered the interdependence of all life forms on the solar-drive chain. By using fossil fuels and creating new electrical and chemical conditions, supposedly to improve the quality of life, we have created an immense unbalance, a situation that the planet will not be able to endure much longer. The Second Law of Thermodynamics also tells us that entropy must increase in all irreversible processes. Life itself is irreversible. No matter what natural evolution or human intervention does to order complexity, the 'net contribution will be an [ultimate] and permanent increase in the entropy and disorder of the Universe' (Adams 1994).

Our duty is to invest the least amount of energy in the physical objects we need for our survival. In this way we will incur the lowest possible entropic debt and extend the viable life of the planet. The alternative is to continue on our present course, investing vast amounts of energy in the maintenance of our present lifestyle, releasing huge quantities of disorganised energy in the form of heat, which eventually becomes part of the permanent heat sink of the planet.

THE GAIAN LIFESTYLE

Unlike other species, humans are equipped with the powers of self-awareness, creativity and language, giving us the capacity to transcend the mere basics of satisfying physiological needs. Yet our total assault on nature has increased exponentially since agricultural settlements first began. Will we continue to mistreat nature, ensuring a quick extermination of our and other species — or will we work towards an infinitely renewable future? If our thought processes had not become so alienated from our feelings and intuition, this would be an insulting question.

Every time we use plastics, insecticides, aluminium, kiln-fired bricks and tiles, chemical paints and cleaners we help push humanity further into the entropic trap. Society's coercion of its members to consume high entropic debt products has been thorough.

For the last 12,000 years, the human race has devised one ideology after another, all of them anthropocentric, showing disregard for nature's requirements. Capitalism, socialism, Marxism, Maoism, monarchy, oligarchy and democracy all represent ideologies based on the control and dominance of human beings. Even the democracy of ancient Greece depended on a slave population. In contrast, the Gaian way of life is based on placing the needs of the Earth organism first and humanity second.

The industrial age has entered every facet of our lives. How can we entirely eliminate all its processes and products? We cannot, but we can make inroads by reviewing our basic needs for shelter, food, drink and bodily functions. Many rural communes have collapsed because they aimed to become self sufficient, when there is no such thing as true and total self sufficiency, as waste heat results from most of life's activities. In the past we thought it was possible — the 'autonomous house' is a manifestation of this. The autonomous house — that is, a house in which all the energy to run and maintain it is generated within the property and all wastes are completely recycled — could be likened to a 'land-based space station' (Vale 1976). But even in space, self-sufficiency is a myth. As Vale has remarked: 'you can't knit light bulbs'.

The Gaian way of life provides an alternative to the concept of autonomy. It has the potential to join and keep together people whose purpose is to live in cooperation with Gaia. Its ideals carry evolutionary potential. By presenting alternatives to industrial society, it could eventually change the economic balance, but it is not a revolution in the usual sense of the word. It is non-violent and does not seek to install another authoritarian system.

The development of computing systems and databases has radically altered the way humans interact with each other; no longer are all daily transactions made face to face. Do you know the name of your bank manager or local government representatives? Does a person living in the suburbs know the neighbours two or three houses away? The Gaian lifestyle provides an alternative to this widespread alienation.

The stated aims of the Gaian lifestyle, based on the premise that no action should be knowingly performed that will adversely affect Gaia's systems, are:

- To develop a way of life based upon minimising entropic debt and energy-use.
- To consume goods as far up the solar-drive chain as possible.
- To reject fossil fuel products wherever possible and rely instead on the solar-drive chain.
- To search for ways of restoring a relationship with the Earth organism, rejecting ideologies requiring that human beings dominate and exploit it.
- To develop a science with its principal premise being that all living things are interrelated in a holocoenotic web of life.

To these principles we add those of Baubiologie™, which relate to how we should design and construct the shelters in which we live:

- Consider geo-biology when selecting building sites. Locate homes at a reasonable distance

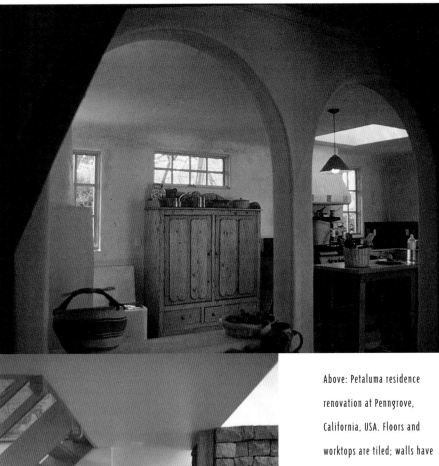

Above: Petaluma residence renovation at Penngrove, California, USA. Floors and worktops are tiled; walls have three coats of natural plaster and a natural-coloured finish (Architect: C. Venolia; Photograph: C. Venolia)

Left: This residence in British Colombia, Canada, has all natural finishes. The rock wall acts as a thermal-storage element and is used in conjunction with a minimal-emission wood-burning enclosed-combustion stove (Photograph: D. Pearson)

from centres of industry and main traffic routes. Create housing developments where dwellings are well separated from one another by green areas.

- Plan homes on an individual basis, considering the family's and the individual's needs.
- Use building materials of natural origin. All wall, floor and ceiling materials should allow air diffusion. Indoor air humidity should be regulated

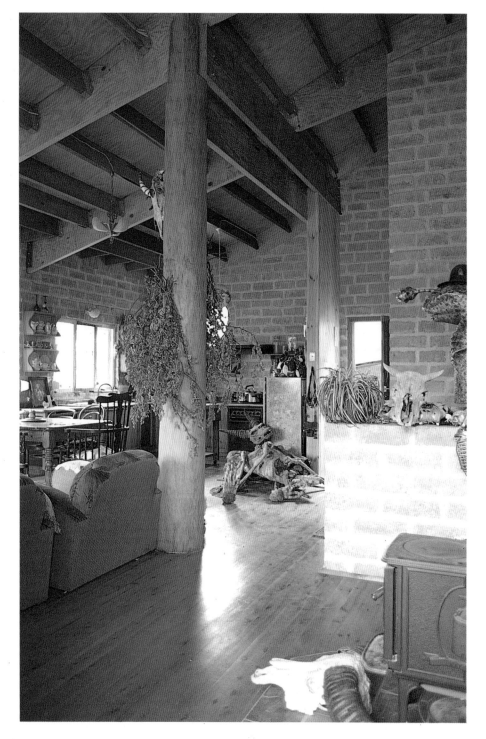

A home with completely natural finishes in the Blue Mountains of NSW, Australia. Elements include Australian eucalypt poles, compressed earth-brick walls, and Australian cypress (termite resistant) flooring (Architect designers: S. and D. Baggs)

• Ensure that buildings either smell pleasant or are neutral in odour; no toxic fumes should be present.

• Use light and colour in accordance with nature. Design with shapes and proportions in harmonic order.

• Provide adequate protection from noise and sound vibrations.

• Use building materials that have little or no radioactivity.

• Preserve natural electric field conditions and physiologically advantageous ionisation on the site. Refrain from altering the natural magnetic fields and minimise artificial electromagnetic fields. Restrict alterations of important cosmic and terrestrial radiation.

• Use ergonomically designed furniture made from appropriate materials.

• Minimise environmental impacts and high energy costs by producing appropriate building materials. All building and production methods should avoid the over-exploitation of limited raw materials as well as minimising harmful side effects and social damage.

◎ The Gaian lifestyle diet ◎

The Gaian attitude to food consumption is based on the solar-drive chain. Plants are considered to be highest on the solar-drive chain, as they are closest to the energy source of the sun, collecting sunlight through their leaves and converting it into energy through photosynthesis and respiration. The plants use this energy to grow and may subsequently become food for animals that are a step down on the solar-drive chain from the plants. These animals may in turn be eaten by other animals (including humans), which are another step down again on the solar-drive chain.

Immense amounts of the sun's original energy are wasted along the way. At every step in the chain around 90 per cent of the energy of the previous step is lost as inefficient chemical transfer in the form of waste heat. For a person to gain 1 kilogram (2¼ pounds) in weight, they would need to eat 10 kilograms (22 pounds) of fish. The fish would need to have consumed around 100 kilograms (220 pounds) of prawns, worms, and other organisms, which in turn would need to have consumed around 1 tonne (2205

naturally by using hygroscopic materials. Neutralise indoor air pollutants by using interior surface materials that are absorbent and hence provide air filtration.

• Consider the balance between indoor heat storage and thermal insulation, as well as the balance between surface temperature and air temperature. Use thermal radiation in heating, employing solar energy as much as possible.

• Through your choice of building methods and materials, encourage low humidity and rapid drying in new buildings.

pounds) of plankton. So, in order for one human being to gain 1 kilogram (2¼ pounds) in weight, 1 tonne (2205 pounds) of these basic lifeforms would be needed (Pedler 1979). The higher up we eat on the solar-drive chain the less energy we waste.

The average meat-eater in the western world consumes an amount of flesh equivalent to approximately 930 kilograms (2050 pounds) of grain per year, while a vegetarian consumes about 180 kilograms (397 pounds). This means that the world provides more than five times the land area to raise crops for carnivores than it does for vegetarians. Vegetarianism is a major change of lifestyle for those who currently eat meat. A decision to become vegetarian should only be undertaken after careful consideration, particularly if you have immune deficiency problems, in which case a compromise diet incorporating fish may be appropriate. This should be discussed with your holistic practitioner.

Wholemeal flour is a nutritionally well balanced foodstuff containing not only a wide range of vitamins, minerals and carbohydrates but also essential fibre. It is high up the solar-drive chain and has a low entropic debt. Processed white flour, on the other hand, lacks many of the nutritional benefits of wholemeal flour. In Greek and Roman times white flour was related to wealth and prestige and in many present-day cultures, whiteness is synonymous with purity, cleanliness and achievement in society. White bread damages our health but conservatism and cultural inertia are formidable influences. Baking your own bread from wholemeal flour is one contribution you can make to the Gaian lifestyle.

THE HEALTHY DIET PYRAMID

The healthy diet can be visualised as a pyramid. At the base are those foods we should eat the most of and at the apex those we should eat the least of. At the bottom of the pyramid, and making up 50 per cent of a healthy dietary intake are the vegetables (except starchy ones like potatoes, sweet potatoes and pumpkin). Next are the complex carbohydrates such as breads, cereals, fruit and starchy vegetables, which should make up about 35 per cent of our diet. Protein from fish, dairy products and eggs should make up about 10 per cent of our daily diet (meat also contains protein, but the serious Gaian avoids meat consumption).

Refined carbohydrates (sugar) and fats should make up only 5 per cent of our daily intake. Refined carbohydrates include cakes, 'health' bars, chocolate and carbonated drinks, all of which should be considered as treats. Fats include butter, margarine, oil, nuts, coconut, cream and mayonnaise. No more than three teaspoons of fats should be consumed in one day. Alcohol also belongs in this part of the pyramid and should be eliminated from the diet or at least mimimised (Doctor N. Malouf, Prince of Wales Hospital, New South Wales, Australia).

THE INSIDE STORY ON VITAMINS

At the beginning of this century only the best land and most fertile soils were farmed and crops were rotated to allow the soil to recover. Today, continuous cropping and the overuse of fertilisers mean that soils have become depleted and loaded with toxic chemicals. These chemicals take over 20 years to weather out of the soil.

Foods grown during the early 20th century were also largely unrefined and unprocessed. Now, crops are prematurely harvested and force-ripened in storage, destroying the natural proteins and enzymes. These inferior foods cause nutritional disorders, deficiencies, lowered immunity and dysfunctions in body chemistry. Vitamin and mineral supplements have become necessary not only to replace those that have been lost from crops but also to help overcome the toxic substances we unintentionally ingest.

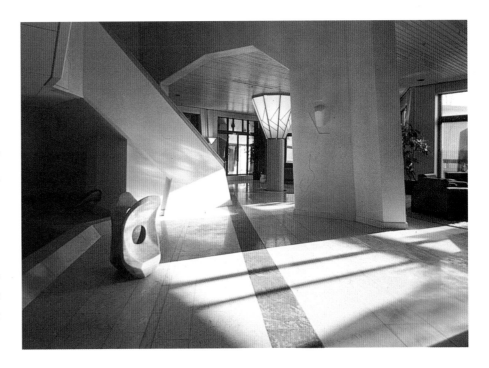

The ING building in Amsterdam, the Netherlands (Architects: T. Alberts and M. van Huut; Photograph: D. Pearson)

As a general rule, most bargain-priced vitamins are comprised of synthetic chemicals. Many medical practitioners claim that the these synthetic chemicals have a molecular structure identical to natural vitamins — similarly, many agriculturalists claim there is no difference between chemical and organic fertilisers. In nature, vitamins do not occur in isolation but in complexes, a quality which is not reproduced by synthetic vitamins. Naturally occurring vitamin C complex is made up of 24 components, vitamin B of 22, vitamin E of nine, and so on. Natural sources also contain a spectrum of yet undiscovered vitamins which synthetic vitamins obviously cannot match. Brewers' yeast, for instance, contains some potent but as yet unidentified 'B-vitamin factors' (Airola 1987) which your body would not get from taking a synthetic vitamin B supplement.

For long-term supplementation of a diet deficient in nutrients, only natural vitamins should be taken, rather than synthetic ones. The only way to tell the difference between synthetic and natural vitamins is to read the label carefully. If it does not specifically state that the vitamin is natural or derived from natural sources, assume it is synthetic. Be on your guard, as the words 'natural' and 'organic' are sometimes misused.

To heal certain ailments, vitamins are sometimes used at doses well above the ordinary requirements of nutritional balance. The stimulating, healing and protective effect they have when used in this way differs completely from their use in correcting nutritional deficiencies. When vitamins are used in higher than recommended doses very specific conditions must be put on their use. Such doses should be approved and strictly supervised by a carefully chosen health practitioner.

FOOD PACKAGING

The packaging on processed food and drink is made using complicated, high entropic debt procedures. The products inside are usually pallid, over-flavoured and far inferior to those prepared in your own kitchen. After consuming the food, the packaging, which took so much energy to produce, is consigned to the garbage dump. Packaging can make up an average of 20 per cent of the price we pay for food (Pedler 1979). When we dispose of the packaging we pay again, for garbage collection and disposal.

Consider a glass bottle of commercial lemonade. No lemons are used in its manufacture, just citric acid, carbonated water, sugar or synthetic sweetener, chemical flavourings, preservatives and perhaps a colouring agent. The glass takes an immense amount of energy to produce, 60 per cent of which enters the environment as waste heat (Bate 1976). This is a complete waste of resources if the container is discarded after use. Recycling is absolutely essential for all containers, whether plastic, glass, steel or aluminium.

If we left every shop as though we had no garbage collection services at home, that is, having removed all excess packaging, a lesson would be learnt by all. Take your own containers and bags when you shop so that you do not need to make use of the shop's plastic bags. If such a procedure were implemented by hundreds of thousands of people, changes *would* occur.

HOME PRODUCE

Why not redefine work by producing what you can from raw materials, primary produce and goods within the home? This may radically reduce your need to work outside the house. If enough people did this, it would not only have an impact on the natural environment by reducing the load on public and private transport but would also improve the quality of home life.

STORING FOOD

Storing food in a refrigerator with a deep-freeze unit built into it is a worthwhile contribution to the Gaian lifestyle because it uses a minimum amount of energy and allows you to store food without preservatives. You can buy produce in bulk at low prices and store it for some months until you are ready to eat it. Choose a refrigerator that contains a non-chlorofluorocarbon (CFC) refrigerant, to help preserve the ozone layer. Most governments provide a ranking system for energy efficiency; choose one with a high rating. Reject the separate freezer cabinet because the heat-pump cycle releases large quantities of irrecoverable waste heat into the atmosphere.

Avoid purchasing deep-frozen food from supermarkets or shops as it has been transported in energy-intensive freezer trucks and stored at low efficiency in banks of deepfreezes. This energy-profligate process delivers a convenience food which has lost most of its flavour.

Dried fruit, herbs and vegetables keep for even longer periods than frozen foods, so consider buying a food drier. Dried fruits are a very useful and nutritious addition to the diet and vegetables dried in season can be used any time of the year in cooking.

A healthy water supply

Our water supplies contain many substances that may adversely affect our health. Chlorine, added as a disinfectant, has been linked to heart disease, the formation of arterial plaque, bladder cancer, bowel and stomach cancer, reduced intake of vitamins C and E by the body and birth abnormalities. Inorganic fluorides, which are the toxic waste products of aluminium production, are added to about 70 per cent of the world's water supplies with the aim of preventing dental caries. According to independent researchers Morton Walker and Kurt Donsback: 'many studies have shown that a level of about one part of fluoride per million parts of water (the concentration added to some of the drinking water) can cause a host of disorders including cancer, allergies, kidney and heart disease'. Aluminium is added to the water supply during the treatment process. It has been linked to cancer, tendonitis and inconclusively to Alzheimer's disease. Radon, which can cause irradiation of the digestive system if taken in sufficiently high doses, is also present in water supplies. The main sources of radon-rich waters for domestic use are deep aquifers, tunnels and spas.

There are a number of methods of reducing the amount of the additives present in water, all of which vary in their degree of success. Water filters reduce the amount of rust particles, dirt, suspended matter and chlorine in water and improve its taste. The most common type of filter utilises a cartridge containing charcoal, the surface of which attracts impurities such as chlorine and the particles that colour the water. These filters are relatively inexpensive but it must be remembered that cartridges need to be changed regularly to maintain their efficiency and stop the growth of bacteria. After filtering it may be necessary to add mineral salts and electrolytes to make up for those removed. We do not recommend the use of jug filters as they do not do much more than improve the taste and colour of the water. Ceramic filters are available but some clog easily and the rate of water flow is usually slow.

In the process of reverse osmosis water passes through a membrane fine enough to stop large molecules including bacteria, viruses, parasites, toxic heavy metals, pesticides, chemical wastes, fluoride, allergens, asbestos, carcinogens and fertilisers. The contaminants are then washed out. As oxygen molecules pass through the membrane faster than water molecules, the filtered water becomes oxygenated. It is a slow process, with around five litres (one gallon two pints) being used to obtain one litre (two pints) of filtered water. Such filters are usually quite expensive.

Distillation involves boiling water and condensing its vapour. It is good for removing chlorine but cannot remove synthetic organic chemicals because they have a much lower boiling point than water, hence reach the vapour state earlier and condense in the distillate. Therefore if the distillation process is to be used the water should be filtered through a carbon filter first. All minerals are removed by the distillation process so electrolyte and mineral supplements should be taken to prevent cramps and other health problems.

Placing water in a clear glass bottle with the lid off in the sunlight for several hours enables chlorine to outgas. Simply boiling your water will also remove chlorine but has the added effect of concentrating the minerals already present.

Purchasing your drinking water in bottles does not necessarily ensure a healthy water supply. Some brands have been found to be more polluted than tap water and all bottled water should be treated as though it is tap water unless the manufacturer can provide a full contents analysis specifying bacterial, mineral and fluoride levels. When the Australian Consumers' Association (ACA) tested 25 bottled non-carbonated waters, they concluded that not one was any safer or healthier than tap water. Only seven complied with the bacterial standards of the Food Code. Particular attention should be given to the radiation levels in all spring or mineral waters. Take care with water collected from metamorphic or igneous rock sources or soils formed from these types of rock. Unless you are prepared to purchase a detector to reveal the extent of radon in your favourite bottled water, the next best thing would be to boycott such products until manufacturers reveal the level of radiation activity along with other

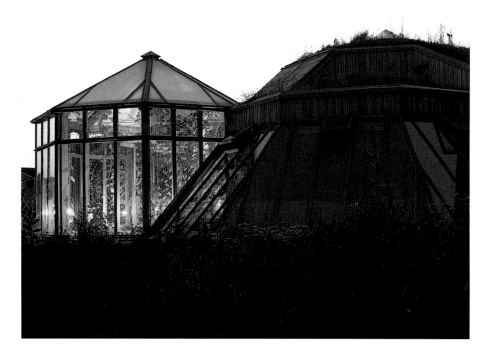

Earth-sheltered house with solarium, Kassel, Germany (Architect: G. Minke; Photograph: D. Pearson)

You should walk with your head erect but relaxed, eyes ahead, shoulders kept low, arms moving vigorously with definite elbow bends and hands slightly clenched, thumbs tucked in and fingers turned inwards.

Oxygen is the essential fuel for every cell in the body so to gain the optimum benefit from walking you need to breathe correctly. With each breath the ribs should move forwards, backwards and sideways, permitting the diaphragm to move downwards and the lungs to fully expand.

Water conservation

To harvest 1 kilogram of wheat, 500 litres (110 gallons) of water are required, while 1 kilogram of rice requires 1919 litres (422 gallons). One kilogram of beef, however, takes 21,000–50,000 litres (4619–11,000 gallons) of water to produce. Compare this with the water needed to manufacture the average car: 23,780–29,060 litres (5230–6392 gallons), just a little more than is required to produce 1 kilogram of beef (Pedler 1979). Industrial production uses up huge quantities of water, with the manufacture of plastics being one of the worst offenders. This is an area of our lives over which we can exercise some individual control, by avoiding as many such manufactured products as possible. We can have the most control, though, by making sure that we use water wisely in our own homes.

TAPS

Aerating taps and spouts are inexpensive, reduce splashing and can reduce flow rates by up to 50 per cent without reducing the effectiveness of the water stream. Five per cent of water can be saved by using quarter-turn taps as they provide better control. Such taps also avoid drip-leaks by having ceramic seat-valves instead of washers. Repair all dripping taps, as a tap leaking one drip each second wastes 1000 litres (264 gallons) of water each year. A single lever or knob control instead of hot and cold taps can avoid people wasting water while they adjust taps to get the water at the right temperature. (They are only suitable for water connected to the mains, not to tanks.)

BATHROOM

Showers, in general, use as much water as a full bath. Install a smaller bathtub, recycle water to the garden and restrict your showers to three or four minutes. Install a flow-control valve to save water in the

pollutants. Generally speaking, you should always try to buy it in glass bottles or remove it from the plastic container as soon as you arrive home.

One way of getting around the problem is to use rainwater run-off from your house's roof so long as the rainwater in your area is not badly polluted. The first portion of run-off is not suitable for drinking and should only be used for flushing toilets, washing and watering the garden. It is wise to place some limestone in the collection tank to counteract acids, metals and salts from the air and roof materials. This need only be one or two brick-size lumps suspended on nylon twine and well secured to the inspection hole at the top of the tank so that all surfaces are exposed.

Exercise

Exercise is a vital part of the healthy Gaian lifestyle. Walking is the best form of exercise, putting the body, mind and spirit in tune with nature. It can be done by anyone, regardless of age, requires no special equipment and helps to achieve aerobic fitness. When your body uses energy quickly, it uses kilojoules (calories) more efficiently and you become more mentally alert.

Pace walking, that is, walking at a rate of around 120 steps per minute, should be undertaken for 30–45 minutes four times a week at least. This will stimulate your endocrine system and increase the rate of your circulation and metabolism.

shower. Choose a toilet with a variable flush, which uses either half or the full cistern of water. If your toilet does not have this facility, place a plastic bag full of water in the toilet cistern to reduce the quantity of water used in flushing. If you put 1 litre (¼ gallon) in the bag, you will save that amount of water per flush. Do not leave the tap running when you brush your teeth as this can waste up to 3.8 litres (¾ gallon) of water. Put the plug in the basin and fill it when you wash your hands as this uses on average 1.9 litres (½ gallon) of water, while leaving the tap running uses about 3.8 litres (¾ gallon). When cleaning the bathroom, use washing soda, sodium bicarbonate or vinegar rather than commercial cleaning products.

KITCHEN

About 10 per cent of all household water use occurs in the kitchen. Dishwashers use excessive quantities of water, averaging 40–50 litres (10½–13¼ gallons) of water per load, whereas dishwashing by hand only uses around 18 litres (4¾ gallons) of water. Waste disposal units use about 30 litres (8 gallons) of water per day and pollute the sewers with organic material.

LAUNDRY

Front-loading machines use approximately 25 per cent less water than top-loading ones. Washing machines with a suds-saver function use about 35 per cent less water than those without. Wear natural fibres such as wool, cotton, silk and linen. Avoid ironing if possible because the process incurs a high entropic debt. Garments should never be dry-cleaned, as the process incurs a high entropic debt and involves toxic chemicals.

Healthy house designed according to Gaian principles, located on the idyllic New Zealand coast (Architects: J. Schulze and F. Poursoltan; Photograph: F. Poursoltan)

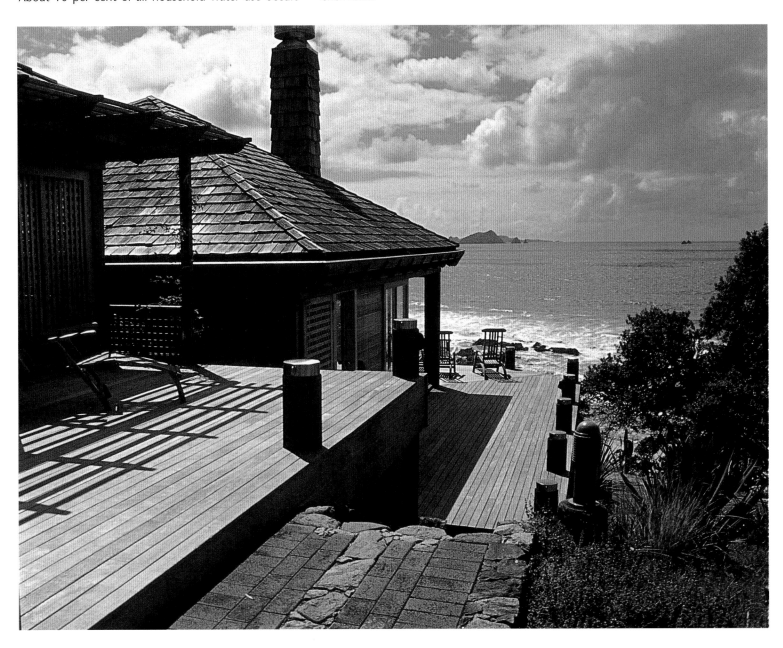

All hot water pipes should be insulated so that you do not waste water by running cold water until hot water can be drawn off. The hot-water unit should be located close to the kitchen, laundry and bathroom.

SOAP AND DETERGENT

Commercial laundry detergents contain dyes, whiteners, brighteners, perfumes and enzymes of bacterial origin. Each ingredient involves separate industrial processes, high entropic debt and pollution. Even 'green' laundry and dishwashing detergents carry a high entropic debt and have a long-term effect on the environment, though they may be labelled 'biodegradable'. It is only possible to use your grey water on the garden when specific brands of detergent have been used. Very few on the market are suitable. It is far better to use plain soap — you will have no problems using your grey water, and less energy is wasted in the manufacture of soap. Try to use soaps based upon vegetable fats such as palm, coconut or soya bean oil rather than those containing tallow, which is derived from animals.

◎ What cost shelter? ◎

If a curtain is hung on a wooden dowel we know that the timber is the product of solar energy, water, nutrients and minerals from the ground, electricity, the human effort taken to operate the machinery that tooled it into shape, and transportation to and from the mill and to the retailer. Imagine that the curtain is hung on a steel rod instead. A huge open-cut mine first yielded iron ore, which was transported to a smelter where it was formed, through heat, into an ingot. The ingot was then transported to a steel mill where, by high energy processes, it was shaped into rods then transported to wholesale and retail outlets. The wood was made by solar energy and the steel by fossil fuel energy. From a Gaian point of view, as long as it was made from plantation timber, the wooden dowel is far preferable to the steel rod.

Oil-fired continuous kilns and huge clay-pits, with their extensive haulage costs, make the cost of fabricating a brick extremely high. Imagine a brick made from timber. Its manufacture would use about one third of the energy that manufacturing a baked clay brick would. As most of the energy in wood comes from the sun, unlike the kiln-baked brick that utilises fossil fuels, its entropic debt would be very low. In addition, kilns release vast quantities of heat and pollutants. The construction of a wood-framed house uses about one third the amount of energy it takes to construct a brick house of the same size (Pedler 1979).

People who choose to build Gaian housing sometimes have difficulty gaining acceptance for their plans from the necessary authorities. Town and urban planners have often only had basic tertiary level training, yet have the power to control the grouping and movement of people and the aesthetics of buildings. Although town and urban planners are not elected representatives, they control the lives and architecture of millions because the elected representatives rely upon their expertise. At the very least, planners should be required to have a second degree in sociology, or the local authority should employ a sociologist. The often idiosyncratic decisions made by local authorities can be challenged in some courts, but this is often a costly procedure. Taxpayers not only pay for their own legal actions in order to achieve a reasonable interpretation of planning laws but also indirectly finance the planners' defences by paying rates.

◎ The rights of other life forms ◎

Viruses, bacteria, protozoa, insects, vertebrates, primates and people have been living together on the planet for a long time. Only humans have the freedom of choice to become farmers, doctors, shopkeepers (and Gaians). With choice comes responsibility — we have enough knowledge to affect the whole world for better or worse. Up until now the general human attitude to other life forms has been dominating and exploitative. Many species have become, or are becoming, extinct. Fur coats continue to be made, epicurean feasts prepared, ivory harvested from elephants and eastern medicines made from endangered species. Industrial agriculture is a perfect example of our species' manipulative behaviour. In particular, the intensive factory style farming of chickens, cattle and pigs is appalling in terms of its confinement of, and cruelty towards, the animals.

The ultimate aim of the Gaian lifestyle is to tread more lightly upon the Earth. The planet on which we all depend for life has one major energy cycle, that is, solar energy absorption, growth, procreation, decay and rebirth. Nothing can change

our dependence on that life cycle. The reason for sustaining the Earth is practical, not romantic or moral, it is simply one of survival. Yet ethics and morality become involved once the Gaian lifestyle has been adopted. If all life forms have basic rights, we should avoid killing. We are all creatures of Gaia.

In the relations of man with the animals, with the flowers, with all the objects of creation, there is a whole great ethic . . . scarcely seen as yet, but which will eventually break through into the light and be the corollary and the complement to human ethics. (Victor Hugo, *La Grande Morale*)

For those who wish to follow Gaian ideals, the way is clear. Society's acceptance is beginning to grow. Some people are preparing for a re-emergence of the Earth-mother, embodied in science as the Gaian movement and the study of ecology. The age of Gaia is beginning, the *gestalten* or symbol of this

new age will be the cave of the heart. Values traditionally seen as female — nurturing, caring, enduring and empathising — will be applied to both sexes. This will be expressed in our dwellings by the gentler forms of architectural enclosure, that is, homes that are of the soil or sheltered within Mother Earth. This is humanity's return to the Earth as one part of Gaia's systems and processes.

One family's or one individual's decision to adopt the Gaian lifestyle has the potential to influence others. In this way, ideas will spread until tens, thousands and perhaps millions of people have come into contact with the principles of the Gaian lifestyle. The decision of one could eventually change the thinking of a whole population. If these ideas spread and millions of people begin to tread more lightly on Gaia's Earth, the world will be a gentler, better place for our children, grandchildren and generations to come.

These ancient standing stones at Carnac, France, remind us of the respect for Gaia's systems that was once an integral part of human nature.

A p p e n d i x a

THE ELECTROMAGNETIC SPECTRUM

(Adapted from Smith and Best, 1989; Elmsley, 1993; Dalton, 1991; Riley, 1995)

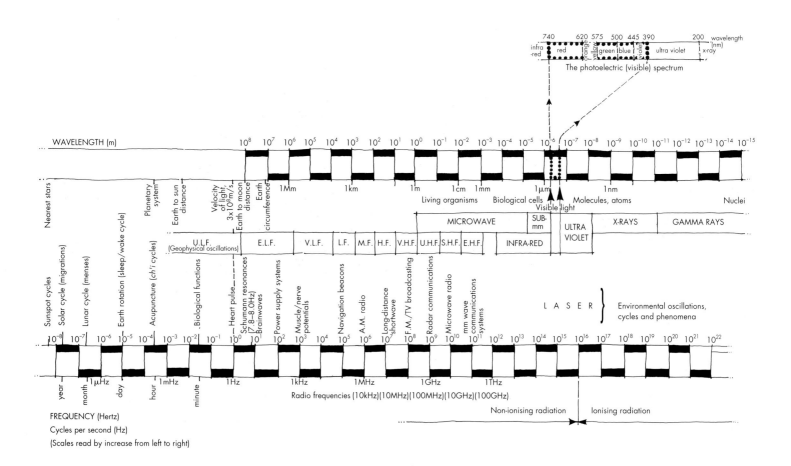

A p p e n d i x b

Calculating the Altitude of the Sun

The following steps will help you to calculate the maximum and minimum angles of sunlight which can be expected on your site. In the southern hemisphere the maximum angle of solar access will occur on 22 December and the minimum angle on 21 June. In the northern hemisphere, the maximum angle will occur on 21 June and the minimum on 22 December.

1. Check in an atlas to find in what latitude (line parallel to the equator) you are located.

2. Face the direction of the sun's zenith, that is, towards the sun's position at noon, when it casts a shadow directly behind you. In the southern hemisphere, this direction is solar north and in the northern hemisphere it is solar south. This direction can also be obtained from a map that shows the angle of deviation of solar north from magnetic north.

3. Find your latitude curve on Figure B.1.

4. Decide for what time of day you wish to calculate the sun's angle and locate it on the bottom horizontal line. In this example, 10:00 am (on the X-axis) in winter, at latitude 40 degrees, has been chosen. A line drawn vertically up from 10:00 am intersects the 40 degree latitude curve at A. Now draw a line horizontally across to B (on the 7-axis). We find that the reading on that axis is about 22 degrees. This means the sun is 22 degrees above the horizon. When it is, for instance, 127 degrees at latitude 5 degrees at 10:00 am, the angle is 37 degrees past 90 degrees.

5. Now we know the altitude of the sun at the 40 degree latitude at 10.00 am, but in which compass direction will the sun lie? Figure B.2 (overleaf) illustrates how the direction of the sun, in relation to the direction of the noonday sun, is different in the northern and southern hemispheres.

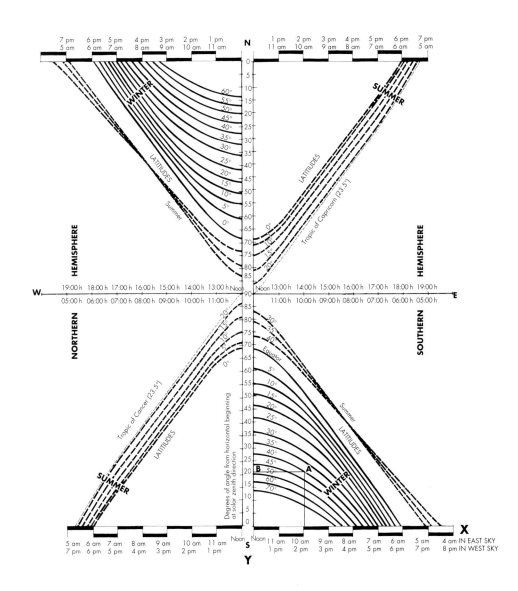

Figure B.1: Solar altitude diagram

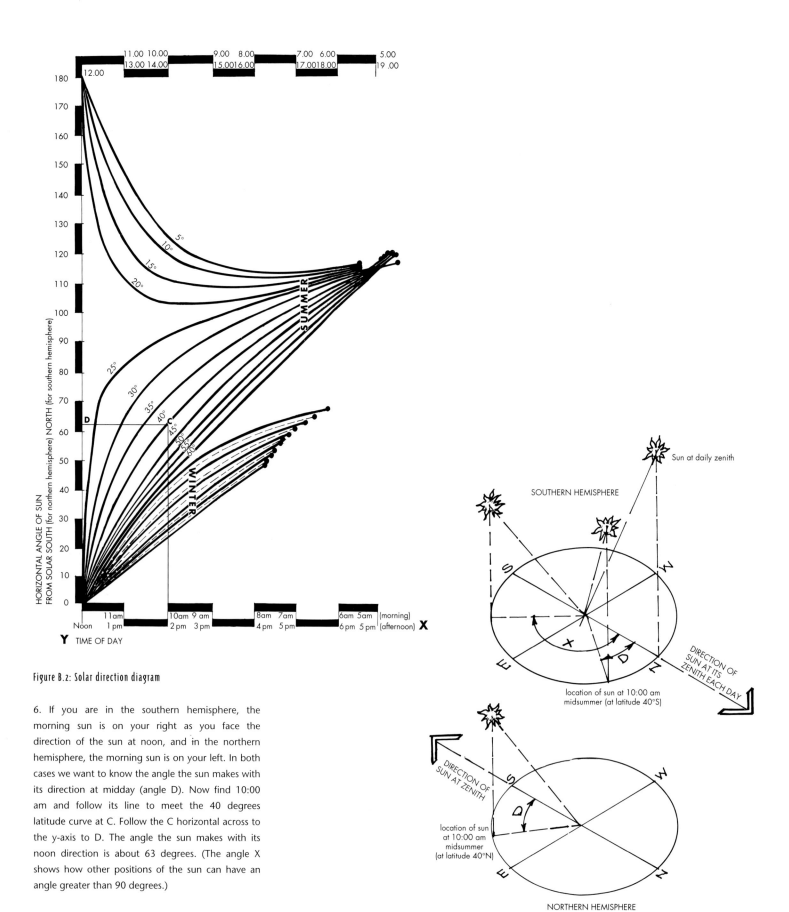

Figure B.2: Solar direction diagram

6. If you are in the southern hemisphere, the morning sun is on your right as you face the direction of the sun at noon, and in the northern hemisphere, the morning sun is on your left. In both cases we want to know the angle the sun makes with its direction at midday (angle D). Now find 10:00 am and follow its line to meet the 40 degrees latitude curve at C. Follow the C horizontal across to the y-axis to D. The angle the sun makes with its noon direction is about 63 degrees. (The angle X shows how other positions of the sun can have an angle greater than 90 degrees.)

SOUTHERN HEMISPHERE

Sun at daily zenith

DIRECTION OF SUN AT ITS ZENITH EACH DAY

location of sun at 10:00 am midsummer (at latitude 40°S)

DIRECTION OF SUN AT ZENITH

location of sun at 10:00 am midsummer (at latitude 40°N)

NORTHERN HEMISPHERE

Figure B.3: Horizontal angle of sun's position for any latitude

A p p e n d i x   c

COPING WITH AIR POLLUTION

Pollution levels are measured in parts per million (ppm) when gas concentrations are being discussed. Particulates, for example lead, are measured by weight per unit volume: microgram per cubic metre ($\mu g/m^3$) or milligram per cubic metre (mg/m^3).

ppm = parts per million
mg/m^3 = milligrams per cubic metre
$\mu g/m^3$ = micrograms per cubic metre

Bq/m^3 = Bequerels per cubic metre
(1 Bq/m^3 = 0.765 picoCurie per cubic foot (pCi/ft^3))
mSv = milliSieverts (1 mSv = 0.1 rem)
ml = millilitres (1 ml = 0.035 fluid ounces)

US EPA = United States of America Environmental Protection Agency
WHO = World Health Organisation
NHMRC = National Health and Medical Research Council of Australia

Table C.1: Air pollutants: problems and solutions

HEALTH EFFECTS OF POLLUTANTS	MAXIMUM EXPOSURE LIMITS	ACTION
CARBON MONOXIDE Carbon monoxide (CO) is a combustion gas which interferes with the delivery of oxygen in the body and can damage lungs. It causes more deaths than all other gases combined. Exposure to 9ppm for several hours may be hazardous to pregnant women and their foetuses, infants, anaemic people and those with respiratory problems; 25ppm in a 24 hour period can hamper vision and brain function; 90ppm causes mild headache, decreased work capacity and alertness, influenza-like symptoms and nausea. Chronic exposure causes decreased ability to exercise and possibly heart attack. Typical indoor concentrations average 0.5–5ppm. The ambient level over a gas stove is 10ppm. Faulty stove burners (usually indicated by a yellow-tipped rather than blue-tipped flame) can increase CO by 30 times. Convection-type kerosene heaters produce an average of 5ppm and radiant-type heaters 13ppm [1].	US EPA: 9ppm for outdoor air (over average 8 hour period, not more than once per year) and 35ppm for one hour (mean). (Any higher may affect those with angina) WHO: as per US EPA [1] NHMRC: interim goals for maximum permissible levels of CO in air (not threshold values): 9ppm (8 hour average not to be exceeded more than once per year) [2]	An exhaust hood and fan over the stove will remove about 70% of pollutants. Check all gas appliances for efficient combustion. Vent gas heaters directly to outside air. Do not have a garage opening off a living space or underground carparking with continuous connections to upper floor. Do not let wood fires smoulder. Remove all sources of tobacco smoke. Only the implementation of transport policies that favour nonpolluting vehicles and the location of airports well away from urban centres will produce major changes to the amount of CO in exterior air [3]. Catalytic converters should be installed in vehicles and regulations should ensure efficiency is maintained to avoid noxious fumes. Avoid sites downwind from airports and highways and downhill from highways.
CARBON DIOXIDE Increasing odours and chemical emissions are noticed when CO_2 rises above 800–1000ppm [2]. The level in unpolluted air is 330ppm and the concentration of CO_2 in exhaled breath is 38,000ppm. CO_2 is not emitted with the combustion of coal gas, but is with natural gas [4].	5000ppm over 8 hours [5]	Buildings can be equipped with CO_2 monitors to control ventilation rate
OXIDES OF NITROGEN Nitrogen dioxide (NO_2) is a combustion gas which affects the body's oxygen supply. Under normal circumstances, lethal levels are not reached in homes [1]. Oxides of nitrogen (NOx) are produced in all combustion reactions involving air. Emissions from idling engines can penetrate indoor spaces. Typical indoor concentrations when stoves, ovens and gas fires are turned on are above 0.05ppm; after an hour or so it spreads throughout the house. Indoor air concentrations can vary from 0.05 to 0.5ppm. Radiant-type kerosene space heaters cause 0.6ppm; convection heaters 1.8ppm [1]. Wood fires and tobacco smoke are also a source of oxides of nitrogen.	US EPA: 0.05ppm in 1 year (annual mean) [1] NHMRC : 0.16ppm (in 1 hour; levels not to be exceeded more than once per month) [1]	Check all gas appliances for efficient combustion. Vent gas heaters directly to outside air. Avoid having a garage opening off a living space and underground carparking with continuous connections to upper floor. Do not let wood fires smoulder. Improve ventilation
HYDROCARBONS Polycyclic aromatic hydrocarbons are complex organic substances released (along with CO and RSPs) when cooking, from wood stoves and fireplaces, vehicular emissions and tobacco smoke. Headaches, depression, mental confusion, physical and mental fatigue, rheumatism, arthritis, myalgic neuralgia and related musculoskeletal and neurological syndromes result from exposure to hydrocarbons		Have correctly designed flues installed, and implement no-smoking rules. We should ultimately move towards non-combustion engine transport to avoid photochemical smog formed from hydrocarbons, nitric oxide which photo-oxidises in air to form ozone, peracalcylnitrates (PANs), oxides of nitrogen and aerosols [11]

COMBUSTION PARTICLES

Factory flues and combustion produce very small particles known as respirable suspended particulates (RSP) which may lodge in the lungs. Incomplete combustion produces tarlike particles called Benzo-(a)-pyrene (BaP). Tobacco smoke is usually the largest indoor source of RSP and BaP followed by wood smoke, unvented gas appliances and kerosene space-heaters [6]. BaP may account for some of the lung cancers in smokers [7]. Cigarette smoking causes emphysema and lung cancer. In the USA, 3% of all deaths are caused by RSPs [8]. Studies showed that the smoking of more than 20 cigarettes a day by men is linked with lung cancer in their non-smoking wives. Most studies of the effect of parental smoking on children show respiratory problems especially in first two years of life [7]. With one smoker in the home, average RSP is 40 $\mu g/m^3$ with 2 or more smokers, 75 $\mu g/m^3$ [7].

US EPA: Total suspended particulates (TSP) are a conservative guide to RSP and are set at 75 $\mu g/m^3$ (annual geometric mean) and 260 $\mu g/m^3$ for a 24 hour period

NHMRC: goal for maximum permissible level of TSP in air is 90 $\mu g/m^3$. This total goal needs to be read in conjunction with sulphur dioxide (SO_2) goal of 260 $\mu g/m3$ in 24 hours [5, 6]

Chimneys and flues should be regularly cleaned and checked for leaks. Vent all combustion appliances (gas stoves, heaters, etc.) to outdoor air. Change or wash filters in equipment regularly. Give up smoking or exclude smoking of tobacco from all but a special area set aside with a separate ventilation system

AEROSOL PARTICLES

Aerosols are a dispersion of solid and liquid matter in air [9]. If fumes, smoke, ash, acid mist or soluble salts are present, health and visibility can be affected. When aerosols form, pollutants enter lungs more deeply than the gas alone can. Most atmospheric aerosols contain 'large' (0.1–1 micrometre) to 'giant' particles (greater than 1 micrometre). The number of particles may increase death rates from heart and lung disease [10] .

Consider prevailing winds when purchasing real estate as a 'river' of aerosols flows from traffic routes and factory flues. (See Hydrocarbons)

RADON

An odourless, colourless gas, radon is a product of the uranium decay chain. It occurs in the soil as a trace element and is present everywhere on the Earth's surface at varying concentrations. It enters buildings through cracks and vents in walls and floors. Water can also be a source as can earth-wall homes and those with rock heat-storage masses. Radon is believed to cause approximately 5–20% of all lung cancer (80% are tobacco-related) [12, 13].

NHMRC : 0.5mSv per year (for school pupils); recommends that action should be taken at 200Bq/m^3 (153 pCi/ft^3) and adopts the International Commission on Radiological Protection (ICRP): 1mSv per year (for the general public) [14]. WHO recommended level: 70Bq/m^3 (53.5 pCi/ft^3)

Increase ventilation by a major flushing of interior air every one to two days while maintaining a continuous room air-exchange rate of 1–2 per hour. Improve sub-floor space ventilation. Install sub-floor fans, weather stripping, weather excluders, caulking, etc. Heat exchangers (mechanical devices used to maintain air-exchange rates while conserving energy) are said to help. Seal off all pathways between soil beneath and interior of a building. Give up smoking. Exclude smoking from all but a special area with a separate ventilation system

OUTGASSING OF PVC PLASTICS

PVC is made from vinyl chloride monomer, a highly toxic carcinogen. Although polymerising the monomer is supposed to remove toxicity, some monomer potentially remains.

Vinylchloride monomer content is limited to 5ppm for food-wrapping and containers (Australian Standard) [15]

Do not use cling-wrap films on oily or alkaline foods. Buy cooking oil in glass bottles. Transfer water purchased in plastic containers to glass. Try to buy foodstuffs in polythene or polypropylene containers (milky white in colour). Do not buy olives in oil in PVC packages. Do not burn PVC containers as vinyl chloride and hydrochloric acid are produced. If inhaled, dizziness and even unconsciousness can result. Liver damage with a delay of some 20 years can also follow [9]

OZONE AND PHOTOCHEMICAL OXIDANTS

Ozone in the stratosphere functions as a screen against UV light, but in the air we breathe, it and other photochemical oxidants have harmful effects on living tissues, particularly plants. Transport and combustion sources emit a mixture of nitrogen oxides and hydrocarbons. These are acted on by strong sunlight to form ozone and other photochemical oxidants. Ozone is also formed during thunderstorms and when photocopying machines are used. 'Brown-air' pollution, which forms over some cities, is caused by photochemical oxidants and many other chemicals, while 'grey-air' pollution is a mixture of sulphur oxides, particulates and moisture. Respiratory and eye irritation result, and emphysema after long-term exposure. Ozone also suppresses the immune response of the lungs and doubles sensitivity to allergens, hence increases the frequency of asthma attacks.

NHMRC : 0.12ppm (goal for maximum hourly average, not to be exceeded more than once a year)
Note: A public warning is required if ozone levels are expected to rise above 0.25ppm [17]

WHO: 0.04ppm [2] ; long-term goal: 0.03ppm (1 hour maximum)

Control measures need to be put in place on combustion-vehicle and industrial-emissions with no exceptions. Make sure that photocopying machines are located in a separate room with ventilation exhaust and air supply separated from other areas. When public warnings are given about air pollution, sensitive people should stay indoors. Vegetation should be planted in cities on a major scale. (NB: Non-medical standard negative ion-generators can emit ozone.)

SULPHUR DIOXIDE

Sulphur dioxide interferes with the cleaning function of the cilia and mucous flow in the lungs, increasing the risk of smokers contracting lung cancer. When sulphur dioxide enters the lungs, it creates sulphuric acid and has been implicated in the increase of asthma, bronchitis and emphysema in people exposed to severe pollution [16]. When sulphur dioxide (and other pollutants) in industrial fumes are diluted by rain, acid rain results.

WHO : 0.48ppm [2]; NHMRC : 0.5ppm (10 minute mean); 0.25ppm (hourly mean) and 0.02ppm (1 year exposure). (NB: 'Levels set in this air quality goal may not be low enough to prevent health effects from this pollutant in the most sensitive members of the population' [17].)

Smokestacks fitted with 'scrubbers' remove SO_2 from the vented waste gases. A direct reading sampling-pump is needed where sensitivity to low levels of SO_2 is a health issue [16]

HEALTH EFFECTS	MAXIMUM EXPOSURE LIMITS	ACTION

PAINT

Some old paint contains the toxic materials Paris-green (copper ethanoato-arsenate) and German vermilion (cinnabar). Even dry paint surfaces can give off fumes for many years after painting [18]. Varnishes take longer to outgas than paints. Solvents cause the most problems (apart from the mercury in some water-based paints). Plasticisers, thickeners, stabilisers, quick-drying and dispersal agents for colouring pigment are also toxic. Chronic poisoning from repeated exposure to low concentrations of fumes can result in damage to the nervous, gastrointestinal and repiratory systems, the liver, kidney, blood and blood-forming tissues and skin.

Check with the painters, signwriters and decorators' union in your country [19]

When removing paints and varnishes, cover face with a mask. Wear long-sleeved clothing and long pants. Before using any paint, obtain a Materials Safety Data Sheet (MSDS) from the manufacturer to determine which of the 600 or more standard chemicals have been used. Preferably, use only non-toxic paints and stains

LEAD

Engine exhaust is the main source of airborne lead dust. Lead from industrial sources is usually well controlled, but renovation of old houses can cause airborne lead paint to be deposited on soil and other surfaces. All roof spaces accessible by trapdoors accumulate lead dust from leaded petrol emissions, industry and unsafe renovation practices. The NHMRC in Australia has stated that: 'within urban populations, young children exposed to high levels of lead may be several points lower on IQ than children with lower exposure' [20]. Lead has a cumulative effect. Fatigue, headache, loss of appetite and memory, lack of coordination, retardation in children, anaemia, and reproductive and kidney problems can result

NHMRC : 25µg per 100 ml of blood (the danger level for the general population) [20];
1.5µg/m^3 (3 month average) [17] (However, it is recommended that children are not exposed to lead at any level.)

0.1 to 0.7 mg/m^3 maximum [12]

WHO: 0.12 mg/m^3 [2]

Hire an expert to vacuum clean your roof space, particularly prior to installing a skylight or otherwise disturbing the roof space. Agitate for a registry of lead-contaminated sites in your region and for the removal of lead from petrol. Conduct tests of the soil around your home and swab tests of surfaces (see Resources List). Regularly wash with soap any surfaces children frequently come into contact with. Avoid disturbing surfaces painted with old lead-based paints.

TOTAL VOLATILE ORGANIC COMPOUNDS (TVOCs)

Formaldehyde is the principal VOC present in indoor environments. Xylene and isobutylaldehyde are also carcinegenous VOCs. Indoor concentrations are usually about four times those outdoors. Sources include paints, solvents, furniture, furnishings (synthetic fabrics), carpets, insecticides, various plastics, fumigants, cleaners, particle board, medium- and high-density fibreboard, plywood, fibreglass and rockwool insulation, wood stoves, kerosene heaters, tobacco smoke, foam insulation and binders in prepasted wallpaper. It is also used to make pigments adhere to fabrics and to make materials flame-resistant. Almost all cottons and linens are made crease-resistant and shrinkproof by the use of formaldehyde [21]. Printing of artwork, film processing and dyeing can produce high concentrations. Formaldehyde causes eye irritation at levels as low as 0.2ppm and begins to effect heart/lung function at 3ppm. As the level rises, symptoms become more severe, and include: sore throat, upper airway irritation, neuropsychological effects, pulmonary oedema, pneumonia and eventually death. Overexposure to VOCs in general can cause abnormal tingling sensations, visual and auditory problems, loss of memory, confusion, disorientation, nervousness, irritability, depression, apathy, compulsive behaviour, weakness in hands, lack of coordination, fatigue and tremor.

In the presence of other pollutants, TVOC levels should be kept below 200µg/m^3 (0.2ppm) (1 hour average) , the interim level at which concern arises, provided no single VOC contributes more than 50% to the total [22]

Isolate, remove or seal off sources of outgassing.
Use second-hand furniture that has already outgassed and that has not been renovated with synthetic materials. Photocopying machines should be isolated in separately ventilated room. Indoor plants can remove many of these pollutants. Be careful not to inhale dust if working with wood-fibre and particle boards. Use PVA glues as all other glues cause problems. Avoid all '2-pot' epoxy systems of coatings, glues, etc.

ASBESTOS

The greatest public risk occurs when buildings constructed with asbestos-based materials are being demolished . Motor vehicle brake linings are another source of airborne asbestos. Exposure to blue asbestos disturbed by demolition causes asbestosis and mesothelioma

US Occ. Safety & Health Admin: Respirators should be worn when exposed to concentrations above 2 fibres per ml of air for an 8 hour period and 10 fibres per ml at any one time [6]. Aust. standards for exposure over not less than 4 hours: Chrysotile (white) 1.0 fibres/ml; Crocidolite (blue) 0.1 fibres/ml; Amosite (brown) 0.1 fibres/ml; Other forms: 0.1 fibres/ml. Any mixture of above or when composition is unknown: 0.1 fibres/ml [23]

Do not sand or scrape old wallboards containing asbestos, asbestos-vinyl tiles, asbestos-backed sheet flooring and insulation coatings, and some old textured surface coatings. Follow health regulations during removal. There are strict regulations governing disposal of asbestos and asbestos-based materials

SYNTHETIC MINERAL FIBRES (SMFs)

SMFs are a range of non-crystalline (amorphous) fibrous materials such as fibreglass, mineral wool and ceramic fibre. SMFs are less potent than white (chrysotile) asbestos but cause irritation of skin, eyes and upper respiratory tract. Long-term exposure slightly increases risk of lung fibrosis and mesothelioma. A slightly increased risk of lung cancer has also been shown in rockwool and slagwool workers [2]

TWA (time-weighted average) exposure of 0.5 respirable fibres per ml of air [2; 24]

In existing buildings, remove all SMF insulation materials and replace with substitute insulation (see Chapter 9)

MICROBIOLOGICAL CONTAMINANTS

Allergic and hypersensitive reactions can be caused by: bacteria like *Legionella pneumophila* and *Flavobacteria, Pseudomonas* spp; fungi such as *Aspergillus* spp, *Aureobasidium* spp, *Penicillium* spp; and protozoa such as *Acanthamoeba polyphhaga* and *Thermoactinomyces* spp [2]. Asthma can be aggravated by the presence of moulds, mites, pollen, algae, insects, animal dander and bird (especially pigeon) droppings

Samples can be taken from interior room air and from supply ductwork if a heating-ventilating air-conditioning (HVAC) system has been installed. Airborne particulate size and concentration is to be measured and HVAC system inspected. (In Australia, samples are assessed by a National Advisory and Testing Authority and a microbial count of aerobic bacteria, moulds and yeasts is taken and dominant genera noted.) Regular cleaning is essential. Remove sources of dampness. Ventilate and admit sunlight. Wash cellular cotton blankets and bed linen in hot water. Use allergy-free, impervious mattresses and pillow covers unless sensitive to the petroleum-based products from which the covers are manufactured. Double covers of japara are far less expensive and will take hot-water washing. Remove carpets, soft toys, curtains and as much furniture as possible. If a vaporiser is used, ventilate the room and change bed linen after airing the mattress.

FUNGICIDES

Fungicides are often used in paint, tiling grout and in the treatment of paper (including wallpaper). Based on toxic organotin compounds and organochlorines, they are used in timber finishes. Sometimes the neurotoxin mercury is used in paints for wood and in plastics. Fungicides are sprayed under buildings to control wet- or dry-rot and termites.

Avoid materials containing fungicides

WOOD PRESERVATIVES

Creosote is still used on fences and posts though it can cause kidney trouble if ingested. (When it is applied, the ground beneath becomes saturated with it.) Pentachlorophenol, the modern equivalent of creosote, is an unacceptable synthetic preservative. It is extremely hazardous if absorbed through skin or inhaled. If treated timber is burnt, the fumes are particularly toxic

Keep children away from soil saturated with creosote. Press for a ban on arsenic preservatives if you live in a country which has not already banned them

PESTICIDES

Pesticides are classified as semi-volatile organic compounds. When pesticides and termiticides are sprayed under buildings they rise up into the interior between floorboards and skirtings. When the soil has been flooded with pesticides the fumes can penetrate concrete floors. Organophosphates interfere with the nervous system as they are rapidly absorbed through the skin and lungs. They cause fatigue, sweating, chest tightness, nausea, dizziness and diarrhoea and are also linked to genetic damage and cancer.

Use non-chemical alternatives for pest control. If sub-floor areas have been sprayed with pesticides, install lights to activate the chemicals to outgas quickly. Install solar-powered ventilators to release fumes to outside air. Arrange frequent inspections by a pest-control firm that uses non-toxic methods to eradicate termites. Call for a total ban on cyclodeines.

POLYCHLORINATED BIPHENYLS

PCBs are toxic organochlorines and are a proven animal carcinogen (causing damage to the foetus) and a suspected human carcinogen. Inhaled or absorbed through the skin or stomach lining, for instance by eating contaminated fish, they are stored in fatty tissue, the liver, thyroid gland, kidneys, lungs, uterus and brain. Although banned in many countries, they still appear in imported paints, adhesives, fire retardants and electric wire and cable insulations. Exposure results in eczema, skin rashes, discolouration of skin, respiratory problems, muscle and joint pains, headache, loss of appetite, nausea, vomiting and abdominal pain [25]. Children exposed to high levels are clumsy, badly coordinated and have poor short-term memory and lowered IQ

Consult authorities when disposing of fluorescent tube ballasts as they contain PCBs. Use non-toxic paints. When removing old paint and electrical installations take care not to inhale or make skin contact with materials. Do not eat fish from PCB-contaminated waters

[1] Department of Energy, Bonneville Power Administration, United States 1983; [2] Gilbert 1992; [3] Ferrari and Johnson 1982; [4] Ferrari, et al 1988; [5] Juriel 1983; [6] California Department of Consumer Affairs 1982; [7] Spengler and Sexton 1983; [8] World Resources Institute Environmental Protection Agency 1992; [9] Kabos 1986; [10] Laura and Ashton 1991; [11] Spedding 1974; [12] General Accounting Office 1980; [13] Division of Energy Conservation, Bonneville Power Administration, United States 1981; [14] National Health and Medical Research Council, Australia 1986; [15] Standards Association of Australia 1992; [16] Ehrlich and Ehrlich 1972; [17] National Health and Medical Research Council, Australia (n/d); [18] Samways 1989; [19] Holmes 1990; [20] 'Sunday spotlight: killer chemicals' 1992; [21] Randolph 1963; [22] Molhave 1990; [23] Worksafe Australia 1988; [24] Worksafe Australia 1990; [25] Randolph 1979

Appendix d

SOIL DEFICIENCIES AND RESULTING DIETARY DEFICIENCIES

If the pH of a soil is too low (acidic) or too high (alkaline) the level of essential minerals is adversely affected, and if nutrients are not available to plants, the deficiency can be passed on to the animals and people who eat them. In alkaline soil, insoluble compounds form and certain fungus diseases develop, concentrating soluble aluminium and iron compounds. Calcium, phosphorus and magnesium become less available. Low pH is unfavourable to most nitrogen-cycle bacteria, resulting in a drop in the amount of accessible nitrogen for plants. Worms, insects, yeasts, moulds, fungi and bacteria are essential for soil richness and the release of nutrients to plants. When a soil's pH falls below 5.5 or rises above 7 (neutral pH), the numbers of these populations begin to fall. [1]

Table D.1: Nutrients which may be deficient in acidic soils (low pH)

MINERAL	FOOD SOURCES	NUTRITIONAL ROLE
Calcium	Dairy products, soybeans, sardines, salmon, peanuts, walnuts, sunflower seeds, green vegetables and dried beans (the drying process concentrates the nutrients)	Needed for bones, teeth, normal growth rates, heart action, muscle activity, blood clotting, healing processes and many enzyme functions. Important during pregnancy and lactation. Assists in maintaining balance between body's use of sodium, potassium and magnesium. Essential for absorption of vitamins A, D and C and phosphorus [2]. If plants (especially dark green, leafy vegetables) cannot access calcium they cannot pass it on to humans. Calcium-deficient pastures affect cows' milk and cheese while beef cattle and sheep pass on the deficiency when consumed. Fats, oxalic acid (in chocolate and rhubarb) and phytic acid (in grains) are capable of preventing calcium absorption. Deficiency can cause rickets, osteomalacia (softening of bones), osteoporosis (brittle bones) and menstrual cramps
Phosphorus	Corn, dried fruits, dairy products, egg yolk, legumes, seeds, nuts, whole grains and fish	A combination of vitamin D, calcium and phosphorus is needed to build bones and teeth. The acid-alkaline balance of blood and tissues, mental activity, nerves and carbohydrate metabolism depend greatly on phosphorus. Deficiency can cause poor mineralisation in bones, diminished sexual capability, general weakness and nervous system deficiencies
Magnesium	Soybeans, nuts, green leafy vegetables, alfalfa, apples, figs, lemons, peaches, whole grains, sunflower seeds, sesame seeds and brown rice	When magnesium is deficient, calcium and potassium cannot be absorbed. Magnesium is an important catalyst in many enzyme reactions. It helps maintain muscle tone, synthesis of protein, and healthy bones and heart function. Involved in lecithin production (used in metabolism of fats by liver) and regulates acid-alkaline balance of body. A natural tranquiliser, it prevents build-up of cholesterol and hence, atherosclerosis. Deficiency can cause kidney damage or stones, muscle cramp, irritability, depression, confusion, impaired protein metabolism, premature wrinkling, atherosclerosis and heart attack [3]

Table D.2: Nutrients which may be deficient in alkaline soils (high pH)

MINERAL	FOOD SOURCES	NUTRITIONAL ROLE
Iron	Egg yolk, liver, kelp, lentils, dried beans, whole rye, sunflower seeds, walnuts, beet tops, alfalfa, spinach, turnip greens, whole-grain cereals, brewer's yeast, raisins, prunes, black molasses, bananas, peaches and apricots [2]	Essential for haemoglobin, which transports oxygen to cells. If iron is not available to plants, beef and sheep carry the deficiency and pass it on to meat-eaters. Vitamin C, as ascorbic acid, aids in absorption of dietary iron. Deficiency can cause anaemia, lowered resistance to disease, low energy, headache, problems with breathing when exercising, lowered interest in sex
Copper	Foods rich in iron are usually rich in copper, eg, whole grains, green leafy vegetables, liver, almonds, prunes, raisins, peas and beans [2]	Essential for absorption of iron and vitamin C. Aids in development of bones, connective tissues, brain and nerves. Present in tobacco, birth-control pills and vehicular emissions. Deficiency may cause anaemia, digestive disturbances, greying and loss of hair, heart and liver damage and impaired respiration. Copper supplements should not be taken as excess copper reduces the level of zinc in the body, resulting in insomnia, depression and irregular menstruation
Manganese	Nuts, green leafy vegetables, peas, beetroot, raw egg yolk, whole-grain cereals, oranges, grapefruit, apricot, bran and wheat germ	Enzymes involved in metabolism of carbohydrates, fats and proteins depend on manganese. Brain and nervous system also need manganese as do the reproduction and mammary glands. Deficiency can cause growth retardation, abnormal bone development, infertility, impotence, digestive disturbances, asthma, temporary paralysis of muscles with eyelid droop, double vision and unclear speech
Zinc	Ground mustard, non-fat powdered milk, eggs, pumpkin seeds, brewer's yeast, wheat germ, round steak, lamb chops and pork loin	Present in over 90 enzymes [4], zinc is needed for protein synthesis, reproductive hormones, sexual maturation and formation of ribonucleic acid (RNA) and deoxyribonucleic acid (DNA). Accelerates healing time for wounds, aids in infertility, helps avoid prostate problems, promotes growth and mental alertness. Most zinc in food is lost in processing. Deficiency can cause possible non-cancerous enlargement of the prostate gland and arteriosclerosis.

[1] Mindell 1985; [2] Airola 1987; [3] Greulach and Adams 1962; [4] Laura and Ashton 1991

Appendix e

SOIL POLLUTANTS

⊛ Neurotoxins ⊛

Neurotoxins cause damage to nerve and brain cells, resulting in loss of appetite and balance, irritability, lassitude, confusion, restlessness, nervousness, clumsiness, dizziness, severe headaches, speech impairment, memory loss, trouble with hearing and eyesight, depression, disturbed sleep, apathy and, in children, hyperactivity accompanied by seizures [1].

Table E.1: The effect of neurotoxins in the environment

NEUROTOXIN	IMPACT ON HEALTH	ACTION
Indigo	Minute doses of indigo accumulate in the soil because of the activities of the dye industry, and can cause the symptoms listed above	Wash your hands and those of your children with a nail brush before meals; wet-mop with sugar soap (rather than sweep) floors, window sills and other areas holding dust. Do not allow pets that spend time outdoors to sleep in the house; wash them regularly. Eat a preponderance of thoroughly washed fruit, vegetables and grains, with calcium and iron supplements. Restrain children from eating outdoors and wash toys regularly. Flush water that has been sitting in pipes overnight into a bucket for use in the garden and never use hot water from the tank for cooking or making tea and coffee
Mercury	Minute doses accumulate in the soil because of hat manufacture, fungicides and pesticides used in horticulture and agriculture	
Lead	Lead from the smelting industry, combustion-engine emissions and lead-based paint can form residues in the soil and cause brain-cell destruction [2], leading to loss of intelligence [3]. Use lead crystal glasses with caution as traces of lead have been found in wine served in lead crystal.	
Pesticides	Pesticides are designed to attack neurological functions in insects, but also affect humans. A major proportion of these chemicals are deposited into the soil after spraying. Organophosphates and carbamates can produce effects ranging from brainwave alteration to severe mental retardation, uncontrollable tremor and crippling nerve damage – and can even cause psychotic, murderous tendencies. Schizophrenic depressive behaviours have been identified in agricultural sprayers, gardeners and others using pesticides and termiticides [1,4]	

⊛ Cadmium ⊛

Table E.2: The effect of cadmium in the environment

IMPACT ON HEALTH	ACTION
It has been argued that cadmium is linked to high blood pressure, impairment of kidney function and the disruption of a number of enzyme systems crucial to health (hence is suspected as a cause of the worldwide increase in diabetes). It affects the function of the testicles and is linked to an increase in prostate cancer and anaemia, emphysema, chronic bronchitis, lung fibrosis and cancer (not yet proven). It accumulates in the body over time. Sources of cadmium include fertilisers, trace elements, batteries, some drinking waters, oysters, processed foods, evaporated milk, tobacco smoke, many ceramics, paint pigments, pesticides, fungicides, electroplating, some rustproofing materials, certain metal welding solders, rubber, many brands of gasoline and lubricating oils, and galvanised and black PVC pipes [5]	Do not drink or cook with the water first drawn from the tap in the morning (use it on the garden). As hot water exacerbates the leaching of cadmium into water, do not use water from the hot water service for cooking or making tea and coffee. Avoid enamelled cooking pots with red, yellow or maroon interiors. Take care that if sewage sludge is used to fertilise soils, it does not originate from sources containing industrial wastes, as vegetables absorb heavy metals. Buy or grow your own organic food. Make sure there is enough zinc in your diet, as zinc deficiency seems to increase toxic levels of cadmium in the blood [6]. Levels of cadmium can be diagnosed by having a hair trace analysis undertaken by a reputable laboratory.

[1] Short 1994; [2] Baghurst, et al 1992; [3] Kostial 1984; [4] Civil Aeromedical Institute (report by A. Revzin) (n/d); [5] 'Guide to low cadmium, phosphate supplements' 1990; [6] Onosoka, et al 1984

Appendix f

Low Allergy Plants

LOW ALLERGEN BIRD- OR INSECT-POLLINATED PLANTS

TREES FOR SHADE AND SHELTER

Agonis flexuosa (Peppermint Tree; Willow Myrtle)
Araucaria heteropylla (Norfolk Island Pine)
Bauhinia blakeana (Deep Purple Orchid Tree)
Carica papaya (Papaw)
Citrus spp (Lemon, orange, lime, grapefruit, mandarin)
Eucalyptus ficifolia (Scarlet Flowering Gum)
Eucalyptus haemostoma (Scribbly Gum)
Eucalyptus nicholii (Peppermint Gum)
Gingko biloba (Maidenhair Tree)
Grevillea robusta (Silky Oak)
Hakea laurina (Pincushion Hakea)
Hakea salicifolia (Willow-leaved Hakea)
Howea forsterana (Kentia Palm)
Lauris nobilis (Sweet Bay)
Acmena smithii, Sysyium spp (Lilly Pilly spp)
Livistona australis (Cabbage Tree Palm)
Magnolia grandiflora (Magnolia)
Malus 'Echtermeyer' (Weeping Crab Apple)
Malus floribunda (Japanese Crab Apple)
Melaleuca quinquinervia (Broad-leafed Paperbark)
Nyssa sylvatica (Tupelo)
Pistacia chinensis (Chinese Pistachio)
Prunus spp (Flowering almond, apricot, cherry)

MEDIUM TO TALL SHRUBS (1-3 METRES (3-10 FEET))

Abelia grandiflora (Glossy Abelia)
Abutilon X frazeri (Chinese Bell Flower)
Baeckia virgata (Twiggy Heath Myrtle)
Banksia ericifolia (Heath Banksia)
Banksia serrata (Old Man Banksia)
Banksia spirulosa 'Giant Candles' (Honeysuckle Banksia)
Boronia heterophylla (Red Boronia)
Brunsfelsia australis (Yesterday, Today and Tomorrow)
Callistemon spp (Bottlebrush spp)
Camellia japonica (Camellia)
Camellia sasanqua (Sasanqua Camellia)
Ceanothus cyaneus 'Blue Pacific' (Californian Lilac)

Epacris impressa (Common White Heath)
Escallonia macrantha (Escallonia)
Gardenia augusta (Gardenia)
Kunzea affinis (Kunzea)
Leptospermum lanigerum v. macrocarpum (Silky Tea Tree)
Melaleuca armillaris (Bracelet Honey Myrtle)
Melaeuca hypericifolia (Red-flowering Paperbark)
Plumbago auriculata (Cape Plumbago)
Rhododendron spp (Azalea, Rhododendron)
Rosmarinus officinalis (Rosemary)
Streptosolen jamesonii (Orange Browallia, Marmalade Bush)
Viburnum upulus (Snowball, Guelder Rose)
Weigela florida 'Variegata' (Weigela)
Westringia fruticosa (Coastal Rosemary)

SMALL SHRUBS AND GROUNDCOVERS (LESS THAN 1 METRE (3 FEET))

Baeckia ramosissima (Rosy Heath Myrtle)
Banksia integrifolia (prostrate) (Coast or White Honeysuckle Banksia)
Bauera rubioides (River Rose, Dog Rose)
Callistemon comboynensis (Callistemon prostrate)
Callistemon pearsonii (Callistemon prostrate forms)
Cerastium tomentosum (Snow-in-summer)
Correa Alba (White Correa)
Cotoneaster conspicuus 'Decorus' (Low-growing Cotoneaster)
Hibbertia pedunculata (Guinea Flower)
Hibbertia serpyllifolia (Guinea Flower)
Juniperus conferta (Juniper)
Kunzea parvifolia (Kunzea)
Lavandula dentata (Toothed Lavender, French Lavender)
Leptospermum spp (Tea Tree spp)
Lobelia trigonacaulis (Lobelia)
Melaleuca hypericifolia (Red-flowering Paperbark)
Micromyrtus ciliata (Fringed Heath-Myrtle)
Pelargonium peltatum (Ivy-leaf Geranium)
Rosmarinus officinalis horizontalis (Rosemary)
Thymus spp (Thyme spp)
Vinca major variegata (Variegated Periwinkle)
Viola hederacea (Native Violet)

CLIMBERS

Actinidia chinersis (Chinese Gooseberry, Kiwi Fruit)
Billardiera cymosa (Sweet Appleberry)
Billardiera longifolia (Purple Appleberry)
Billardiera scancens (Climbing Appleberry)
Campsis grandiflora (Trumpet Vine)
Clematis Montana 'Rubens' (Clematis)
Hardenbergia viciacea (Purple Coral Pea)
Kennedya rubicunda (Dusky Coral Pea)
Pandorea pandorana (Wonga Vine)
Passiflora aurantia (Passion Flower)
Mandevilla laxa (Chilean Jasmine)
Passiflora edulis (Passionfruit)
Rosa banksiae (Banksia Rose)
Rosa spp (Climbing Rose)
Solanum jasminoides (Jasmine Nightshade)

GRASSES

Microlaena stipoides (Rice Grass, Weeping Grass)
Themeda australis (Kangaroo Grass)
Cynodin dactylon spp (Greenlees Couch, low-pollinating)
Stenotaphrum secundatum (Buffalo Grass, low-pollinating)

ANNUAL AND PERENNIAL FLOWERS

Ageratum spp (Ageratum)
Alyssum spp (Alyssum)
Anemone spp (Anemone)
Aquilegia spp (Aquilegia (Columbine))
Begonia spp (Begonia)
Campanula medium (Canterbury Bells)
Digitalis spp (Foxglove)
Clarkia spp (Clarkia)
Coleus spp (Coleus)
Centaurea cyanis (Cornflower)
Delphinium spp (Delphinium)
Lunaria biennis (Honesty)
Impatiens spp (Impatiens)
Nemesia spp (Nemesia)
Nasturtium spp (Nasturtium)
Viola spp (Pansy)
Petunia spp (Petunia)
Phlox spp (Phlox)
Salvia spp (Salvia)

Antirrhinum majus (Snapdragon)
Dianthus barbatus (Sweet William)
Verbena spp (Verbena)

PLANTS THAT MAY CAUSE ALLERGIES

WIND-POLLINATED TREES

Acacia spp (Acacia, Wattle)
Acer spp (Maple spp)
Alnus spp (Alder spp)
Betula spp (Birch spp)
Callitris glaucophylla (White Cypress Pine, Murray Pine)
Cupressus macrocarpa (Monterey Pine)
Cupressus sempervirens (Cypress Pine)
Fraximus spp (Ash spp)
Juglans spp (Walnut spp)
Ligustrum spp (Privet)
Liquidambar styraciflua (Liquidambar)
Melia asedarach (White Cedar)
Olea spp (Olive spp)
Populus deltoides (Poplar)
Prosopis juliflora (Mesquite)
Quercus spp (Oak spp)
Salix spp (Willow spp)
Ulmus spp Elm spp

FLOWERS

All of the *Asteraceae* family (Daisy, Chrysanthemum, Calendula, Marigold)

Bass, D. (n/d) The Low Allergen Garden (pamphlet), Concord Hospital, Sydney.

A p p e n d i x   g

POISONOUS PLANTS

*** deaths reported

** toxic but no deaths and/or poisoning reported

* can cause dermatitis or irritate skin on contact

Sources: 'Pretty but dangerous' 1983; Sutherland 1993

Table G.1: Plants poisonous to humans and animals

BOTANICAL NAME	COMMON NAME	PARTS THAT ARE TOXIC	LEVEL OF TOXICITY
Abrus precatorius	Crab's eye, Gidee-gidee, Jequirity bean	seeds	***
Achillea millefolium	Yarrow or Milfoil	all	*
Acokantera spectabilis	Wintersweet	fruit and plant	***, *
Aconitum napellus	Aconite or Monkshood	all	***
Agapanthus orientalis	Agapanthus or African Blue Lily	sap	*
Aleurites fordii	Tung-oil Tree	fruit kernel	**
Allamanda spp	Allamanda	fruit	**
Alocasia macrorrhiza	Cunjevoi, Elephant Ear	all	***, *
Amanita spp	Toadstools	all	***
Amaryllis belladonna	Belladonna Lilly	bulb	**
Anacardium occidentale	Cashew Tree	leaves	*
Anemone spp	Windflower	all	**
Aquilegia spp	Columbine	seeds	**
Artemisia absinthium	Wormwood	all	*
Asclepias fruticosa	Swan Plant	pods	**
Atropa belladonna	Deadly Nightshade	berries	***
Brugmansia candida	Angel's Trumpet	seeds, leaves, flowers	**
Caladium spp	Caladium	all	*
Carissa spectabilis	Wintersweet	fruit and plant	***
Castanospermum australe	Black Bean or Moreton Bay Chestnut	seeds	**
Cestrum spp	Green Cestrum, Cestrum, Jessamine or Green Poison Berry (orange fruit)	all, especially fruit	**
Chrysanthemum coccineim	Pyrethrum	all	*
Chrysanthemum maximum	Shasta Daisy	all	*
Chrysanthemum morifolium	Florist's Chrysanthemum	all	*
Chrysanthemum parthenium	Feverfew	all	*
Clematis spp	Traveller's Joy	all	*
Colocasis esculenta	Elephant's Ears, Taro	root	**
Conium maculatum	Hemlock Weed, Carrot fern	all	**
Consolida ambigua	Larkspur	Seeds and young plants	**
Convallaria majalis	Lilly of the Valley	all	*
Cosmos bipinnatus	Cosmos	all	**
Cotoneaster spp	Cotoneaster	all	*
Crataegus spp	Hawthorn	fruit	**
Cycas spp	Zamia Palm or Tree Zamia, Sago Palm	seeds, fresh or improperly prepared	**
Cydonia oblonga	Quince	seeds, fresh leaves	**
Daphne spp	Daphne	berries	***, *
Datura arborea	Angel's Trumpet	nectar, seeds	***
Datura metel (weed)	Hairy Angel's Trumpet	all	***
Datura stramonium (weed)	Thornapple	all	***

Botanical name	Common name	Parts that are toxic	Level of toxicity
Dendrochide photinophylla	Shining Leaf or Mulberry Leaf Stinging Tree	leaf	*
Dieffenbachia spp	Dumb Cane	berries	***
Digitalis purpurea	Foxglove	all	**
Duranta repens	Duranta or Golden Dewdrop	berries	***
Ervatamia coronaria	Crepe Jasmine	all	***
Euonymus europaeus	Spindle tree	all, especially fruit and seeds	**
Euphorbia marginata	Snow-on-the-mountain	sap	**
Euphorbia milii	Crown of Thorns	sap	*
Euphorbia pulcherrima	Poinsettia	sap	*
Euphorbia tirucalli	Naked lady, Pencil bush	sap	* (temporary blindness)
Exocaria agallocha	Milky mangrove	sap	*
Gelsemium sempervirens	Yellow Carolina Jasmine	leaves, flowers, nectar and honey	**
Gloriosa superba	Glory Lily	all especially root	***
Hedera helix	English Ivy	all, especially berries	**, *
Helenium autumnale	Sneezeweed	all	*
Helianthus annuus	Sunflower	all	*
Helleborus niger	Christmas rose	all	**
Iris germanica	Flag Iris, Flag Lily or Fleur de Lis	all	**
Jatropha curcas	Physic Nut	seeds	**
Kalmia latifolia	Calico Bush	all	**
Lantana camara (weed) and all spp	Lantana	unripe berries	**
Lathyrys spp and Lathyrus odoratus	Sweet pea	seeds	**
Lepidozamia peroffskyana	Giant Burrawang	seeds	***
Ligustrum vulgare	Common Privet	leaves, fruit, berries	**
Lobelia cardinalis	Cardinal Flower	all	***
Macrozamia communis	Common Burrawong	seeds	**
Malus spp	Apple	leaves, seeds in large amounts	***
Mangifera indica	Mango	sap	*
Manihot esculenta	Cassava	raw roots	**
Melia azedarach australasica	Cape Lilac or White Cedar	fruit, leaf, bark and flowers	***
Melianthus comosus	Cape Honey Flower	root	**
Monstera deliciosa	Fruit Salad Plant, Swiss Cheese Plant	ripe fruit	*
Moraea spp	Butterfly Iris	all	**
Narcissus pseudonarcissus	Daffodil	sap and bulb	**, *
Nerine spp	Spider Lily	bulb	**
Nerium oleander (Thevetia peruviana)	Common Oleander	all	***
Ornithogalum thjyrsoides	Star-of-Bethlehem or Chincherinchee	bulb and flower spike	**
Plumeria spp	Frangipani	sap	**, *
Poinciana gilliesii	Bird of Paradise	unripe seed pod	**
Primula obconia	Primula	all	*
Prunus armeniaca	Apricot	kernels (if consumed in large quantities)	***
Prunus cerasus	Cherry	kernels	**
Prunus dulcis	Almond	unripe, bitter kernels	***
Prunus laurocerasus	Cherry laurel	bruised leaves	**
Ranunculus spp	Buttercups	all	*
Rheum rhaponticum	Rhubarb	leaf	***
Rhodomyrtus macropcarpa	Native Loquat, Finger Cherry	fruit	blindness
Rhus cotinus	Smoke Tree, Rhus Tree	sap	*
Ricinus communis	Castor Oil Plant	seeds (if 2–8 are consumed)	***
Robinia pseudoacacia	Black Locust, Robinia	all	**
Rudbeckia hirta	Black-eyed Susan	all	*
Sarcostemma australie	Caustic Bush, Caustic Vine	sap	*
Scilla nonscripta	Bluebell	bulb	**
Semecarpus australiensis	Tar Tree, Marking Nut	sap	*

BOTANICAL NAME	COMMON NAME	PARTS THAT ARE TOXIC	LEVEL OF TOXICITY
Senecio cineraria	Dusty Miller	all	*
Solandra spp	Golden Chalice, Chalice Vine	sap, leaves, flowers	**,*
Solanum dulcamara	Woody Nightshade	berries	**
Solanum mammosum	Cow's Udder Plant	unripe fruit, leaves	**
Solanum nigrum	Black Nightshade, Blackberry Nightshade	green fruit	***
Solanum sodomaeum (hermannii)	Apple-of-Sodom	fruit	***
Solanum tuberosum	Potatoes	green skin, berries	***
Synadenium grantii	African Milk Bush	sap	**,*
Tanacdgum vulgare	Common Pansy	all	*
Taxus baccata	Yew	seed in pod, leaves	***
Thevetia peruviana (also see Nerium oleander)	Yellow Oleander	all, especially seed in kernel	***
Toxicodendron succedaneum	Scarlet Rhus, Kuntze, Japanese Wax Tree, Sumach	all, as well as smoke	**,*
Triunia youngiana	Red Nut	seeds	**
Urtica spp	Stinging Nettle, Scrub Nettle	all	*
Wilkstroemia indica	Tie Bush	fruit	***
Wisteria floribunda, W. sinensis	Wisteria	seeds and pods	**
Zantedeschia aethiopica	Calla Lily, White Arum lily	all, especially the spike	***

*** deaths reported
** toxic but no deaths and/or poisoning reported
* can cause dermatitis or irritate skin on contact
Sources: 'Pretty but dangerous' 1983; Sutherland 1993

A p p e n d i x h

BUSHFIRE RESISTANT VEGETATION

The following is a list of fire-retardant tree species, with their common names and the height to which they grow. We have included species that do not significantly increase the rate of combustion during a fire, but have not included those that recover quickly, because they do not provide effective resistance to fire.

BUSHFIRE RESISTANT VEGETATION

Acacia baileyana (Cootamundra Wattle), evergreen, 6 m (20 ft)

Acacia botrycephala (see *Acacia terminalis*)

Acacia cultriformis, (Knife-leaf or Golden Glow Wattle), evergreen, 2–4 m (6½–13 ft)

Acacia cyanophylla (see *Acacia saligna*)

Acacia cyclops (Western Coastal Wattle), evergreen 2–2.5 m (6½–8 ft)

Acacia dealbata (Silver Wattle), evergreen, 6–30 m (20–100 ft)

Acacia decurrens (see *Acacia normalis*)

Acacia discolor (see *Acacia terminalis*)

Acacia glandulicarpa (Hairy-pod Wattle), evergreen, 0.6–1.2 m (2–4 ft)

Acacia howitii (Sticky or Glenfalloch Wattle), evergreen, 2.6–6 m (8½–20 ft)

Acacia iteaphylla (Willow Leaf Wattle), evergreen, 2–3 m (6½–10 ft)

Acacia longifolia (see *Acacia sophorae*)

Acacia ligulata (Umbrella bush), evergreen, 2.5–5 m (8–16½ ft)

Acacia melanoxylon (Blackwood), evergreen, 6–30 m (20–100 ft)

Acacia normalis (Sydney Green Wattle), evergreen, 6–12 m (20–40 ft)

Acacia pravissima (Ovens Wattle), evergreen, 3–6 m (10–20 ft)

Acacia prominens (Gosford Wattle), evergreen, 4–10 m (13–33 ft)

Acacia retinodes (Wirilda), evergreen, 3–6 m (10–20 ft)

Acacia saligna (Golden Wreath or Orange Wattle), evergreen, 1–8 m (3–26 ft)

Acacia sentis (see *Acacia victorae*)

Acacia sophorae (Sydney Golden Wattle), evergreen, 3–5 m (10–16½ ft)

Acacia sowdenii (Western Myall), evergreen, 3.5 m (11½ ft)

Acacia terminalis (Sunshine or Cedar Wattle), evergreen, 2.5–6 m (8–20 ft)

Acacia trineura (Three-nerve Wattle), evergreen, 2–3 m (6½–10 ft)

Acacia vestita (Hairy Wattle), evergreen, 3 m (10 ft)

Acacia victorae (Bramble Wattle), evergreen, 2.5–6 m (8–20 ft)

Acer pseudoplatanus (Sycamore Maple), deciduous, 12–18 m (40–60 ft)

Acmena smithii (Lilly-pilly), evergreen, 6–18 m (20–60 ft)

Agonis juniperina, evergreen, 6–12 m (20–40 ft)

Ajuga australis (Australian Bugle), perennial form, 0.1–0.3 m (4–12 in)

Angophora costata (Smooth-bark Apple-myrtle, Sydney Red Gum, Rusty Gum), evergreen, 15–24 m (50–80 ft)

Atriplex cinerea (Coast Saltbush, Grey Saltbush), evergreen, 0.6–1.5 m (2–5 ft)

Atriplex nummularia (Old-man Saltbus)h,evergreen, 1–2.5 m (3–8 ft)

Atriplex vesicaria (Saltbush), evergreen, 1–2.5 m (3–8 ft)

Banksia marginata (Silver Banksia), evergreen, 2.5–10 m (8–33 ft)

Brachychiton populneus (Kurrajong), evergreen, 6–15 m (20–50 ft)

Bursaria spinosa (Sweet Bursaria or Prickly Box), evergreen, 2–8 m (6½–26 ft)

Carpobrotus glaucescens (Angular Pigface), perennial, prostrate

Carpobrotus modestus (Pigface), perennial, prostrate

Carpobrotus rossii (Pigface), perennial, prostrate

Carpobrotus virescens (Pigface), perennial, prostrate

Casuarina cunninghamiana (River She Oak), evergreen, 10–15 m (33–50 ft)

Casuarina obesa, evergreen, 2–3 m (6½–10 ft)

Ceratonia siliqua (Carob, St John's Bread), evergreen, 5–10 m (16½–33 ft)

Chaemaecytisus prolifer (False Tree Lucerne/Tagasaste), evergreen, 3–6 m (10–20 ft)

Coprosma baueri (see *Coprosma repens*)

Coprosma repens (Looking Glass Plant, Mirror Bush, Taupata), evergreen, 2.5–3 m (8–10 ft)

Coprosma retusa (see *Coprosma repens*)

Corynocarpus laevigatus (New Zealand Laurel, Karaka), evergreen, 6–12 m (20–40 ft)

Cotoneaster lacteus (Cotoneaster), evergreen, 2.5–4 m (8–13 ft)

Cotoneaster glaucophyllus serotina (Cotoneaster), evergreen, 2.5–5 m (8–16½ ft)

Cotoneaster serotinus (see *Cotoneaster glaucophyllus serotina*)

Cytisis prolifer (see *Chaemaecytisus prolifer*)

Echium candicans (Pride of Madeira), evergreen, 1–2.5 m (3–8 ft)

Einadia hastata, evergreen, 0.5 m (20 in)

Einadia nutans, evergreen, 0.5 m (20 in)

Elaegnus pungens, evergreen, 3–5 m (10–16½ ft)

Enchylaena tomentosa (Ruby or Barrier Saltbush), evergreen, 0.6 m (24 in)

Eriobotrya japonica (Loquat), evergreen, 3–6 m (10–20 ft)

Eucalyptus bauerana (Blue Box), evergreen, 3–6 m (10–20 ft)

Eucalyptus kondininensis (Stocking Gum), evergreen, 13–15 m (43–50 ft)

Eucalyptus lehmannii (Bush Yeate), Lehmann's Gum, evergreen, 5–8 m (16½–26 ft)

Eucalyptus maculata (Spotted Gum), evergreen, 18–30 m (60–100 ft)

Eucalyptus occidentalis (Flat-topped Yate), evergreen, 18–24 m (60–80 ft)

Eucalyptus sargentii (Salt River Mallet), evergreen, 8–10 m (26–33 ft)

Eugenia smithii (see *Acmena smithii*)

Ficus spp. (Moreton Bay Fig and other native figs), evergreen, height varies from 3–7 m (10–23 ft) for *Ficus robinignosa* 'variegata' (Variegated Rusty Fig), through 6–18 m (20–60 ft) for *Ficus eugeniodes* (Small-leaf Fig), to 15–30 m (50–100 ft) for *Ficus macrophylla* (Moreton Bay Fig)

Fraxinus spp. (Ash), deciduous, height varies from 6 m (20 ft) for *Fraxinus chinensis* (Chinese Ash) to 15–24 m (50–80 ft) for *Fraxinus americana* (White Ash), to 25 m (80 ft) for *Fraxinus excelsior* (English Ash)

Grevillea aquifolium, evergreen, 0.3–1.5 m (1–5 ft)

Grevillea barklyana (Jervis Bay form) (Large Leaf Grevillea), evergreen, 2–6 m (6½–20 ft)

Grevillea shiressii, evergreen, 1–4 m (3–13 ft)

Grevillea 'Poorinda Constance', evergreen, 1–3 m (3–10 ft)

Grevillea 'Poorinda Queen', 'Poorinda Queen', evergreen, 1.5–3 m (5–10 ft)

Grevillea victoriae (Royal Grevillea), evergreen, 1–3 m (3–10 ft)

Grevillea victoriae 'Murray Queen', evergreen, 1–3 m (3–10 ft)

Hakea elliptica (Oval-leaf Hakea), evergreen, 2.5–5 m (8–16 ft)

Hakea salicifolia (Willow Hakea), evergreen, 3–6 m (10–20 ft)

Hakea saligna (see *Hakea salicifolia*)

Hakea suaveolens, evergreen, 2–4 m (6½–13 ft)

Hymenosporum flavum (Native Frangipani, Wing-seed Tree), evergreen, 5–12 m (16½–40 ft)

Jacksonia scoparia (Winged Broom Pea, Dogwood), evergreen, 1.5–4 m (5–13 ft)

Juglans nigra (Black Walnut), deciduous, 15–24 m (50–80 ft)

Juglans regia (Persian Walnut), deciduous, 10–15 m (33–50 ft)

Lagunaria patersonia (Pyramid Tree, Norfolk Island Hibiscus, Whitewood), evergreen, 6–12 m (20–40 ft)

Lasiopetalum macrophyllum (Shrubby Velvet-bush), evergreen, 1.5–3 m (5–10 ft)

Lasiopetalum schulzenii (Drooping Velvet-bush), evergreen, 1 m (3 ft)

Laurus nobilis (Bay Laurel, Sweet Bay, Grecian Laurel), evergreen, 15–30 m (50–100 ft)

Melia azedarach var. australasica (White Cedar), deciduous, 6–12 m (20–40 ft)

Morus alba (White Mulberry), deciduous, 5–11 m (16½–36 ft)

Morus nigra (Black Mulberry), deciduous, 7–8 m (23–26 ft)

Morus rubra (Red Mulberry), deciduous, 12–18 m (40–60 ft)

Myrtus communis (Common Myrtle), evergreen, 2–4 m (6½–13 ft)

Myoporum insulare (Boobialla), evergreen, 2.5–6 m (8–20 ft)

Myoporum serratum var. obovatum (see *Myoporum insulare*)

Photinia serrulata (Chinese Hawthorn), evergreen, 4–8 m (13–26 ft)

Pinus canariensis (Canary Islands Pine), evergreen, 15–24 m (50–80 ft)

Pinus halepensis (Aleppo Pine, Calabrian Pine), evergreen, 10–12 m (33–40 ft)

Pittosporum undulatum (Sweet Pittosporum), evergreen, 6–12 m (20–40 ft)

Platanus orientalis (Plane/Sycamore, Oriental Plane), deciduous, 23–24 m (75–80 ft)

Populus alba (White or Silver Poplar), deciduous, 15–22 m (50–72 ft)

Prunus spp (stone fruits, eg plum, peach, apricot), deciduous, 10–18 m (33–60 ft)

Pyracantha spp. (Firethorn), evergreen, 2–5 m (6½–16½ ft)

Quercus spp. (Oak), deciduous, 6–30 m (20–100 ft)

Salix spp. (Willow), deciduous, 3–20 m (10–66 ft)

Schinus molle (Pepper Tree), evergreen, 6–15 m (20–50 ft)

Schinus terebinthifolus (Brazilian Pepper Tree), evergreen, 5–8 m (16½–26 ft)

Sterculia diversifolia (see *Brachychiton populneus*)

Tamarix articulata (see *Tamarix aphylla*)

Tamarix aphylla (Tamarisk, Athel Tree), evergreen, 6–10 m (20–33 ft)

Tamarix parviflora (Early Tamarisk), deciduous, 4–5 m (13–16½ ft)

Tilia europaea (Common Linden, Common Lime), deciduous, 18–30 m (60–100 ft)

Tilia vulgaris (see *Tilia europaea*)

Ulmus spp (Elm), deciduous, 10–30 m (33–100 ft)

Anderson 1968; Australian Plant Study Group 1990; Blomberg 1972; Country Fire Service (n/d); Cunningham, et al 1981; Forestry Commission of New South Wales 1980; Forestry and Timber Bureau 1972; Francis 1989; Kreviter and Tardif 1986; Molnar 1974; Morley and Toelken 1983; Williams 1966

Glossary

ANTHROPOGEOGRAPHY: The study of the relationship between people and geography; the distribution of populations on the basis of geography and climate.

BAUBIOLOGIE™: 'Building biology'; the application of holistic principles to the construction of healthy living and working environments, based on an understanding of the relationship between people's health and the built environment.

BIOCLIMATE: The atmospheric conditions and processes affecting plant, animal and human biology.

BIOENERGETICS: The study of the biological energy fields associated with all living organisms.

BIOHARMONIC: In harmony with nature; supporting a healthy flow of energy.

CH'I: The energy which, according to ancient Chinese thought, breathes life into the natural world, producing growth and harmony. The beneficial circulation of *ch'i* is the aim of *feng shui*.

COLLECTIVE UNCONSCIOUS: The world spirit believed by Swiss psychologist Carl Jung to connect all human beings, living and dead; rocks, water and other components of the earth are said to be points of contact that allow communication to occur.

CURRY NET: The pattern of the Earth's geomagnetic field as described by Curry, a German medical practitioner, who believes that geomagnetism occurs in 75 centimetre (30 inch) wide strips 3.5 metres (11 feet 6 inches) apart, running northeast to southwest and northwest to southeast around the globe.

DIFFUSION: The mixing of vapours, gases and liquids and their penetration of solid permeable materials. The rate at which diffusion takes place is dependent upon temperature, air moisture content and vapour pressure. Diffusive (or 'breathing') building materials prevent the build-up of condensation and in some cases help to filter out pollutants in the air.

DOWSING: The locating of subterranean water, minerals or ley lines using a Y-shaped twig, L-shaped metal rod, pendulum, etc, with the human body acting as a form of antenna.

EARTH-ENERGIES: The energy forces arising from the Earth. The Earth's surface contains many sites which emit high concentrations of energy.

ECOSYSTEM: Organisms interact with both the living and non-living elements of their immediate environment, forming an ecosystem. Matter and energy circulate continuously between the various components of an ecosytem.

ELECTRIC FIELD: A field of force created by electric charges or by a variation in magnetic intensity.

ELECTROCLIMATE: The combination of natural electrical and low frequency fields from the atmosphere with artificial low and high frequency radiation and electrostatic fields created by a building, electrical appliances, etc. The aim is to maintain an electroclimate which is as close as possible to the natural state of the site.

ELECTROMAGNETIC FIELD: A force field that combines both a magnetic and an electric field; present with electrical current.

ELECTROSTATIC: Pertaining to static electric force fields, rather than those taking the form of waves (such as electromagnetism). Electrostatic effects tend to occur in dry weather and may be experienced as a slight shock when a discharge passes between two surfaces of opposite charge, through the body, to earth.

ELF: See Extremely Low Frequency.

ENTROPIC DEBT: The amount of waste heat generated by manufacturing and extraction processes. A product which took a large amount of energy to produce — for example, aluminium — can be said to have a high entropic debt.

EXTREMELY LOW FREQUENCY (ELF): This band of frequencies occurs at the lower end of the electromagnetic spectrum and can be present in the fields produced by power lines, microwave transmissions, and electrical equipment such as microwave ovens, computer terminals and those which have built-in transformers.

FENG SHUI: A Chinese practice blending geomancy and astrology, based on the principle that location in the universe affects destiny. Its goal is to situate buildings in tune with nature and the universe so that harmony, happiness and prosperity prevail for the inhabitants.

FIELD: The area around a source of energy within which a measurable force exists. Electric or magnetic fields are sometimes termed radiation because electromagnetic forces radiate out from their source.

GAIAN HYPOTHESIS: The idea put forward by Doctor James Lovelock that the Earth is a single organism, a living entity made up of interlinked life systems. 'Gaia' is the name of the ancient Greek goddess of the Earth.

GEOENERGETICS: See Earth-energies.

GEOMAGNETIC FIELD (GMF): The Earth's magnetic field.

GEOMANCY: The art of divination through the observation of signs on the Earth.

GEOPATHOGENIC ZONES: Places on the Earth's surface which are capable of causing disease or ill health.

GMF: See Geomagnetic Field.

HARTMANN EARTH GRID: The pattern of the Earth's geomagnetic field as described by Hartmann, a German medical practitioner, who believes that geomagnetism occurs in 20 centimetre (8 inch) wide strips, separated from each other by 2 metres when running north/south and by 2.5 metres (8 feet 2 inches) when running east/west around the globe.

HEALTHY HOUSE: A low-allergy house in which the structure, finishes and furnishings have been selected for their diffusive qualities; such a building breathes, the materials absorb and filter interior and external air pollutants, and there is minimal distortion to the natural electroclimate.

HOLISTIC: The tendency in nature for the formation of wholes that are greater than the sum of their parts. For example, according to holistic medicine one should consider the whole person, including psychological and spiritual factors, when treating an illness.

HOLOCOENOTIC: The holocoenotic principle asserts that an ecosystem should be treated as a whole unit because its components are continuously interacting with one other.

HYGROSCOPIC: Able to absorb moisture from the air.

ION: An atom or molecule that has acquired an electric charge by gaining or losing an electron.

Ionising radiation: Electromagnetic radiation which is high enough in energy to cause an atom or molecule to gain or lose an electron, creating an ion. Ionising radiation occurs above the ultraviolet band of the electromagnetic spectrum.

Ley lines: A term used by Alfred Watkins (1855–1935) to describe the alignment of prehistoric and historic monuments in the British landscape. These lines are claimed by dowsers to radiate powerful forces which can affect our wellbeing.

Low-allergy house: A house in which chemical outgassing, dust-creating and dust-holding materials and disruption to the natural electroclimate are minimised.

Materialism: The doctrine that matter is the only reality and that all questions can be settled by observation, but not by intuition.

Microclimate: The climatic factors prevailing in a small space, which differ from the general climate (macroclimate) of the area.

Microwave: The band of electromagnetic radiation used for cooking (by energy absorption), radar and telecommunications, because it can be formed into narrow beams.

Ming t'ang: The Chinese name for a semi-circular pool, sunken garden or ceremonial area on the south side of a building.

Morphic resonance: The effect of pattern and shape on our lives and wellbeing.

Morphogenic: Shapes or forms arising from inherited characteristics that are not necessarily physical. Rupert Sheldrake hypothesises that morphogenic fields are responsible for a system's characteristic form and organisation.

Negion: An ion formed when an electron (carrying a negative charge) that has been displaced from an air molecule becomes attached to another molecule, giving it a negative charge. An excess of negions compared with posions is considered to be beneficial to wellbeing. (See Posion.)

Outgassing: The spontaneous release of gases (toxic or non-toxic) by a material as it dries out or ages.

Parascience: A practice combining both the controlled experimental procedures of science and the mysticism and occultism of protoscience. Many of the activities of parascience are subjective, intuitive and difficult to measure.

Passive-solar design: An integrated system of building design and materials that utilises natural climatic conditions to maintain the internal climate of the building without utilising additional energy. (Active solar design uses purpose-designed and manufactured systems in addition to the design of the building to make use of solar energy.)

Photosynthesis: The process by which plants use sunlight and carbon dioxide to produce carbohydrates, which release energy when the plant takes in oxygen and respires.

Photovoltaic: Solar panels comprise a number of photovoltaic cells which produce an electric current when photons from the sun hit their surfaces.

Phyllotaxis: The laws governing the arrangement of leaves on the stems of plants; the geometry of growth.

Posion: An ion formed when an electron (carrying a negative charge) is displaced from an air molecule, leaving it with a positive charge. An excess of posions compared to negions in the air is considered to be detrimental to wellbeing.

Protoscience: The mystical practices which form the historic background to modern-day science; many of these practices are not measurable or repeatable in experiments, as required by modern science.

R-Value: Measure of a material's resistance to heat loss or gain. The higher the R-value, the greater a material's insulation capacity.

Radiation: See Field.

Radon (Rn_{222}): A radioactive gas which is produced in the earth during the decay process of uranium. One of the daughter products of radon attaches to dust particles in the air and can be breathed in, remaining radioactive for 20 minutes after its release.

Telluric: Of the Earth; of the soil.

Thermal mass: High density components of a building (for example, concrete floor pads near windows) that store heat to later be released (at night, for instance). The higher the conductivity of a material, the greater its capacity to store heat.

Yin and Yang: The two polar energies which Chinese philosophy teaches are the cause, through their interaction, of the universe. *Yin* is feminine, passive and dark while *yang* is masculine, active and bright.

Resources list

This directory has been compiled to assist readers in their search for healthy materials and suitable services. Not all the products listed comply with every criterion required of a healthy building, but we have included them because they are better than any other products currently available. Acceptable natural materials that are universally available have not been included. The list is not exhaustive, but provides a representative sample of products and services available in Australia, New Zealand, the United Kingdom, the United States of America and Asia.

Note: Australia is undergoing a gradual changeover to eight digit telephone and fax numbers. Please check with the directory information service if calls to any of the numbers provided can not be connected.

CONTENTS

SECTION 1: BUILDING MATERIALS, PRODUCTS AND TRADES

ADHESIVES, WOODWORKING

AUSTRALIA

Bostik Australia Pty Ltd (Bostik™ PVA water emulsion 4101)
191 O'Riordan St Mascot NSW 2020
Ph (02) 317 5088

UNITED STATES

AFM Industries, Inc (Adhesives, sealers and paints)
350 West Ash St, Suite 700 San Diego CA 92101
Ph 619 239 0321 Fax 619 239 0565

Franklin International (Titebond ES747, solvent-free adhesive)
2020 Bruck St Columbus OH 43207
Ph 1 800 347 4583 Fax 1 800 879 4553

W.F. Taylor Co.
11545 Pacific Ave Fontana CA 92337
Ph 1 800 397 4583 Fax 1 800 310 802 2831

ADOBE
(SEE SECTION 8)

ASBESTOS REMOVAL

AUSTRALIA

Middlemass Industrial Services
PO Box 745 Revesby NSW 2212
Ph (02) 773 8133 Fax (02) 773 8448

UNITED STATES

Call your regional Environmental Protection Agency (EPA) office, the State Occupational Safety & Health Administration (OSHA) or the American Lung Association (Ph 1 800 LUNGUSA)

ASPHALTIC BITUMEN FELT
(SEE ROOFING)

BAMBOO
(SEE FLOORING)

BRICKS
(SEE EARTH CONSTRUCTION)

BUILDING PAPER

NEW ZEALAND

Duroid Ltd ('GreenWrap', Heavyweight 'GreenWrap' and 'GreenCap', fire-retardant, breathing building papers which permit moisture permeability and retard air/water penetration)
Pte Bag 82822 Penrose Auckland Ph (9) 579 8859
Fax (9) 579 9126

UNITED KINGDOM AND EUROPE

British Sisalcraft Ltd (VLC Grade 411, lowest vapour-resistant building paper)
Commissioners Rd Strood, Kent ME2 4ED

Excel Industries (BI Natur Dampf-bremspappe vapour-control paper)
13 Rassau Industrial Estate, Ebbw Vale, Gwent NP3 5SD

Klober Plastics Ltd (Tyvek sarking felt)
Unit 3B Pear Tree Industrial Estate, Upper Langford, Avon BS 18 7DJ

UNITED STATES

Denny Sales Corporation
3500 Gateway Dr Pompano Beach FL 33069
Ph 1 800 327 6616 Fax 305 972 5794

CLEANING SYSTEMS

AUSTRALIA

Breville (Vaporapid Steam Cleaner, which cleans fats and limescale from ovens, sinks, etc)
149 Pyrmont St Pyrmont NSW 2009
Ph (02) 660 6144 Fax (02) 660 0229

Environmental Health Systems (Ducted vacuum system which vents to outside air)
PO Box 733 Chatswood NSW 2067
Ph (02) 413 3805 Fax (02) 413 3735

CONCRETE, REINFORCED

NEW ZEALAND

Pultrusion Technology (Reinforced concrete with glass fibre)
PO Box 323 Gisborne Ph (06) 867 8582
Fax (06) 867 8542

UNITED STATES

Fibermesh Company (Polypropylene-fiber reinforced concrete)

4019 Industry Dr Chatanooga TN 37416
Ph 615 892 7243 Fax 615 892 8080

DISABLED ACCESS

AUSTRALIA
A.P.Morling Pty Ltd (Wheelchair lifts for porches, stairways, etc)
305 Dandenong Valley Highway Dandenong Vic 3175
Ph (03) 9213 3500 Fax (03) 9213 3599
Freecall: 1800 65 3500

UNITED STATES
Access Specialists Inc
4366 Edgewood Ave Oakland CA 94602
Ph 510 548 5752

DRAINAGE

AUSTRALIA
Everhard Industries (Stormwater detention system)
405 Newman Rd Geebung Qld 4034
Ph (07) 265 3999; Cairns, Qld Ph (070) 31 3558;
Sydney, NSW Ph (02) 757 2799; Melbourne, Vic
Ph (03) 553 0899; Adelaide, SA Ph (08) 212 1700;
Perth, WA Ph (09) 328 6644; Hobart, Tas
Ph (002) 73 3455

Johnson Filtration Systems (Aust) Pty Ltd (Anti-static grating)
88 Brickyard Rd Geebung Qld 4034
Ph (07) 867 5555 Fax (07) 265 2768

Stormtech Drains
35 Portman St Zetland NSW 2017 Ph (02) 699 3519

NEW ZEALAND
Everhard Industries
Wellington Ph (644) 569 3513 Fax (644) 569 3300

UNITED STATES
Aquapore Moisture Systems (Porous irrigation pipes made of recycled materials)
610 S. 80th St Phoenix AZ 85043
Ph 1 800 635 8379 Fax 602 936 9040

Structural Plastics Corp (Tree grates made of recycled plastic)
2750 Lippincott Boulevard, Flint MI 48507
Ph 1 800 523 6899

EARTH CONSTRUCTION

AUSTRALIA
Earth Bricks
899 Pittwater Rd Collaroy NSW 2097
Ph (02) 9971 8974

Earthwise Constructions
PO Box 170 Kangaroo Flat Vic 3355 Ph (03) 45 3136

Engineered Aggregates Australia Pty Ltd (CEAC) (Rammed-earth walls)
20 Brisbane Rd Mooloolaba Qld 4556
Ph (074) 447 877 Fax (074) 443 909

Georgica Earthbricks
Lane Rd Georgica via Lismore NSW 2480

Hipwell Mud Bricks
PO Axedale Vic 3551 Ph (054) 336 370

Ramtec Pty Ltd (Rammed-earth walls)
105 Forrest St Cottesloe WA 6011 Ph (09) 384 5777

Self-sufficiency Supplies
Forth and Clyde Sts Kempsey NSW 2440

NEW ZEALAND
Alan Drayton Builders Ltd
74 Kohu Rd Titirangi Ph (09) 817 7177

Building Biology & Ecology Services of New Zealand
PO Box 2764 Auckland Ph/Fax (64–99) 358 2202

Terry Wood
PO Box 31079 Milford Auckland Ph (09) 478 6668

UNITED KINGDOM AND EUROPE
British Earth Sheltering Association
The Caer Llan Berm House, Lydart Nr. Monmouth, Gwent NP5 3JJ

Centre of Earthen Architecture, University of Plymouth School of Architecture
The Hoe Centre, Notte St Plymouth PL1 2AR

CRATerre–EAG
BP 53 F–38090, Villefontaine, France

UNITED STATES
California Earth Art and Architecture Institute
10177 Baldy Ln Hesperia CA 92345
Ph 619 956 7533

The Cob Cottage Company
PO Box 123 Cottage Grove OR 97424
Ph 503 942 3021

Southwest Solaradobe School
PO Box 153 Bosque NM 87006 Ph 505 252 1382

The Terra Group
1058 Second Ave Napa CA 94558 Ph 707 224 2532

ELECTRICAL EQUIPMENT

AUSTRALIA
ATCO Controls (Constant voltage transformers and controls for low voltage lighting)
130 Melrose Dr Tullamarine Vic 3043
Ph (03) 338 2333 Fax (03) 330 3595

Commercial Lighting Improvements Pty Ltd (Longlife incandescent lights)
11/365 West Botany St Rockdale NSW 2216
Ph (02) 597 5900 Fax (02) 599 3320

Heim Lighting Pty Ltd (Energy-saving lights)
11/26 Megalong St Katoomba NSW 2780
Ph (047) 82 5599 Fax (047) 82 5621

Osram Australia Pty Ltd (Low-wattage incandescent tungsten lights)
423 Pennant Hills Rd Pennant Hills NSW 2020
Ph (02) 481 8399 Fax (02) 481 9468

Rojen Consultancies (Demand switches)
5 Elizabeth Rd Wanneroo WA 6065
Ph (09) 306 3816 (After hours)

NEW ZEALAND
Building Biology and Ecology Services of New Zealand
PO Box 35921 Browns Bay Auckland
Ph/Fax (09) 479 3161

Elec-Technique Ltd (Demand switches)
37 Roslyn Tce Devonport NZ Ph (09) 445 9118

UNITED KINGDOM AND EUROPE
Natural Therapeutics (Demand switches and electromagnetic shielding devices)
25 New Rd Spalding, Lincolnshire PE11 1DQ

UNITED STATES
Duro-Lite Lamps Inc. (Vita-Lite full-spectrum fluorescent tubes)
9 Law Dr Fairfield NJ 07004 Ph 1 800 526 7193
(ext. 5316)

Enterpriser Lighting Inc (100-year light bulb)
12509 Patterson Ave Richmond VA 23233
Ph 1 800 394 2852 Fax 804 784 0334

Environmental Systems Inc (Full-spectrum Ott-Lite fluorescent tube)
204 Pitney Rd Lancaster PO 17601 Ph 717 394 3182

Healthful Hardware (Chromalux full-spectrum incandescent bulbs)
PO Box 3217 Prescott AZ 86302 Ph 602 445 8225

International Institute for Bau-Biologie & Ecology
PO Box 387 Clearwater FL 34615
Ph 813 461 4371 Fax 813 441 4373

National Cathode Corp. (Cold cathode tube lighting)
252 W. 29th St New York NY 10001
Ph 212 594 1960 Fax 212 563 1249

The Ion & Light Company (Duro-Lite tubes, full-spectrum Neodymium bulbs)
2263–1/2 Sacramento St San Francisco CA 94115
Ph 415 346 6205

ELECTRICIANS (BIOELECTRICIANS)

AUSTRALIA
P.R. McBride & Co. Pty Ltd
5 Panaview Cres. North Rocks NSW 2152
Ph (02) 872 1492

NEW ZEALAND

Gary Beck
Elec-Technique Ph (09) 445 9118

Reinhold Huber
Lonely Track Rd Albany Ph (09) 473 1637

UNITED STATES

Environmental Electrics (Electrical contracting, EMF surveys)
PO Box 10284 San Rafael CA 94912 Ph 415 721 1515

Environmental Risk Testing
1155 N. Slate St, #420 Bellingham WA 98225
Ph 206 734 6777

International Institute for Bau-Biologie and Ecology
PO Box 387 Clearwater FL 34615
Ph 813 461 4371 Fax 813 441 4373

Land & Sea Electric (Electrical contracting, EMF testing and mitigation)
444 Brickell Ave Plaza 51–273 Miami FL 33131
Ph 305 674 9716

EXHAUST FANS
(SEE VENTILATION)

FIBRE-CEMENT PRODUCTS
(INTERNAL AND EXTERNAL LININGS, FLOORING, ROOFING, PIPES FOR IRRIGATION, STORM WATER, SEWAGE, ELECTRICAL CONDUITS)

AUSTRALIA

James Hardie & Co Pty Ltd
PO Box 219 Granville NSW 2142 Ph (02) 638 9999
Fax (02) 638 9778

UNITED STATES

American Cemwood (Shingles)
PO Box C, Albany OR 97321 Ph 1 800 367 3471

Cal-Shake (Shingles)
0PO Box 2265 Irwindale CA 91706
Ph 1 800 736 7663 Fax 818 969 7520

Faswall Concrete Systems (Concrete/mineralised wood blocks)
1676 Nixon Rd Augusta GA 30906
Ph 706 793 8880 Fax 706 793 3311

FiberCem (Shingles)
PO Box 411368 Charlotte NC

James Hardie Building Products (Shingles, siding)
10901 Elm Ave Fontana CA 92335
Ph 1 800 426 4051

Supradur (Shingles)
PO Box 908 Rye NY 10580
Ph 1 800 223 1948; Fax 914 967 8344

Tectum Inc (Building panels)
PO Box 920 Newark OH 43058
Ph 614 345 9691 Fax 1 800 832 8869

FLOORING

ASIA

Ever Talent Ltd (Bamboo; tongue and grooved; can be supplied unsealed for natural finish)
12th Floor, 3 Matheson St Causeway Bay Hong Kong
Ph (852) 573 3066 Fax (852) 573 730

AUSTRALIA

Duroloid Pty Ltd (Linoleum)
236 Wickham Rd Moorabbin Vic 3189
Ph (03) 555 9921 Fax (03) 553 2131

Forbo Australia Pty Ltd (Marmoleum)
15 Ferndell St Granville NSW 2142 Ph (02) 738 4800
Freecall 008 888 344 Fax (02) 645 4270

Heritage Contract Systems (Natural rubber and polyolefine flooring)
16 Wetherill St Silverwater NSW 2128
Ph (02) 648 5599 Freephone 1800 242 660
Fax (02) 649 6760

Natural Floor Covering Centre
5 Salisbury Rd Stanmore NSW 2048
Ph (02) 569 6999 Fax (02) 550 9196

Natural Floors
33 Henry St Stepney SA 5069
Ph (08) 363 2828 Fax (08) 363 1039

UNITED KINGDOM AND EUROPE

Crucial Trading Ltd (Natural fibre flooring)
Unit 8 Treowain Industrial Estate, Machynlleth, Powys SY20 Wales

DLW Floorings & Forbo-Nairn Ltd (Linoleum)
Centurion Court, Milton Park, Nr. Abingdon, Oxfordshire OX14 4RY

UNITED STATES

Dodge-Regupol Inc (Cork and recycled rubber flooring)
PO Box 989 Lancaster PA 17608
Ph 1 800 322 1923 Fax 717 295 3414

Forbo North America (Natural linoleum)
PO Box 667 Hazelton PA 18201 Ph 1 800 0475

Gerbert Ltd (Natural linoleum)
PO Box 4944 Lancaster PA 17604 Ph 717 299 5083
Fax 717 394 1937

GTE Products (Recycled-content ceramic tiles)
Ph 717 724 8322

Hendriksen Naturlich
7120 Keating Ave Sebastopol CA 95472
Ph 707 829 3959 Fax 707 829 1774

Ipocork (Cork flooring)
1280 Roberts Boulevard, Suite 403 Kennesaw GA
30144 Ph 1 800 828 2675

Reliance Carpet Cushion (Non-allergenic)
15700 S. Main St Gardena CA 90248
Ph 213 321 2300 Fax 213 523 1807

Smith & Fong (Bamboo flooring)
222–1/2 Winfield St South San Francisco CA 94110
Ph 415 285 8230

Stoneware Tile Company (Recycled-content ceramic tiles)
1650 Progress Dr Richmond IN 47374
Ph 317 935 4760

GLASS

AUSTRALIA

Cydonia, The Glass Studio Pty Ltd (Stained glass and slumped, textured glass panels)
17Cnr Station and Wilford Sts Newtown NSW 2042
Ph (02) 557 5898 Fax (02) 550 5670

DGI (Dale Glass Industries)
93 Wetherill St Silverwater NSW 2128
Ph (02) 647 2911 Fax (02) 748 3443

Glass Brick Company
19 Graham Rd Clayton South Vic 3169
Ph (03) 547 4556 Fax (03) 558 5620

Ha'fele Australia Pty Ltd (Combination hopper and casement sash windows)
8 Monterey Rd Dandenong Vic 3175
Ph (03) 212 2000 Fax (03) 212 2002

Miglas Australia Pty Ltd (Double-glazed timber windows)
57–59 Canterbury Rd Montrose Vic 3765
Ph (03) 728 3999 Fax (03) 728 3555

Pilkington (Australia) Ltd
Glass Products Division
35–45 Malta St Villawood NSW 2163
Ph (02) 726 6688

UNITED KINGDOM AND EUROPE

Pilkington Glass Ltd
Victoria House, Cowley Hill Works, St Helens, Merseyside WA10 3TT

The Swedish Window Co Ltd
Milbank, Earls Colne Industrial Park, The Airfield, Earls Coln, Colchestee, Essex CO6 2NS

UNITED STATES

Andersen Windows Inc. (Highly insulative windows, water-based finishes)
100 Fourth Ave North, Bayport MN 55003
Ph 612 439 5150

Southwall Technologies (Solar control and insulating glass)
1029 Corporation Way, Palo Alto CA 94303
Ph 1 800 365 8794 Fax 415 967 0182

INSULATION

AUSTRALIA
Cellulose Insulation Manufacturing Co
PO Box 1153 Cooparoo Qld 4151
Ph (07) 3397 9154

Golden Fleece Insulation Pty Ltd (Wool insulation)
Broadway Ct Cobram Vic 3644 Ph (058) 711 233
Fax (058) 722 336

Higgins Wool & Textiles Pty Ltd (Wool insulation)
469 Greenwattle St Toowoomba Qld 4350
Ph (076) 332 600 Fax (076) 332 429

UNITED KINGDOM AND EUROPE
Excel Industries Ltd (Cellulose insulation)
13 Rassau Industrial Estate, Ebbw Vale, Gwent
NP3 5SD

Isolfloc UK Ltd (Cellulose insulation)
Ecological Building Technology
31 Heathfield, Stacey Bushes, Milton Keynes
MK12 6HR

Rockwool Products Ltd (Mineral wool fibre insulation)
Pencoed, Bridgend CF35 6NY

Vencil Resin Ltd ('Jablite', CFC-free, expanded polystyrene sheet)
Arndale House, 18–20 Spital St Dartford, Kent
DA1 2HT

UNITED STATES
Cellulose Insulation Manufacturers' Assoc.
136 S. Keowee St Dayton OH 45402
Ph 513 222 2462

Greenwood Cotton Insulation Products Inc.
PO Box 1017 Greenwood SC 29648
Ph 1 800 546 1332 Fax 1 800 942 4814

Icynene Inc. (Non-outgassing insulation)
376 Watline Ave Mississauga ON L4Z 1X2 Canada
Ph 1 800 758 7325 Fax 905 890 7784

Palmer Industries
10611 Old Annapolis Rd Frederick MD 21701
Ph 301 898 7848

LANDSCAPE CONSTRUCTION

AUSTRALIA
Higgins Landcare (Wool and jute mulch matting and erosion control)
469 Greenwattle St Toowoomba Qld 4350
Ph (07) 33 2600

UNITED STATES
Presto Products Corp. (Geoweb system for retaining walls and erosion control)
PO Box 2399 Appleton WI 54913
Ph 1 800 548 3424

Wood Recycling Inc. (Recycled hydromulch for erosion control)
PO Box 6087 Peabody MA 01961
Ph 1 800 982 8732 Fax 508 535 4252

LIGHTING
(SEE ELECTRICAL INSTALLATIONS)

LOUVRES
(SEE SUN-CONTROL LOUVRES)

MUDBRICKS
(SEE EARTH CONSTRUCTION)

PAINTERS (BIOPAINTERS)

AUSTRALIA
Environmental Painting
2/19 Tobruk Ave Cremorne NSW 2090
Ph (02) 953 4918

The Natural Paint Company
89 Cary St Leichhardt NSW 2040
Ph (02) 569 9892 Fax (02) 569 3762

The Painting Team
24 Old Beecroft Rd Cheltenham NSW 2119
Ph (02) 869 0077 Fax (02) 869 0199

PAINTS

AUSTRALIA
Bio Products Australia Pty Ltd
25 Aldgate Terrace Bridgewater SA 5155
Ph (08) 339 1923 Fax (08) 267 5156

Clean House Effect
345 King St Newtown NSW 2042 Ph (02) 516 4681
Fax (02) 699 1035

Dulux Australia
McNaughton Rd Clayton Vic 3186 Ph (03) 542 5678

Livos Plant Chemistry Paint Products
6/26 Megalong St Katoomba NSW 2780
Ph/Fax (047) 82 6155

Murobond Coatings
PO Box 487 Newtown NSW 2042 Ph (02) 962 9243

Nucletron Pty Ltd
PO Box 979 Bondi Junction NSW 2022
Ph (02) 369 1990 Fax (02) 369 1994

Organoil Pty Ltd (for interior timber finishes)
PO Box 377 Byron Bay NSW 2481 Ph (066) 858 836

Porter's Paints
895 Bourke St Waterloo NSW 2017
Ph (02) 698 5322 Fax (02) 698 5449;
Shop 8 Westgate Mall Cantonment St WA 6160
Ph (09) 430 5054 Fax (09) 430 6933

Star Cooling Paint
SCI Industries Pty Ltd
156 Ryans Rd Nundah Brisbane Qld 4012
Ph (07) 266 6677

NEW ZEALAND
Auro Organic Paints
Weleda NZ Ltd
PO Box 8132 Havelock North Ph (06) 877 7394

Bio Paints (Agents)
Box 7 Upper Moutere Nelson Ph (03) 543 2951

Breathe Easy Homes
PO Box 37 Silverdale Ph (09) 426 3189

Building Biology & Ecology Institute of New Zealand
Floor 1, 22 Customs St West Auckland New Zealand
Ph (09) 358 2202

NVF Paints Ltd
PO Box 261 Whangaparaoa Auckland
Ph (09) 424 0237

UNITED KINGDOM AND EUROPE
Auro Organic Paint Supplies Ltd
Unit 1, Goldstones Farm, Ashdon, Saffron Walden,
Essex CB10 2LZ

Ecos Environmental Paints Ltd
11 Dunscar Industrial Estate, Blackburn Rd Egerton,
Bolton BL7 9PQ

Keim Paints Ltd
Muckley Cross, Morville, Nr. Bridgend, Shropshire
WV16

Nutshell Natural Paints
Newtake, Staverton, Devon TQ9 6PE

Ostermann & Scheiwe UK Ltd
26 Swakeleys Dr Ickenham, Middlesex UB1 8QD

UNITED STATES
AFM Enterprises Inc.
350 West Ash St, Suite 700 San Diego CA 92101
Ph 619 239 0321 Fax 619 239 0565

Chem-Safe Products
PO Box 33023 San Antonio TX 78265
Ph 210 657 5321

Eco-Design Company (Bio-Shield and Livos natural paints)
1365 Rufina Circle, Santa Fe NM 87501
Ph 1 800 621 2591 Fax 505 438 6315

Miller Paint Company (Low-biocide paints)
317 SE Grand Ave Portland OR 97214
Ph 503 233 4491

Sinan Company (Auro natural paints)
PO Box 857 Davis CA 95617 Ph 916 753 3104

PERGOLAS
(SEE SUN-CONTROL LOUVRES)

PLUMBING

AUSTRALIA

Mora Thermostatic Mix Valve (Hot water temperature control)
PO Box 287 Mordialloc Vic 3195 Ph (039) 587 5811
Fax (039) 587 5822

PM Industries (Bathroom fittings)
PO Box 180 Brookvale NSW 2100
Ph (02) 9905 3244 Fax (02) 9905 0833

Ryemetal Holdings Pty Ltd (Hot water temperature control)
16–18 Malcolm Rd Braeside Vic 3195
Ph (03) 587 5811 Fax (03) 587 6875

Tersia Australia Pty Ltd (Polypropylene piping)
55 Bignell St Illawong NSW 2234 Ph (02) 543 6643
Mobile 018 219 649

Tomco International Pty Ltd (Tomus safety tap system)
PO Box 1814 Coffs Harbour NSW 2450
Ph (066) 53 8424

UNITED STATES

Controlled Energy Corporation (Tankless gas water-heating system)
Fiddler's Green, Waitsfield VT 05673
Ph 1 800 642 3111 Fax 802 496 6924

Pesco Distribution Center Inc. (Future-Flush, dual toilet retrofit)
2570 Industry Ln Norristown PA 19403
Ph 1 800 441 5114 Fax 215 630 8569

21st Century Water Systems (Divert-It Undersink water efficiency system)
1314 Main St Morro Bay CA 93442
Ph 1 800 369 4444 Fax 805 772 1709

PLYWOOD
(SEE TIMBER)

PUMPS
(SOLAR ENERGY POWERED – SEE SECTION 7)

RAINWATER TANKS

AUSTRALIA

Sydney Rainwater Tanks
1 Colt Ct, Penrith NSW 2760 Ph (mobile): (018) 44
4644 Ph (after hours) (047) 32 1720

UNITED STATES

Living Structures (Roof catchment)
PO Box 6447 Santa Fe NM 87502 Ph 505 438 0888

RECYCLED BUILDING MATERIALS

AUSTRALIA

'Country Dream' Renowned Furniture (Natural finished, recycled timber kitchens)
Shop 6b, MegaCentre, Blacktown Rd Blacktown
NSW 2148 Ph (02) 831 6411

Rock and Dirt Pty Ltd (Recycled fill, sand, road base, aggregates for concrete)
11 Lancelly Pl Artarmon NSW 2065 Ph (02) 439 8888

Rozelle Recycled Building Centre Pty Ltd
88–90 Lilyfield Rd Rozelle NSW 2039
Ph (02) 818 1166 Fax (02) 818 1112

Second Hand Building Centre
211 Bay St Brighton-le-Sands NSW 2216
Ph (02) 599 4765 Fax (02) 597 1782

UNITED KINGDOM AND EUROPE

SALVO
PO Box 1295 Bath, Avon BA1 3TJ

J.R. Nelson (Reclaimed, converted pitch pine)
The Sawmill, Newchurch, Romney Marsh, Kent
TN29 ODT

Zedcor (Recycled plastic damp-proof membranes)
Bridge Street Mill, Bridge St Witney, Oxfordshire
OX8 6LJ

UNITED STATES

Berkeley Architectural Salvage
722 Folger Ave Berkeley CA 94710 Ph 510 849 2025

California Resource Recovery Assoc.
4395 Gold Trail Way, Loomis CA 95650
Ph 916 652 4450

Urban Ore
1333 6th St Berkeley CA 94710 Ph 510 559 4460

ROOFING

AUSTRALIA

Sealex Industries NSW (Asphaltic bitumen felt roofing — not polypropylene modified)
20 Bessemer St Blacktown NSW 2148
Ph (02) 621 1433

Shingles Australia Pty Ltd
PO Box 750 Murwillumbah NSW 2484
Ph (066) 79 9150

NEW ZEALAND

New Zealand Shakes & Shingles Ltd
13 Jays Rd Woodlands Park Auckland
Ph (09) 817 2301

UNITED KINGDOM AND EUROPE

Dunstable Rubber (Roof linings for use under turf roofs)
Eastern Ave, Luton Rd Dunstable, Bedfordshire
LU5 4JY

Erisco-Bauder Ltd (Turf roof systems)
Broughton House, Broughton Rd Ipswich,
Suffolk IP1 3QS

Eternit UK Ltd (Fibre-reinforced tiles and corrugated sheets)
Meldreth, Royston, Hertfordshire SG8 5RL

National Society of Master Thatchers
High View, Little St, Yardley, Hastings,
Northamptonshire

Onduline (Bitumen fibre corrugated sheets)
Eardley House, 182–184 Camden Hill Rd Kensington,
London W8 7AS

UNITED STATES

Gerard Roofing Technologies (Slate-look recycled steel shingles)
955 Columbia St Brea CA 92621
Ph 714 529 0407 Fax 714 529 6643

Post Harvest Developments (Slate-look roofing made from recycled tyres)
PO Box 11 Ottawa ON Canada K1P 6C3
Ph 613 722 4548 Fax 613 722 5548

Tread Mill Inc. (Roofing made from cut, flattened tyres)
PO Box 407 Williams OR 97544 Ph 503 846 7385

Zappone (Recycled and recyclable aluminium and copper shingles)
2928 North Pittsburg, Spokane WA 99207
Ph 1 800 285 2677

SARKING
(SEE BUILDING PAPER)

SECOND-HAND MATERIALS
(SEE RECYCLED BUILDING MATERIALS)

SEWERAGE

AUSTRALIA

Garry Scott Compost Toilet Systems (Clivus Multrum dry toilet system)
Mullumbimby NSW 2482 Ph (066) 84 3468;
Melbourne, Vic Ph (03) 557 6943
Fax (03) 557 4786; Brisbane, Qld Ph (07) 279 3409
Fax (07) 376 2061

Dowmus Pty Ltd
Waste Management Systems
PO Box 51 Mapleton Qld 4560 Ph (074) 414 144
Fax (074) 414 653

Envirolet
PO Box 189 Bentleigh Vic 3201 Ph (03) 557 6943

Nature Loo
PO Box 1213 Milton Qld 4064 Ph (07) 3367 0601

UNITED KINGDOM AND EUROPE

Ecoclear (Clivus Multrum dry toilet system)

c/o Southern Water, Otterbourne, Winchester, Hampshire SO21 2SW

IFO Products Manufacture (Low-flush toilets)
S–29500 Bromealla, Sweden

UNITED STATES
Biological Mediation Systems Inc. (Biological Toilet)
PO Box 8248 Fort Collins CO 80526
Ph 1 800 524 1097 Fax 970 221 5748

Clivus Multrum Inc (Dry toilet system)
21 Canal St Lawrence MA 01840 Ph 1 800 962 8447

SHINGLES
(SEE ROOFING)

SHUTTERS
(SEE TIMBER)

SKYLIGHTS
(SEE VENTILATION)

SOLAR ENERGY SYSTEMS
(SEE SECTION 4)

STORM WATER
(SEE DRAINAGE)

SUN-CONTROL LOUVRES

AUSTRALIA
John Waters Industries (JWI Sunshield Louvre Systems)
31 Prime Dr Seven Hills NSW 2147
Ph (02) 674 3600 Fax (02) 674 3530

Steelbond (Sydney) Pty Ltd (Eclipse Opening Roof)
2/363 Horsley Rd Milperra NSW 2214
Ph (02) 772 1677 Freecall 1800 801 572

UNITED STATES
Phifer Wire Products Inc. (Sun-control fabric and screens)
PO Box 1700 Tuscaloosa AL 35403
Ph 1 800 633 5955 Fax 205 759 4450

Zomeworks Corp.
PO Box 25805, 1011 A Sawmill Rd NW,
Albuquerque NM 87125 Ph 1 800 279 6342
Fax 505 243 5187

TERMITE CONTROL

AUSTRALIA
Granitgard (Crushed granite termite-barriers)
141 King George St Cohuna Vic 3568
Ph (03) 2549 Fax (03) 417 6008

**Systems Management Pty Ltd (R.Verkerk)
(Holistic termite control)**

4 Jarrett La Leichhardt NSW 2040 Ph (02) 564 1614

Termi-Mesh Australia (Anti-termite mesh)
10 Westchester Rd Malaga WA 6062
Ph (09) 249 3868 Fax (09) 249 1021

UNITED STATES
Bio-Integral Resource Center (BIRC)
PO Box 7414 Berkeley CA 94707 Ph 510 524 2567

Estex Ltd
3200 Polaris Ave #9 Las Vegas NV 89102
Ph 1 800 543 5651 Fax 702 364 8894

Isothermics Inc (Heat fumigation)
9311 Loma Ave Villa Park CA 92667
Ph 714 974 0987

Live Oak Structural Inc.
801–B Camelia St Berkeley CA 94710
Ph 510 524 7101 Fax 510 524 7240

Tallon Termite & Pest Control Co.
1949 E. Market St Long Beach CA 90805
Ph 310 422 1131 Fax 310 423 6146

TIMBER

AUSTRALIA
Bio Products Australia Pty Ltd (Timber preservatives)
25 Aldgate Terrace Bridgewater SA 5155
Ph (08) 339 1923

Carter Holt Harvey (Australia) Pty Ltd (Plywood, Ecoply Texture 2000)
PO Box 180 Mt Ommaney Qld 4074
Ph (07) 3376 7222 Fax (07) 3274 0061

CSR Softwoods (Plantation Pine treated with Ammoniacal Copper Quaternary, or ACQ)
Level 6, 9 Help St Chatswood NSW 2067
Ph (02) 372 5777 Fax (02) 372 5750

CSR Timber Products
Level 7, 9 Help St Chatswood NSW 2067
Ph (02) 372 5800 Fax (02) 372 5827

Eco-Timber Co of Australia Pty Ltd
PO Box 5091 South Murwillimbah NSW 2484 Ph (066) 77 7420 Fax (066) 77 7108

Forward Products Pty Ltd (Hybeam floor joists containing no metal)
PO Box 794 Mt Waverley Vic 3149
Ph (03) 886 3299 Fax (03) 886 3250

Timber Shutter Co
PO Box 5338 Gold Coast Mail Centre Qld 4217
Ph (075) 913 282 Fax (075) 913 759

NEW ZEALAND
Koch Timber Processing
PO Box 8091 Kensington Ph (09) 479 3161

UNITED KINGDOM AND EUROPE
Ecological Trading Company Ltd
659 Newark Rd Lincoln LN6 8SA

Ecotimber Products
Unit 10, Allens Corporate Park, Skellingthorpe Rd
Saxilby, Lincolnshire LN1 2LR

Milland Fine Timber Ltd
The Working Tree, Milland, Nr. Liphook, Hampshire GU30 7JS

REMTOX (Boron rods and boron/glycol treatments for rot)
Spring Ln, Smethwick, Warley, West Midlands B66 1PE

Timber Research and Development Association (TRADA)
Stocking Ln, Hughenden Valley, High Wycombe, Bucks HP14 4ND

UNITED STATES
Big Timberworks Inc. (Recycled lumber)
PO Box 368 Gallatin Gateway MT 59730
Ph 406 763 4639 Fax 406 763 4818

Conklin's Antique Barnwood (Salvaged woods)
R.R.1, Box 70 Susquehanna PA 18847
Ph 717 465 3832

Eco-Timber International Inc. (Sustainable tropical hardwoods)
350 Treat Ave San Francisco CA 94110
Ph 415 864 4900 Fax 415 864 1011

Edenshaw Woods (Sustainable wood from Peru and Mexico)
211 Seton Rd Port Townsend WA 98368
Ph 1 800 950 3336 Fax 206 385 7870

Forest Trust Wood (Hand-peeled logs and poles)
PO Box 519 Santa Fe NM 87504 Ph 505 983 8992
Fax 505 986 0798

Goodwin Heart Pine Company (River-recovered heart pine and cypress)
Route 2, PO Box 119–AA Micanopy FL 32667
Ph 1 800 336 3118

Jefferson Lumber Company (Recovered lumber)
PO Box 696 McCloud CA 96057 Ph 916 235 0609
Fax 916 235 0434

Menominee Tribal Enterprises (Sustained yield eastern hardwoods)
PO Box 10 Neopit WI 54150 Ph 715 756 2311

Mountain Lumber (Recycled lumber)
PO Box 289 Ruckersville VA 22968
Ph 1 800 445 2671

Sea Star Trading Company (Sustainable tropical hardwoods)
PO Box 513 Newport OR 97365 Ph 503 265 9616
Fax 503 265 3228

Wise Wood
Box 1271 McHenry IL 60050 Ph 815 344 4943

VENTILATION

AUSTRALIA

Breeze Power Natural Cooling Pty Ltd
2/10 Pioneer Ave Thornleigh NSW 2120
Ph (02) 484 8188 Freecall 1800 637 175
Fax (02) 484 8382

John Richmond Manufacturing (Ceiling exhaust fans)
18 Downard St Braeside Vic 3195 Ph (03) 9580 4388
Fax (03) 9580 7421

Ozone Manufacturing Pty Ltd
212 Silverwater Rd Silverwater NSW 2141
Ph (02) 748 7748 Fax (02) 748 7749

Repelec (Aust) Pty Ltd (Manrose range of extractor fans)
PO Box 6046 Silverwater Business Centre Silverwater NSW 2128

Solarlite Industries Pty Ltd (Exhaust fans, skylights, heating and cooling)
2/10 Pioneer Ave Thornleigh NSW 2120
Ph (02) 484 8188 Fax (02) 484 8382

UNITED KINGDOM AND EUROPE

Willan Building Services Ltd ('Passivent' ventilation system)
2 Brooklands Rd Sale, Cheshire M33 3SF

UNITED STATES

Aldes (Air inlets)
4537 Northgate Court, Sarasota FL 34234
Ph 1 800 255 7749 Fax 813 351 3442

Resource Conservation Technology Inc. (Fantech bathroom exhaust fans)
2633 N. Calvert St Baltimore MD 21218
Ph 301 366 1146

Therma-Store Products (Heat recovery ventilators)
PO Box 8050 Madison WI 53708
Ph 1 800 533 7533 Fax 608 222 1447

Vent-Aire Systems (Heat recovery ventilators)
4850 Northpark Dr, Colorado Springs CO 80918
Ph 719 599 9080 Fax 719 599 9085

WALL CLADDING

AUSTRALIA

CSR Wood Panels (Hardboard Weathertex planks, sheets and shingles)
9 Help St Chatswood NSW 2067 Ph (02) 372 5800
Fax (02) 372 5822

James Hardie Building Systems Pty Ltd (Hardboard)
260 Musgrave St Coopers Plains Qld 4108
Ph (07) 864 7800 Fax (07) 875 1652

James Hardie & Co Pty Ltd (Moulded Glass Reinforced Cement Panels)
PO Box 219 Granville NSW 2142 Ph (02) 638 9999
Fax (02) 638 9778

UNITED KINGDOM AND EUROPE

Falcon Panel Products ('Bitroc' and 'Bivent' bitumen-impregnated fibreboard)
Walton Bridge Rd Walton Bridge, Shepperton, Middlesex TW17 8NA

Heraklith Ltd (woodwool/magnesite sheathing and infill board)
21 Broadway, Maidenhead, Berkshire SL6 1JK

Karlit Sales Co Ltd (Medium board structural sheathing)
Ash House, Ash Rd New Ash Green, Dartford KT24 6TU

L. Slack & Son ('Minerit', cement and vegetable fibre board)
Courthouse St Pontypridd, Glamorgan CF37 1JX

UNITED STATES

Abtco (Hardboard siding)
PO Box 98, Highway 268 Roaring River NC 28669
Ph 910 696 2751

James Hardie Building Products (Fiber-cement siding)
10901 Elm Ave Fontana CA 92335 Ph 1 800 426 4051

WATER FILTRATION

AUSTRALIA

Australian Water Ventures Pty Ltd (Culligan reverse-osmosis system)
Level 5, 61 Macquarie St Sydney NSW 2000
Ph (02) 252 2500 Fax (02) 252 2515

Blackwattle Environmental (Water disinfection and odour control)
Unit 24B, 1–3 Endeavour Rd Caringbah NSW 2229
Ph (02) 525 9778

Environmental Health Systems (Water filtering systems)
PO Box 733 Chatswood NSW 2067
Ph (02) 413 3805 Fax (02) 413 3735

UNITED STATES

Coast Filtration (Water Safe)
142 Viking Ave Brea CA 92621 Ph 714 990 4602

Nigra Enterprises (Cuno and General Ecology 'Spark L Pure' filters)
5699 Kanan Rd Agoura CA 91031 Ph 818 889 6877

WATERPROOFING

AUSTRALIA

Colloid Australia Pty Ltd (Volclay self-sealing, non-coated panels for walls)

PO Box 362 North Geelong Vic 3215
Ph (052) 72 1090 Fax (052) 78 5833

UNITED STATES

Thoro System Products (Thoroseal cement-based coating)
7800 NW 38th St Miami FL 33166 Ph 305 592 2081
Fax 305 592 9760

WHITE ANT CONTROL
(SEE TERMITE CONTROL)

WINDOWS
(SEE GLASS)

SECTION 2:
CONSULTANTS AND CONSULTING SERVICES

AIR POLLUTION

AUSTRALIA

Division of Building, Construction and Engineering (Testing of materials for outgassing)

Commonwealth Scientific and Industrial Research Organisation
PO Box 56 Highett Victoria 3190 Ph (03) 9252 6000
Fax (03) 9252 6244

Hans Jakobi (Interior pollution testing)
34 Osprey Dr Illawong NSW 2234 Ph (02) 543 2350

Roger L. Price
PO Box 733 Chatswood NSW 2067
Ph (02) 413 3805 Fax (02) 413 3735

UNITED STATES

A Room of One's Own
12439 Magnolia Boulevard, #263 Valley Village CA 91607 Ph 818 981 7245 Fax 818 766 5882

Ecologically Safe Homes
7471 North Shiloh Rd Unionville IN 47468
Ph 812 332 5073

Ideal Environments
401 West Adams, Fairfield IA 52556
Ph 515 472 6547

Interagency Indoor Air Council
1200 6th Ave Seattle WA 98101 Ph 206 442 2589

David Kibbey (Environmental Building Consultant)
1618 Parker St Berkeley CA 94703 Ph 510 841 1039

Hal Levin & Associates
2548 Empire Grade, Santa Cruz CA 95060
Ph 408 425 3946
(Also call your regional Environmental Protection Agency (EPA) office, the State Occupational Safety & Health Administration (OSHA) or the American Lung

Association (Ph 1 800 LUNGUSA)

ARCHITECTS

Australia

David W. Baggs Pty Ltd (Environmental, energy efficient architecture, earth-sheltered, earth-brick and straw-bale buildings)
9 Featherwood Way Castle Hill NSW 2154
Ph (02) 9899 2003 Fax (02) 9894 9168

ECA Space Design Pty Ltd (Environmental architecture, bioenergetics, building biology and ecology, healthy buildings, earth-sheltering, landscape and environmental urban design)
9 Featherwood Way Castle Hill NSW 2154
Ph (02) 9899 2003 Fax (02) 9894 9168

ECO Design Foundation Incorporated (Energy efficient ecological design)
PO Box 369 Rozelle NSW 2039 Ph (02) 555 9412
Fax (02) 555 9564

The Manly Studio (Biological architecture based on the principles of Rudolf Steiner)
37–39 The Corso Manly NSW 2095
Ph (02) 977 7648 Fax (02) 977 0295

Neal Mortensen (Biological architecture and complete CAD services)
50 Felton Rd Carlingord NSW 2118
Ph (02) 872 5871

David Oliver (Environmental, rammed earth, small and large scale building design)
Greenway Australia
PO Box 648 Mooloolabah Qld 4557
Ph (074) 44 6211 Fax (074) 44 3909

Graham Osborne
Arkishop & Colour Consultancy (Environmental, rammed earth building design)
Shop 3/11 Fletcher St Byron Bay NSW 2481
Ph (066) 85 8558 Fax (066) 85 5645

Craig and Sue Pattinson
Arcoessence Pty Ltd (Environmental architecture, healthy buildings and interior design)
PO Box 28 Beechwood NSW 2446 Ph (065) 85 6010

The PEOPL Group (Biological and ecological urban design, bio-architecture, bio-engineering, environmental planning and design)
39 Cheryl Cres, Newport Beach NSW 2106
Ph (02) 9999 4883 Fax (02) 9979 7397

Gerhard Schurer (Environmental architect)
PO Box 251 Belair SA 5052 Ph (08) 302 6458
Fax (08) 302 6911

New Zealand

Reinhard Kanuka-Fuchs
Director, Building Biology & Ecology Institute of New Zealand

PO Box 35921 Browns Bay Auckland
Ph (09) 479 3161

United Kingdom and Europe

Neville Churcher
County Architects Dept.
76 High St Winchester, Hampshire, England

Christopher Day (Steiner-inspired design)
Pen-Y-Lyn, Brynberian, Cymych, Dyfed SA41 3TL
Walesar

John Doggart (Energy-conscious design)
ECD, 11 Emerald St London WC1N 3QL

Bruno Erat
Ekosolar Oy
Kilo gård 02610 Espoo, Finland Ph 90 513 200

Prof. Declan Kennedy
Planungsbüro Kennedy
Ginsterweg 4–5 D–31595 Steyerberg Germany
Ph 5764 2158 Fax 5764 2368

Paul Leech (Environmental architecture)
Gaia Associates
11 Upper Mount St Dublin 2 Ireland

Howard Liddell (Environmental architecture)
Gaia Architects
Aberfeldy Studios, Chapel St Aberfeldy, Perthshire
PH15 2AW Scotland

David Pearson (Environmental architecture)
Gaia Environments Ltd
20 High St Stroud, Gloucestershire GL5 1AS

Prof. P. Schmid
Faculty of Architecture and Building Science,
Tue-Eindhoven University of Technology
Tue Postvak 8/ PO Box 513/ 5600 MB Eindhoven,
The Netherlands Ph: (040) 472 373

Floyd K. Stein
Atelier ISLY, Lystrupmindevej 12, Lystruphave 8654
Bryrup Denmark Ph/Fax: 7575 7508

Brenda and Robert Vale (Environmental architecture)
28 Lower Kirklington Rd Southwell, Nottinghamshire
NG25 ODN

United States

Gregory Acker
ECO+TECH Construction
720 NW 23rd Ave Portland OR 97210
Ph 503 222 4143

Architects/Designers/Planners for Social Responsibility (ADPSR)
Nor Cal Chapter
PO Box 9126 Berkeley CA 94709 Ph 510 273 2428

Tom Bender
38755 Reed Rd Nehalem OR 97131
Ph 503 368 6294

Paul Bierman-Lytle
Environmental Construction Outfitters
44 Crosby St New York NY 10012
Ph 1 800 238 5008

Boston Society of Architects/Architects for Social Responsibility
52 Broad St Boston MA 02109 Ph 617 951 1433

Richard L. Crowther
401 Madison St, Unit A, Denver CO 80206
Ph 303 388 1875

Croxton Collaborative Architects
1122 Madison Ave New York NY 10028

Design Harmony
16 N. Boylan Ave Raleigh NC 27603
Ph 919 755 0300

Clint Good
PO Box 143 Lincoln VA 22078 Ph 703 478 1352

William McDonough & Partners
410 E. Water St Charlottesville VA 22902
Ph 804 979 1111

NACUL Center
592 Main St Amherst MA 01002 Ph 413 253 8025

The CoHousing Company
1250 Addison St, Suite 113 Berkeley CA 94702
Ph 510 549 9980

Bob Theis
DS&A Architects
1107 Virginia St Berkeley CA 94702
Ph 510 526 1935 Fax 510 526 1961

Sim van der Ryn & Associates
55C Gate Five Rd Sausalito CA 94965
Ph 415 332 5806

Carol Venolia
PO Box 4417 Santa Rosa CA 95402
Ph 707 579 2201

ELECTRONICS AND ELECTROMAGNETIC POLLUTION

New Zealand

Albino Gola (Electromagnetic pollution and dowsing)
39 Ellerton Rd Mt Eden Auckland 1003
Ph (09) 638 8622

Danny McBride, Electronic Engineer
Alpha-Eagle Research Laboratory
PO Box 34–333 Birkenhead Auckland 1310
Ph/Fax (09) 483 5655

United States

Mr Craig D. Smith (Technological strategies for avoiding electromagenetic fields)
Certified EM Compatibility Engineer
National Assoc. Radio & Telecommunications

Engineers, BS, UCSB
Northwest Scientific, 1325 Imola West Suite 628
Napa Calif 94559 USA

FENG SHUI

AUSTRALIA
Feng shui **Society of Australia**
PO Box 597 Epping NSW 2121

Juergen Schmidt (*Feng shui***, geobiology, electropollution)**
PO Box 891 Mt Barker SA 5251 Ph/Fax (08) 398 3626

NEW ZEALAND
Michael Chin
PO Box 100516 NSMC Auckland

UNITED KINGDOM AND EUROPE
International *Feng Shui* Society
Lazenby House, 2 Thayer St London W1M 5LG

UNITED STATES
GEO (Geomancy education)
205 – 35th St San Francisco CA 94116
Ph 415 753 6408

Geomancer's Booksource
American School of Geomancy
PO Box 1039 Sebastopol CA 95473
Ph 707 829 8413

Yun Lin Temple (*Feng shui*** classes)**
2959 Russell St Berkeley CA 94705
Ph 510 841 2347 Fax 510 548 2621

LANDSCAPE ARCHITECTURE

AUSTRALIA
Earthscape Consultants
5 Blair Ave Croydon NSW 2132
Ph (02) 747 4439 Fax (02) 744 5676

UNITED KINGDOM AND EUROPE
Michael Brown & Partners (Landscape consultants)
9 Dowry Square, Hotwells, Bristol BS8 4SH

Henry Doubleday Research Association
National Centre for Organic Gardening, Ryton-on-Dunsmore, Coventry CV8 3LG

Michael Littlewood (Landscape and Permaculture consultant)
Troutwells, Higher Hayne, Watchet, Somerset TA23 ORN

Permaculture Association (Britain)
PO Box 1, Buckfastleigh, Devon TQ11 OLH

Tony Thapar (Landscape architect)
27 Dillotford Ave Coventry CV3 5DR

The Works Landscape Services
144 Wood Vale, London SE23 3EB

LIFE-CYCLE COSTING OF BUILDINGS

AUSTRALIA
Dr Selwyn Tucker
Div. of Building & Construction Engineering, CSIRO
PO Box 56 Highett Vic 3190 Ph (03) 9252 6000
Fax (03) 9252 6244

TERMITES

AUSTRALIA
CSIRO Division of Entomology
GPO Box 1700 Canberra City ACT 2601

WATER DIVINING

AUSTRALIA
Mr R. Latcham
Water Divining Association
Bribie Island Qld 4507

UNITED KINGDOM AND EUROPE
British Society of Dowsers
Tamley Ln, Hastingleigh, Ashford, Kent

UNITED STATES
American Society of Dowsers
Danville VT 05828 Ph 802 684 3417

SECTION 3:
INSTRUMENTS AND
EQUIPMENT

AIR, WATER AND SOIL QUALITY

ASIA
Eutech Cybernetics Pty Ltd (pH testing)
55 Ayer Rajah Cres No.04–21/24 Singapore 0513
Ph 778 7995 Fax 773 0836

Hanna Instruments (S) Pty Ltd (Total dissolved solids pocket meter)
514 Chai Chee La 07 07, Bedik Industrial Estate Singapore Ph 242 3806 Fax 442 8005

AUSTRALIA
Air-met Scientific Pty Ltd (Surface testing kits for mercury, lead, formaldehyde, arsenic, chromium, lead, carcinogenic amines, radionuclides, corrosives and dust; air-pollution test kits; flow and pressure meters; anenomoters; manometers)
PO Box 133 Nunawading Vic 3131
Ph (03) 877 1422 Fax (03) 894 4642

Arthur Bailey Surgico Pty Ltd (Pocket-size thermo-hygrometer for measuring air temperature and humidity)
PO Box 222 Leichhardt NSW 2040 Ph (02) 555 1588
Fax (02) 555 9130

Blackmore & Singleman Pty Ltd (Dehumidifiers – sales and rental)
59 Anzac St Greenacre NSW 2190 Ph (02) 708 6322

Cornell Group ('Tramex' Moisture Encounter)
PO Box 87 Killara NSW 2071 Ph (02) 418 1002
Fax (02) 498 8576

Dry Home Dehumidifiers
Sydney NSW Ph (02) 9988 4222 Fax (02) 449 8947

Duff and McIntosh Pty Ltd (Thermal flux meter for heat energy conservation monitoring and testing)
13/45 Leighton Place Hornsby NSW 2077
Ph (02) 482 1411 Fax (02) 482 1489

John Morris Scientific Pty Ltd (Moisture content meters for concrete, timber and air (Protimeter); dissolved oxygen monitor ; flowmeters; waste water testing; hygrometers)
61–63 Victoria Ave Chatswood NSW 2067
Ph (02) 417 8877 Fax (02) 417 8855 Vic
Ph (03) 816 9444 Fax (03) 816 9135; Qld
Ph (07) 854 1713 Fax (07) 252 1067; SA
Ph (08) 362 5809 Fax (08) 363 0781

Hannah Instruments Inc (pH testing)
Australian Agents: Surgico Pty Ltd 55 Lilyfield Rd
Rozelle NSW 2039 Ph (02) 555 1588
Fax (02) 555 9130)

Selby Scientific and Medical
32 Birnie Ave Lidcombe NSW 2141
Ph (02) 643 2666 Fax (02) 643 2596

Sensatronics (Meters for detecting LPG, propane, refrigerants or natural gases, eg, radon, carbon monoxide)
13 Rosella St East Doncaster Vic 3109
Ph (03) 841 4220 Fax (03) 841 7520

Tech-Rentals (Air velocity meters; noise level/dose meters; temperature/humidity monitors; oscilloscopes; pH meters, etc)
18 Hilly St Mortlake NSW 2137 Ph (02) 736 2066
Fax (02) 736 1491; Melbourne, Vic
Ph (03) 879 2266 Fax (03) 879 4310; Adelaide, SA
Ph (08) 344 6999 Fax (08) 269 6411; Brisbane, Qld
Ph (07) 875 1077 Fax (07) 277 3753

NEW ZEALAND
Tech-Rentals (Air velocity meters; noise level/dose meters; temperature/humidity monitors; oscilloscopes; pH meters, etc)
19 Mauranui Ave Newmarket Ph (9) 520 4759
Fax (9) 524 4280; 271 Willis St Wellington
Ph (04) 384 4833 Fax (04) 384 4677

UNITED KINGDOM AND EUROPE
Institute of Water and Environmental Management
15 John St London WC1N 2EB

National Society for Clean Air
136 North St Brighton, Sussex BN1 1RG

Soil Association
86 Coulston St, Bristol BS1 5BB

Soil Survey and Land Research Centre
Cranfield Institute of Technology, Silsoe Campus,
Bedford MK45 4DT

UNITED STATES
Healthful Hardware (Radiation-free, photoelectric smoke detectors; water filter quick-test kits; ultraviolet sensometers)
fi720PO Box 3217 Prescott Arizona 86302 USA
Ph (602) 445 8225

Hannah Instruments Inc (pH testing)
PO Box 849 Woosocket Rhode Island 02895 USA
Ph (401) 765 7500 Fax (401) 765 7575

International Institute for Bau-Biologie & Ecology
PO Box 387 Clearwater FL 34615 Ph 813 461 4371
Fax 813 441 4373

National Testing Laboratories Inc 'Watercheck' (Complete water analysis)
556 South Mansfield St Ypsilanti Michigan 48197
USA (216) 449 2525

ELECTROMAGNETIC FIELDS, RADIATION AND RADON

AUSTRALIA
Geoinstruments Pty Ltd (Geomagnetic Field Proton Magnotometer G856 – for Hire)
348 Rocky Point Rd Ramsgate NSW 2219

Nucletron Pty Ltd (Geiger counters for measuring alpha, beta and gamma radiation)
PO Box 979 Bondi Junction NSW 2022
Ph (02) 369 1990 Fax (02) 369 1994

Radshield (Australia) Pty Ltd (Radiation detectors)
PO Box 6528 Bundall Qld 4217 Ph (075) 711 297
Fax (075) 711 381 Freecall 1800 641 118

Rohde & Schwarz (Australia) Pty Ltd (Portable radio frequency analyser)
PO Box 6105 Silverwater NSW 2141
Ph (02) 748 0155 Fax (02) 748 1836

NEW ZEALAND
Building Biology and Ecology Services of New Zealand
PO Box 35921 Browns Bay Auckland
Ph/Fax (09) 479 3161

UNITED STATES
Healthful Hardware (Electric shielding aprons; electrical field wall coverings; computer shields; radon monitors; radon test kits for earth, air and water and alpha, beta and gamma radiation)
PO Box 3217 Prescott Arizona 86302 USA
Ph (602) 445 8225

Environmental Testing & Technology
PO Box 369 Encinitas CA 92924 USA
Ph (619) 436 5990

International Institute for Bau-Biologie & Ecology Inc
PO Box 387 Clearwater FL 34615 USA
Ph (813) 461 4371 Fax (813) 441 4373

International Medcom (Geiger counters for measuring alpha, beta and gamma radiation)
7497 Kennedy Rd Sebastapol CA 95472 USA
Ph 707 823 0336

Magnetic Sciences International
2425B Channing Way Suite 489 Berkeley CA 94704
USA Ph/Fax (510) 205 5080

Radiation Technology Inc (Tracer 3D Magnetometer for measuring pulsed electromagnetic fields)
600 N. Hametown Rd Akron Ohio 44333 USA
Ph (216) 666 7710 Fax (216) 666 6208

Safe Environments
2512 Ninth St #17 Berkeley CA 9410 USA
Ph (510) 549 9693 Fax (510) 849 4465

Safe Technologies Corporation
154 Rosemary St Needham MA 02174 3258 USA
Ph (617) 444 7778

Terradex Corporation (Track Etch detectors for long-term radon detection)
460 N. Wiget La Walnut Creek CA 94598 USA
Ph (415) 938 2545 Telex 33 7793

FENG SHUI

ASIA
Lo P'an **Compass**
Kwok Chi Wan
F020 1st Floor SG Wang Plaza 55100 Kuala Lumpur
Malaysia

NOISE LEVEL MEASUREMENT

AUSTRALIA
Rohde & Schwarz (Australia) Pty Ltd (Noise monitoring sound-level monitor)
PO Box 6105 Silverwater NSW 2141
Ph (02) 748 0155 Fax (02) 748 1836

RTA Technology Pty Ltd (Environmental Noise Logger – for hire)
1st floor 160 Castlereagh St Sydney NSW 2000
Ph (02) 267 5939 Fax (02) 261 8294

PESTS

AUSTRALIA
Pest-Free
Level 10, 24 Market St Sydney NSW 2000 Freecall
1800 678 673

UNITED STATES
Weitech Inc (Transonic heavy-duty pest repeller for most fleas, spiders, bats, rodents and squirrels)
PO Box 1659
310 Barclay Way, Sisters OR 97759 USA
Ph (503) 549 0205 Toll-free 1 800 343 2659
Fax (503) 549 8154

SECTION 4: ALTERNATIVE ENERGY EQUIPMENT

BATTERIES

AUSTRALIA
Century Yuasa Solar Sun SSR (Batteries for use in solar and remote area power supply systems
13 Tarlington Place Smithfield NSW 2164
Ph (02) 725 5244
(Offices in every state)

IEI (Aust) Pty Ltd (Solar block batteries)
15–17 Normanby Rd Clayton Vic 3168
Ph (03) 544 8411 Fax (03) 544 8648
(Offices in five states)

UNITED STATES
Christie Electric Corp. (Rechargers for batteries with analysers and sequencers)
18120 S. Broadway Gardens Ca 90248 USA (310)
715 1402 Fax (310) 618 8368

PUMPS

AUSTRALIA
B/W Solar
9 Newborough St Scarborough WA 6019
Ph/Fax (09) 341 8711

Suntron Power Products Pty Ltd
2/66–70 Railway Rd Blackburn Vic 3130
Ph (03) 894 2544 Fax (03) 894 3370

Synergy Power Corporation Pty Ltd (Wind-powered water pump)
53 McCoy St Myaree WA 6154
Ph (09) 330 2877 Fax (09) 330 3278
Freecall 1 800 672877

REMOTE-AREA POWER SYSTEMS

AUSTRALIA
Platypus Power Micro-Hydro generation-system and Pyramid Power Solar/Diesel Hybrid system
Agent: Illawarra Electricity, Southeastern Renewable Energy
Locked Bag 8849 South Coast Mail Centre NSW
2521 Ph (042) 282 999 Fax (042) 282 890

SINE-WAVE INVERTERS (CONVERT DIRECT CURRENT (DC) INTO ALTERNATING CURRENT (AC))

AUSTRALIA
CSA Energy-technique
PO Box 2207 Shepparton Vic 3630
Ph (058) 311 518 Fax (058) 311 518

Mechron Australia
PO Box 376 Campbelltown SA 5074
Ph 018 81 7516 Fax (08) 396 4493

Selectronic Components Pty Ltd
25 Holloway Dr Bayswater Vic 3153
Ph (03) 762 4822 Fax (03) 762 9646

Siemens Ltd
Power Engineering & Automation Systems Dept
544 Church St Richmond Vic 3121
Ph (03) 420 7111 Fax (03) 420 7477

SOLAR ENERGY SYSTEMS

AUSTRALIA
BP Solar Australia Pty Ltd
100 Old Pittwater Rd Brookvale NSW 2100
Ph (02) 938 5111 Fax (02) 939 1548

Rainbow Power Company Ltd
1 Alternative Way Nimbin NSW 2480
Ph (066) 89 1430 Fax (066) 89 1109

Solar Energy Industries Assoc. of Australia Inc
505 St Kilda Rd Melbourne Vic 3004
Ph (03) 866 8977 Fax (03) 866 8922

Solarex Pty Ltd
78 Biloela St Villawood NSW 2163
Ph (02) 727 4455 Fax (02) 727 7447

UNITED KINGDOM AND EUROPE
Solar Products International Ltd (Solar technology catalogue)
4 The Mount, Guildford, Surrey GU2 5HN

UNITED STATES
American Solar Network
12811 Boxhill Court, Herndon VA 22071
Ph 703 620 2242

Independent Energy Systems
14306 Batten Rd NE, Duvall WA 98019
Ph 206 788 4569 Fax 206 839 9361

Integral Energy Systems
109 Argall Way, Nevada City CA 95959
Ph 1 800 735 6790

Zomeworks Corporation
PO Box 25805, 1011 A Sawmill Rd NW,
Albuquerque NM 87125 Ph 1 800 279 6342
Fax 505 243 5187

SOLAR-OPERATED FANS

AUSTRALIA
Environmental Health Systems (Solarfan)
PO Box 733 Chatswood NSW 2067
Ph (02) 413 3805 Fax (02) 413 3735

SOLAR HOT-WATER SYSTEMS

AUSTRALIA
Edwards Energy Systems Pty Ltd
109 Vulcan Rd Canning Vale WA 6155
Ph (09) 455 1999 Fax (09) 455 1201
(Offices in four states)

Quantum Link Energy Systems Pty Ltd
109 Long St Smithfield NSW 2164 Ph (02) 725 2944
Fax (02) 725 3490

Solahart Industries Pty Ltd
112 Pilbara St Welshpool WA 6106 Ph (09) 458 6211
Fax (09) 458 7640

UNITED KINGDOM AND EUROPE
Solar Energy Services
Freepost, Eastbourne, East Sussex BN22 7BR

Sunuser Ltd
157 Buslingthorpe Ln, Leeds LS7 2DQ

Thermomax Ltd
15 Stockwood Rise, Camberley, Surrey GU15 2EA

UNITED STATES
Sage Advance Corporation
1001 Bertelson Rd, Suite A, Eugene OR 97402
Ph 503 485 1947

Sun Quest Inc.
1555 Rankin Ave Newton NC 28658
Ph 704 465 6805 Fax 704 465 7370

Sun Utility Network
5741 Engineer Dr, Huntington Beach CA 92649
Ph 1 800 822 SOLAR

SOLAR TRACKING SYSTEMS

AUSTRALIA
Suntron Power Products Pty Ltd (Suntracker)
2/66–70 Railway Rd Vic 3130 Ph (03) 894 2544
Fax (03) 894 3370

UNITED STATES
Zomeworks Corporation
PO Box 25805, 1011 A Sawmill Rd NW,
Albuquerque NM 87125 Ph 1 800 279 6342
Fax 505 243 5187

SECTION 5: HEALTH PRODUCTS, EQUIPMENT AND SERVICES

BACK SUPPORT

AUSTRALIA
The Bad Back Centre Pty Ltd (Back-care furniture)
223 Edgecliff Rd Woollahra NSW 2025
Ph (02) 387 6997

Sun Medical Equipment Centre (Back supports and cushions)
14 Pound Rd Hornsby NSW 2077 Ph (02) 476 2605

UNITED KINGDOM AND EUROPE
Scan-sit Ltd (Balans chairs)
Unit 4, 111 Mortlake Rd Kew, Richmond TW9 4AB

HOUSEHOLD PRODUCTS

UNITED KINGDOM AND EUROPE
The Healthy House (Mail order catalogue)
Cold Harbour, Ruscombe, Stroud GL6 6DA

UNITED STATES
Healthful Hardware (Healthy cleaning products)
PO Box 3217 Prescott Arizona 86302 USA
Ph (602) 445 8225

Nontoxic Environments Inc.
PO Box 384 Newmarket NH 03857 Ph (603) 659 5919

The Living Source
7005 Woodway Dr, Suite 214 Waco TX 76712
Ph 1 800 662 8787 Fax 817 776 9392

MEDICAL PRACTITIONERS AND CLINICS

AUSTRALIA
Allergy Aids Centre of Australia
28 Martha St Granville NSW 2142
Ph (02) 637 8122

Allergy Information Network and Allergy Prevention Clinic
370 Victoria Ave Chatswood NSW 2067
Ph (02) 419 7731

Allergy, Sensitivity and Environmental Health Association Queensland (Inc)
PO Box 45 Woody Point Qld 4019 Ph (07) 284 8742

Australian Natural Therapists Association
PO Box 522 Sutherland NSW 2232

The Australian Traditional Medicine Society Ltd
PO Box 1027 Meadowbank NSW 2114
Ph (02) 809 6800 Fax (02) 809 7570

Dr Mark Donohoe, Principal Consultant
Environmental Health Consulting Division, Clean

House Effect
29 Raglan St Mosman NSW 2088 Ph (02) 9968 1087

Environmental Medical Clinic
Sydney Natural Medical Centre
15 South Steyne Manly NSW 2095
Ph (02) 9977 7888 Fax (02) 9977 3436

Food Allergy Clinic
Royal Prince Alfred Hospital
Missenden Rd Camperdown NSW 2050
Ph (02) 515 6111

Sydney Colon Health Clinic
50 Nicholson St, St Leonards NSW 2065
Ph (02) 906 5288 Fax (02) 906 7688

UNITED KINGDOM AND EUROPE

Association of General Practitioners of Nature Medicine
38 Nigel House, Portpool Ln, London EC1N 7UR

Institute of Complementary Medicine
PO Box 194 London SE16 1QZ

London Hazard Centre
Headland House, 308 Grays Inn Rd London WC1X 8DS

National Institute of Medical Herbalists Ltd
9 Palace Gate, Exeter EX1 1JA

UNITED STATES

American Academy of Environmental Medicine
Ph 303 622 9755

National Association of Physicians for the Environment
Ph 301 571 9750

NEGATIVE ION GENERATORS

AUSTRALIA
Bionic Products Pty Ltd (Elanra negative-ion generator)
PO Box 686 Surfers Paradise Qld 4217
Ph (075) 92 1522 Fax (075) 38 2243

UNITED KINGDOM AND EUROPE
Mountain Breeze
6 Priorswood Place, Skermersdale, Lancashire WN8 9QB

UNITED STATES
The Ion & Light Company
2263–1/2 Sacramento St San Francisco CA 94115
Ph 415 346 6205

PYRAMIDS

AUSTRALIA
Mystique Pyramid Design (Pre-fabricated)
PO Box 118 Palmyra WA 6157 Ph (09) 342 9478

WATER FLOWFORMS
(FOR WATER FILTRATION SEE SECTION 1)

Virbela Flowforms induce a vortex into water flow, cleansing and improving microclimates.

AUSTRALIA
Mark Baxter
Flow Research Group
The Manly Studio
37–39 The Corso Manly NSW 2095
Ph (02) 977 7648 Fax (02) 977 0295

NEW ZEALAND
Flow Research Group
PO Box 1255 Hastings Hawkes Bay

UNITED KINGDOM AND EUROPE
Virbela Flowform Research Group
Emerson College, Forest Row, Sussex RH18 5JX

UNITED STATES
Waterforms Inc.
Route 177, PO Box 930 Blue Hill ME 04614
Ph 207 374 2384 Fax 207 374 2383

SECTION 6:
HOME FURNISHINGS AND
NATURAL FABRICS

AUSTRALIA
Community Aid Abroad One-world Shop (Home furnishings, clothing, etc)
Shop CM–05, Mezzanine Level, Centrepoint, Sydney NSW 2000 Ph/Fax (02) 231 4016;
Freecall 1800 088 455 (mail order catalogue available)

'Country Dream' Renowned Furniture (Natural finished recycled timber)
Shop 6b, MegaCentre, Blacktown Rd Blacktown NSW 2148 Ph (02) 831 6411

Futon Express
554 Oxford St Bondi Junction NSW 2022
Ph (02) 369 1244

Futon Furniture Australia
59 Campbell St, St Peters NSW 2044
Ph (02) 550 4042

Laura Ashley (Aust) Pty Ltd
100 Market St Sydney NSW 2000 Ph (02) 232 2829

Maud N. Lil (Organic cotton products)
5/126 Glenayr Ave Bondi NSW 2026
Ph (02) 306 243 Fax (02) 331 1938

Mother Nature Babywear
PO Box 266 Double Bay NSW 2028
Ph (02) 380 6854 Fax (02) 331 7360

Ozzie Mozzie Nets (100% cotton bed-linen, 100% cotton flannelette sheets, cellular blankets)
678 Barrenjoey Rd Avalon NSW 2107
Ph (02) 918 0414 Fax (02) 973 1701

Sheridan and Actil Cotton Collection
Wholesaler: Textiles Industries (Aust) Ltd
12–28 Arncliffe St Arncliffe NSW 2205
Ph (02) 597 7855

Sydney Greencloth Australia (Environmental couture, custom-made clothing)
25 Meagher St Chippendale NSW 2008
Ph (02) 318 2336

NEW ZEALAND
Futon Ya San (Futons, slat beds and accessories)
PO Box 80069 Green Bay Ph (09) 828 0122

UNITED KINGDOM AND EUROPE
Alphabeds (Solid wood beds and futons)
Pencader, Dyfed SA39 9JD Wales

The Chartwell Design Co
Brook Ln, Plaxtol, Nr. Sevenoaks, Kent TN15 0QR

Global Village Crafts Ltd (Sustainable bamboo, rattan and teak furniture)
Sparrow Works, Bower Hinton, Martock, Somerset TA12 6LF

The Treske Shop
5 Barmouth Rd London SW18 2DT

Wesley-Barrell (Traditional upholstery)
52 Regent St London SW14

UNITED STATES
Crown Sleep Shops (Cotton/innerspring beds)
250 South San Gabriel Boulevard, San Gabriel CA 91776 Ph 213 681 6356 Fax 818 796 9101

DesignTex Inc. (Fabrics)
200 Varick St, 8th Floor, New York NY 10014
Ph 212 886 8100 Fax 212 886 1111

Dona Designs (Organic cotton futons and bedding)
825 Northlake Dr, Richardson TX 75080
Ph 214 235 0465

Furnature (Chairs and couches)
310 Washington St Boston MA 02135
Ph 617 783 4343 Fax 617 787 0350

Heart of Vermont (Nontoxic furniture)
The Old Schoolhouse, Route 132, PO Box 183 Sharon VT 05065 Ph 1 800 639 4123 Fax 802 763 2075

House of Hemp (Hemp fabrics)
PO Box 14603 Portland OR 97214 Ph 503 232 1128
Fax 503 232 0239

Natural Cotton Colours Inc. (FoxFibre organically grown cotton)
PO Box 66 Wickenburg AZ 85358 Ph 602 684 7199

Ocarina Textiles (FoxFibre bedspreads)
16 Cliff St New London CT 06320 Ph 203 437 8189

The Natural Bedroom (Natural fibre bedding and bedroom furniture)
PO Box 3071 Santa Rosa CA 95402
Ph 1 800 365 6563

SECTION 7:
COMPUTER EQUIPMENT

HARDWARE

AUSTRALIA
Apple Australia (Safe terminals/monitors)
16 Rodborough Rd Frenchs Forest NSW 2086
Ph (02) 452 8000 Fax (02) 452 8160

NEC Home Electronics Australia Pty Ltd (Terminals/monitors with magnetic and electric field screening)
Sydney NSW Ph (07) 868 1811;
New Zealand Ph (09) 579 8444

NEW ZEALAND
NEC Home Electronics (Terminals/monitors with magnetic and electric field screening)
Auckland Ph (09) 579 8444

UNITED STATES
Safe Computing Pty Ltd
33 William St Needham MA USA 02194 Ph (617) 444 7778 Fax (617) 444 9528

SOFTWARE

AUSTRALIA
Australian Health (Chem Alert for Windows, a program that traces the chemical content of products and their effect on human health)
18 Hardy St South Perth WA 6151 Ph (09) 368 1711 Fax (09) 474 1794

Medline Knowledge Finder (Program that develops a medical database for an individual)
JAM Software Pty Ltd
3 Foster St Leichhardt NSW 2040 Ph (02) 550 0884

UNITED STATES
Occupational Safety & Health Administration (Information manual of 1400 chemicals, available on disk)
Government Institutes
4 Research Place Maryland USA 20850–3226
Ph (301) 921 2300 Fax (301) 921 0373

SECTION 8:
USEFUL ORGANISATIONS

CONSTRUCTION

AUSTRALIA
CSIRO Bookshop (Booklet available: Bulletin No 5 (pise, adobe, CINVA-ram construction))
PO Box 310 North Ryde NSW 2113
Ph (02) 934 3444 Fax (02) 934 4555

National Building Technology Centre (Earth construction information)
PO Box 30 Chatswood NSW 2065

Special Housing Branch (Adobe construction guidelines)
Ministry of Housing and Construction (Vic)
GPO Box 16570N Melbourne Vic 3001

Victoria Self-Build Housing Scheme (Earth construction information)
Ministry of Housing, 13th Floor, 250 Elizabeth St Melbourne Vic 3000

NEW ZEALAND
Earth Building Association of New Zealand
PO Box 1452 Whangarei

Earthbuilding South Pacific (Education service)
Unit 11/1 Turner St Auckland 1001
Ph (09) 302 3521 Fax (09) 309 9759

Eco Design Shop
Willis St Village, 142 Willis St Wellington
Ph (04) 382 9802

UNITED KINGDOM AND EUROPE
The Building Centre
26 Store St London WC1E 7BT

Building Research Establishment
Bucknalls Ln, Garston, Watford WD2 7JR

Cork Industry Federation
67 Leavesden Rd Weybridge, Surrey KT13 9BX

National House-Building Council
Chiltern Ave Amersham, Buckinghamshire HP6 5AP

UNITED STATES
Builders for Social Responsibility
RR1, Box 1953 Hinesburg VT 05461
Ph 802 482 3295

Center for Maximum Potential Building Systems
8604 F.M. 969 Austin TX 78724 Ph 512 928 4786

International Institute for Bau-Biologie & Ecology
PO Box 387 Clearwater FL 34615 Ph 813 461 4371 Fax 813 441 4373

Natural Building Network
PO Box 1110 Sebastopol CA 95473
Ph 707 823 2569

Out On Bale (Un)Ltd
1037 East Linden St Tucson AZ 85719
Ph 520 624 1673

The Splinter Group
5521 Marshall St Oakland CA 94608
Ph 510 654 2746

ELECTROMAGNETIC FIELDS

AUSTRALIA
Association of Citizens against Telecommunication Towers (ACATT) (Kate Barrett)
2/91 Henley Beach Rd Henley Beach South SA 5022
Ph (03) 356 4408

Powerline Action (Vic) Inc
3/247 Flinders La Melbourne Vic 3000
Ph (03) 654 4512 Fax (03) 650 3689

NEW ZEALAND
Adopt Radiation Controls Inc (ARC)
C/- Bruce Morrison
PO Box 21113 Henderson Auckland

Environmental Protection for Children Trust (EPC)
393 Ilam Rd Christchurch Ph (03) 351 7329
Fax (03) 343 3693

ENERGY

AUSTRALIA
Dept of Primary Industries and Energy
GPO Box 858 Canberra ACT 2601 Ph (06) 272 4588
Fax (06) 273 1232

Energy Information Centre
18 Hickson Rd The Rocks NSW 2000
Ph (02) 247 1144 Fax (02) 247 1438; Melbourne,
Vic Ph (03) 650 1195 Freecall 1800 13 6322
Fax (03) 650 2338; Brisbane, Qld Ph (07) 234 9807
Freecall 1800 17 5518 (Qld country only)
Fax (07) 234 9969; Adelaide, SA Ph (08) 204 1888
Fax (08) 204 1880

Energy Information Service
Murdoch University Energy Research Institute
Murdoch University Murdoch WA 6150
Ph (09) 360 2868 Fax (09) 310 6094

The Integrated Energy Mangement Centre
163–169 Main Rd Moonah Tas 7009
Ph (002) 71 6460 Fax (002) 73 3420

Office of Energy
PO Box 536 St Leonards NSW 2065
Ph (02) 901 8888 Fax (02) 901 8777

Renewable Energy Group
SECWA 363–365 Wellington St Perth WA 6000
Ph (09) 326 6034 Fax (09) 326 4600

Solar Energy Industries Assoc. of Australia Inc.
505 St Kilda Rd Melbourne Vic 3004
Ph (03) 866 8977 Fax (03) 866 8922

UNITED KINGDOM AND EUROPE

Building Energy Research Enquiry Service (BRESCU)
Bucknalls Ln, Garston, Watford WD2 7JR

Centre for Alternative Technology
Llwyngwern Quarry, Machynlleth, Powys SY20 9AZ
Wales

The Ecology Building Society
8 Station Rd Cross Hills, Keighley, West Yorkshire
BD20 7EH

Ecological Design Association
The British School, Slad Rd Stroud, Gloucestershire
GL5 1QW

Energy Efficiency Office
Dept of the Environment, 1 Palace St London
SW1E 5HE

**Renewable Energy Enquiries Bureau, Energy
Technology Support Unit**
Building 156 Harwell Laboratory, Oxfordshire
OX11 0QR

The Solar Energy Society (UK–ISES)
King's College London, Campden Hill Rd London
W8 7AH

Walter Segal Self-Build Trust
57 Charlton St London NW1 1HU

UNITED STATES

American Solar Energy Society
2400 Central Ave, G–1, Boulder CO 80301
Ph 303 443 3130 Fax 303 443 3212

Energy Information Administration
U.S. Department of Energy
Forrestal Building, El–231 Washington DC 20585
Ph 202 252 6411

Northeast Sustainable Energy Association
50 Miles St Greenfield MA 01301 Ph 413 774 6051

Rocky Mountain Institute
1739 Snowmass Creek Rd Snowmass CO 81654
Ph 970 927 3851 Fax 970 927 4178

SECTION 9:
JOURNALS AND OTHER
PUBLICATIONS

BBE Monographs
Building Biology & Ecology Institute
PO Box 2764 Auckland New Zealand
Ph (09) 358 2202

Building with Nature
PO Box 4417 Santa Rosa CA 95402
Ph 707 579 2201

Clean Slate
Centre for Alternative Technology
Llwyngwern Quarry, Machynlleth, Powys
SY20 9AZ Wales

Earthword
580 Broadway, #200, Laguna Beach CA 92651

EcoDesign
Ecological Design Association
The British School, Slad Rd Stroud, Gloucestershire
GL5 1QW

Environ
PO Box 2204 Fort Collins CO 80522
Ph 303 224 0083

Environmental Building News
RR1, Box 161 Brattleboro VT 05301
Ph 802 257 7300

Home Power Magazine
PO Box 520 Ashland OR 97520 Ph 916 475 3179

Interior Concerns
PO Box 2386 Mill Valley CA 94941
Ph 415 389 8049 Fax 415 388 8322

Permaculture
Permaculture International Journal
PO Box 6039 South Lismore NSW 2480 Australia
Ph (066) 220020 Fax (066) 220579

**Report: Non-ionizing Electromagnetic Fields and
Human Health: Are Current Standards "Safe"?**
Don Maisch
PO Box 96 North Hobart Tas 7002 Aust

Resurgence
Ford House, Hartland, Bideford, Devon

References

INTRODUCTION

Mygind, N. (1986) *Essential Allergy*, Blackwell Scientific, Oxford.

CHAPTER 1:
GAIA AND THE FIVE ELEMENTS

Alexandersson, O. (1982) *Living Water*, Turnstone Press, Wellingborough, Northamptonshire UK.

Bachler, K. (1980) *Erfahrungen einer Rutengangerin*, Veritas Verlag, Linz.

Baggs, S.A., Baggs, Joan C., & Baggs, D.W. (1991) *Australian Earth-covered Building*, 2nd edn, New South Wales University Press, Kensington NSW.

Blavatsky, Helena P. (1950) *The Secret Doctrine: The Synthesis of Science, Religion and Philosophy*, 4th Adyar edn, Theosophical Publishing House, London, 6 vols.

Butti, K., & Perlin, J. (1981) *A Golden Thread*, Marion Boyars, London.

Delpech, V. (1992) *Indoor Air Pollution and Health: A Literature Review*, Health Promotion Unit, Hornsby NSW/Hillview Commission, Health and Information Centre.

Eastland, B.J. (1990) 'Applications of in situ generated relativistic electrons in the ionosphere', *ESEC Technical Report*, vol. 136, 13 December.

Ehrlich, P., & Ehrlich, Anne (1972) *Population Resources Environment: Issues in Human Ecology*, Freeman, San Francisco.

Endros, R. (1981) *Die Strahlung der Erde*, Paffrath, Remscheid.

Ferguson, D. (1987) *Indoor Air Pollution: The Concern of Architects*, dissertation no. 2, Royal Australian Institute of Architects Practice Division, Sydney.

Gartner, K. (1980) *Brauchl-Natur-Wohnen in Biologischen Fertighaus*, Peter Brauchl, Vienna.

Gilbert, D. (1992) 'Ensuring a healthy indoor environment', *Geotecture*, vol. 9, no. 1, pp. 13–29.

Hardy, D., et al (1987) *Pyramid Energy: The Philosophy of God, The Science of Man*, Delta K, Michigan.

Hartmann, E. (1976) *Krankheit als Standortproblem*, 2 Aufl., Haug-Verlag, Heidelberg.

Leviton, R. (1988) 'Under the weather', *Journal of Natural Health and Living*, vol. 1, no. 2.

Mackay, A. (1992) *Ecological living: a guide towards holistic living*, Institut fur Baubiologie und Oikologie, Rosenheim.

Myers, N. (ed.) (1985), *The Gaia Atlas of Planet Management*, Pan, London.

Oberbach, J. (1980) *Fire of Life*, DBF Publishers, Grunwald.

Pedler, K. (1979) *The Quest for Gaia*, Souvenir Press, London.

Robins, D. (1985) *Circles of Silence*, Souvenir, London.

Schneider, A. (trans. H. Ziehe) (1988) *Building Biology Correspondence Course*, International Institut fur Baubiologie™ und Oikologie, Neubeuern.

Schumacher, E.F. (1973) *Small is Beautiful*, Sphere Books, London.

Smith, C.W., & Best, S. (1989) *Electromagnetic Man: Health Hazards in the Electrical Environment*, Dent, London.

Soyka, F. & Edmonds, A. (1978) *The Ion Effect*, Bantam/E.P. Dutton & Co., New York.

Talbot, M. (1991) *The Holographic Universe*, Grafton (Harper Collins), London.

van der Leeuw, J. (1976) *The Fire of Creation*, Theosophical Publishing House, Wheaton, Illinois.

CHAPTER 2:
CHOOSING A HEALTHY LOCATION

Bureau of Meteorology, Australia (1991) *Climatic Survey of Sydney*.

Cook, D. (1993) 'Toxic dump may breach water act', *Sydney Morning Herald*, 27 November, p. 7.

Curson, P., & Siciliano, F. (1992) *Atlas of Premature Mortality in New South Wales, 1981–1988*, Commonwealth Department of Community Services and Health/Australian Government Publishing Service, Canberra ACT, April.

Federal Airports Corporation, Australia (1990) *Proposed Third Runway: Sydney (Kingsford Smith) Airport*, draft environmental impact statement by Kinhill Engineers Pty Ltd, Federal Airports Corporation, Mascot.

Gauquelin, M. (1980) *How Atmospheric Conditions Affect Your Health*, ASI, New York.

Hecht, J. (1993) 'The changeable past of the world's climate', *New Scientist*, 24 July.

Huntington, E. (1947) *The Mainsprings of Civilisation*, Wiley, New York.

Leviton, R. (1988) 'Under the weather', *Journal of Natural Health and Living*, vol. 1, no. 2.

New South Wales State Pollution Control Commission (1991) *Reducing Traffic Noise*, Roads and Traffic Authority/New South Wales Department of Housing, Sydney, August.

Pearce, F. (1992) 'A plague on global warming', *New Scientist*, 12–26 December, p. 12.

Phillips, R.O. (1992) *Sunshine and Shade in Australasia*, 6th edn, technical report 92/2, Commonwealth Scientific and Industrial Research Organisation Division of Building Construction and Engineering.

Ramsay, G.C., & Dawkins, D. (1993) *Building in Bushfire-prone Areas: Information and Advice*, SAAHB36–1993, Commonwealth Scientific and Industrial Research Organisation & Standards Australia, Sydney.

Standards Association of Australia (1987) *Acoustics — Room Design, Sound Levels and Reverberation Times for Building Interiors* (AS2107), Standards Association of Australia, Sydney.

Sowers, G.F. (1979) *Introductory Soil Mechanics: Geotechnical Engineering*, Macmillan, New York.

Soyka, F., & Edmonds, A. (1978) *The Ion Effect*, Bantam/E.P. Dutton & Co, New York.

Tietze, H. (1988) *Earthrays*, Tietze Publishers, Bermagui NSW.

United States Department of Energy (1981) *Building in expansive clays*, earth-sheltered structures fact sheet 11, US Department of Energy, Buildings Division Stillwater/Division of Engineering, Oklahoma State University.

United States Environment Protection Agency (1974), *Information on levels of Environmental Noise Requisite to Protect Public Health and Welfare with an Adequate Margin of Safety*, US Environment Protection Agency report no. 550/9–74–004.

CHAPTER 3:
WHAT IS A HEALTHY HOUSE?

Higgins, E. (1989) 'White-anting the environment', *The Weekend Australian*, 25 November.

Sweet, F. (1994) 'Building on natural forms', *New Scientist*, 22 January.

CHAPTER 4:
THE IDEAL FORM FOR THE HEALTHY HOUSE

Blavatsky, Helena P. (1960) *Isis Unveiled*, Theosophical University Press, Pasadena, California, vol. 1.

Brooker, C. (1988) 'The Earth's magnetic field and its effect on the animal nervous system', in *Energy Medicine Around the World*, ed. T. Srinivasan, Gabriel Press, Phoenix.

Burr, H.S. (1972) *The Fields of Life*, Ballantyne, New York.

Hall, M. (1962) *The Secret Teachings of All Ages*, Phil. Res. Society, Los Angeles, California.

Hardy, D., et al (1987) *Pyramid Energy: The Philosophy of God, The Science of Man*, Delta K, Michigan.

Kanuka-Fuchs, R., & Rattenbury, Jenny (eds) (1993) *Building and Renovation*, Building Biology and Ecology Institute, Auckland NZ, BBE no. 14, Spring.

Kerrill, B., & Coggin, K. (1975) *The Guide to Pyramid Energy*, Pyramid Power, Santa Monica, California.

Leadbeater, C. (1926) *Glimpses of Masonic History*, Theosophical Publishing House, Adyar, Madras, India.

Robins, D. (1985) *Circles of Silence*, Souvenir, London.

Schul, W., & Pettit, E. (1986) *Pyramid Power: A New Reality*, Stillpoint, Walpole, New Hampshire.

Sheldrake, R. (1987) *A New Science of Life*, Blond & Briggs, London.

Sheldrake, R. (1989) *The Presence of the Past*, HarperCollins, London.

Smith, C.W., & Best, S. (1989) *Electromagnetic Man: Health Hazards in the Electrical Environment*, Dent, London.

Smuts, J.C. (1926) *Holism and Evolution*, Macmillan, London.

Stanway, A. (1979) *Alternative Medicine: A Guide to Natural Therapies*, MacDonald & Jane's, London.

Toth, M., & Nielsen, G. (1985) *Pyramid Power*, Aquarian, Wellingborough UK.

CHAPTER 5:
USING *FENG SHUI* IN THE HEALTHY HOUSE

Blavatsky, Helena P. (1950) *The Secret Doctrine: The Synthesis of Science, Religion and Philosophy*, 4th Adyar edn, Theosophical Publishing House, London, 6 vols.

Darras, J.C. (1986) *Isotopic and Cytologic Assays in Acupuncture*, World Union of Acupuncture, Paris.

Feuchtwang, S.D.R. (1974) *An Anthropological Analysis of Chinese Geomancy*, Southern Materials Center, Taipei.

Lip, Evelyn (1990a) *Feng Shui for Business*, Heian International, Union City, California.

Michell, J. (1975) *The Earth Spirit*, Thames & Hudson, London.

O'Brien, Joanne, & Ho, K.M. (1991) *The Elements of Feng Shui*, Element, Dorset.

Skinner, S. (1983) *The Living Earth Manual of Feng Shui*, Graham Brash, Singapore.

Too, Lillian (1993) *Feng Shui*, Konsep Books, Kuala Lumpur, Malaysia.

Walters, D. (1987) *Ming Shu: The Art and Practice of Chinese Astrology*, Pagoda, London.

Walters, D. (1988) *Feng Shui*, Pagoda, London.

Walters, D. (1991) *The Feng Shui Handbook*, Aquarian, London.

CHAPTER 6:
FENG SHUI AND HOLISTIC DESIGN PRINCIPLES

Combs, A. (1992) 'The meeting ground of science and spirit: New themes for a new science' in *Holistic Science and Human Values*, Burnier, et al (eds), Theos. Science Centre, Adyar, Madras, India (53–59)

Eberhard, W. (1989) A Dictionary of Chinese Symbols, Routledge, London.

Kanuka-Fuchs, R. (1994) 'Tui Community, Golden Bay, Nelson', Building Biology and Ecology Institute, Auckland NZ, BBE no. 18, Spring.

Lip (1993) *Feng Shui for Business*, Time Books International, Singapore.

CHAPTER 7:
A HEALTHY GARDEN FOR THE HEALTHY HOUSE

Bernatzky, A. (1966a) 'Climatic influences of greens and city planning', *Anthos*, vol 1., p. 23.

Bernatzky, A. (1966b) 'The performance and value of trees', *Anthos*, vol. 1, p. 125.

Clifford, D. (1966) *A History of Garden Design*, Faber & Faber, London.

Fromm, E. (1973) *The Anatomy of Human Destructiveness*, Fawcett Crest, New York.

Geiger, R. (1966) *The Climate Near the Ground*, Harvard University Press, Cambridge, Massachusetts.

Jane, Pamela (1987) 'Garden pests at bay, the natural way', *Sun Herald*, 29 March, p. 127.

Lip, E. (1990b) *Feng Shui for the Home*, Heian International, Union City.

Meyer, W. (1973) 'Man–and–plant communication: interview with Marcel Vogel', *Unity*, vol. 153, no. 1, p 96.

Mollison, W. (1992) *Permaculture: A Designer's Manual*, Tagari, Tyalgum NSW.

Myers, N. (ed) (1990) *The Gaia Atlas of Future Worlds*, Gaia/Penguin, London.

'Pretty but dangerous' (1983) *Choice*, April, vol. 24, no. 4, pp 3–7.

Retallack, Dorothy (1973) *The Sound of Music and Plants*, De Vorsse & Co, Santa Monica, California.

Robinette, G.O. (1970) Can plants filter noise from our environment?, unpublished manuscript, New Haven.

Robinette, G.O. (1972) *Plants, People and Environmental Quality*, United States Department of Interior, National Parks Service, Washington DC.

Searles, H. (1960) *Non-human Environment in Normal Development and its Schizophrenia*, International University Press, New York.

Short, Kate (1994) *Quick Poison, Slow Poison*, Envirobook Publishers, St Albans NSW.

Simonds, J. (1961) *Landscape Architecture*, Iliffe, London.

Singh, T.C.N. (1962) 'On the effect of music and dance on plants', *Bihar Agricultural College Magazine*, Sabour, Bhagalpur, India, vol. 13, no. 1.

Thoreau, Henri (1845) Journal, 5 July.

Tompkins, P., & Bird, C. (1974) *The Secret Life of Plants*, Penguin, Harmondsworth UK.

Too, Lillian (1993) *Feng Shui*, Konsep Books, Kuala Lumpur, Malaysia.

Ulrich, R. (1983) 'View through a window may influence recovery from surgery', *Science*, vol. 224, 24 January, pp. 420–21.

Walters, D. (1988) *Feng Shui*, Pagoda, London.

White, R. (1954) *Effects of Landscape Development on the Natural Ventilation of Buildings and their Adjacent Areas*, research report 45, A & M College System, Eng. Exp. College Station, Texas.

CHAPTER 8:
BUILDING BIOLOGY AND ECOLOGY

Baldwin, M., & Farant, J. (1990) 'Study of selected volatile organic compounds in office buildings at different stages of occupancy', *Proceedings, Fifth International Conference on Indoor Air Quality and Climate*, 29 July–3 August, Canada Mortgage and Housing Corporation, Ottowa.

Craig, P. (1986) *Organometallic Compounds in the Environment: Principles and Reactions*, Longmans, London.

Haghighat, F., & Donnini, G. (1993) 'Emissions of indoor pollutants from building materials: state of the art review', *Architectural Science Review*, vol. 36, pp. 13–22.

Laura, R. S., & Ashton, J. F. (1991) *Hidden Hazards*, Bantam, Moorebank NSW.

Plehn, W. (1990) 'Solvent emission from paints', *Proceedings, Fifth International Conference on Indoor Air Quality and Climate*, 29 July–3 August, Canada Mortgage & Housing Corporation, Ottowa.

Randolph, T. (1970) 'Domiciliary chemical air pollution in the etiology of ecologic mental illness', *International Journal of Social Psychology*, vol. 16, pp. 223–65.

Richardson, B.A. (1991a) 'Humidity in buildings, microorganisms and toxic gas generation', *Complementary Medical Research*, vol. 5, no. 2, pp. 116–19.

Richardson, B.A. (1991b) *Defects and Deterioration in Buildings*, E. & F.N. Spon, London.

Rodgers, S. (1987) 'Diagnosing the tight-building syndrome', *Environmental Health Perspectives*, vol. 76, p. 195.

Schneider, A. (trans. H. Ziehe) (1988) *Building Biology Correspondence Course*, International Institut fur Baubiologie™ und Oikologie, Neubeuern.

Thompson, P., O'Brien, R., & editors of *Life* (1966), *Weather*, Time-Life International, The Netherlands.

Tucker, W. (1988) 'Air pollution from surface materials: factors influencing emissions and predictive models', *Healthy Buildings '88, State of the Art Reviews*, Stockholm, vol. 1, pp. 149–57.

Wright, D. (1978) *Natural Solar Architecture*, Van Nostrand, New York.

Wolverton, B.C., McDonald, R.C. & Watkins, E.A. Jnr (1984) 'Foliage plants for removing indoor air pollutants from energy efficient homes', *Econ. Bot.* vol. 38, no. 2, pp. 224–229.

Wolverton, B.C., Johnson, M.S. & Bounds, K. (1989) 'Interior landscape plants for indoor air pollution abatement', *Interiorscape*, September, special report supplement.

CHAPTER 9:
CONSTRUCTING THE SAFE AND HEALTHY HOUSE

Armstrong, S. (1988) 'Marooned in a mountain of manure', *New Scientist*, 26 November.

Brown, S. (1994) 'World markets want pollutant-free interior paints', *Building Innovation and Construction Technology*, 1 December, pp. 5–7.

Croft, P.H.W., et al (1984) 'Seasonal arsenic exposure from burning chromium-copper-arsenate treated wood', *Journal American Medical Association*, vol. 251, no. 18, pp. 2393–6.

CSR Ltd (1993), *Material Safety Data Sheet: CSR Wood Panels*, no. 530:2, CSR Ltd, Chatswood NSW, May.

Faecham, P., et al (1990) *Health Aspects of Excreta and Sullage Management*, World Bank, Washington.

Handreck, K. (1980) *Soils: An Outline of Their Properties and Management*, Discovering Soils no. 1, Commonwealth Scientific and Industrial Research Organisation Division of Soils in association with Rellim Technical Publishers, Melbourne.

Hartog, B.J., & Pouw, H.J. (1994) *Antimicrobial effects of linoleum*, TNO Nutrition and Food Research, Ultrecht Deweg, Aelst, The Netherlands, 2 June.

Holmes, Noni (1990) *Painters Hazard Handbook*, Operative Painters and Decorators Union of Australia, Crows Nest NSW.

James Hardie & Co Pty Ltd (1994a), *Material Safety Data Sheet: Moulded Glass Reinforced Cement Panels*, no. 0002:1, James Hardie & Co Pty Ltd, Camellia NSW.

James Hardie & Co Pty Ltd (1994b), *Material Safety Data Sheet: Building Boards*, no. 0006:1, James Hardie & Co Pty Ltd, Camellia NSW.

Johnson, J.A. (1981) 'The etiology of hyperactivity', *Exceptional Children*, vol. 47, no. 5, p. 352.

Kabos, Adrienne (1986) *A–Z of Chemicals in the Home*, Total Environment Centre, Sydney.

Kanuka-Fuchs, R. (ed.) (1991) 'Cellulose fibre insulation', *Natural Insulation*, Building Biology and Ecology Institute of New Zealand, BBE no. 7, Summer.

Livos Australia, brochure on natural paint.

Myers, N. (ed.) (1985), *The Gaia Atlas of Planet Management*, Pan, London.

Northcote, K. (1974) *A Factual Key for the Recognition of Australian Soils*, 4th edn, Rellim, Adelaide.

NSW State News Building Industry Connection (1994a), 'Keeping your cool on insulation', 30 August.

NSW State News Building Industry Connection (1994b), 'Working with asbestos: ways to keep safe', 24–27 August.

Ott, J.N. (1982) *Light, Radiation and You*, Devin-Adair, Old Greenwich, Connecticut.

Ozanne-Smith, Joan (1993) 'Architectural glass injuries in the home', *Glass Australia*, 2 July.

Pedals, P. (1992) *Energy from Nature: Renewable Energy Handbook*, 6th edn, Rainbow Power Co, Nimbin NSW.

Plywood Association of Australia (1994) *Material Safety Data Sheet: Plywood/Laminated Veneer Lumber (LVL)*, Plywood Association of Australia, Newstead Qld, 30 October.

Reidel, D.P., et al (1991) *Residues of Arsenic, Chromium and Copper on and Near Playground Structures Built of Wood Pressure-coated with CCA-*

type Preservatives, Environmental Health Center, Health and Welfare, Ottawa.

Schneider, A. (trans. H. Ziehe) (1988) *Building Biology Correspondence Course*, International Institut fur Baubiologie™ und Oikologie, Neubeuern.

von Pohl, G.F. (1978) *Georadiation: Source for Illnesses and Cancer*, 2nd edn, Verlag Feucht.

Wieslander, G., et al (1993) 'Emission of volatile organic compounds (VOC) from water based paints: a contributing cause of respiratory symptoms and bronchial hyperresponsiveness', *Proceedings*, International Conference on Volatile Organic Compounds in the Environment, London, 27–28 October, eds G. Leslie & R. Perry, pp. 447–63.

Wilson, P. (1988) *The Good Wood Guide*, Wilderness Society, Sydney.

CHAPTER 10:
SPECIAL HEALTH AND SAFETY ISSUES

Baggs, S.A., & Wong, C.F. (1987) 'Survey of radon in Australian residences', *Architectural Science Review*, vol. 30, pp. 11–22.

Child Accident Prevention Foundation of Australia (1992) *A Safer Home for Children*, Child Accident Prevention Foundation, Sydney.

Clarensjo, K., & Kumlin, P. (1984) *Radon in Dwellings: Remedial Action for New and Reconstructed Dwellings*, R90, Swedish Council for Building Research, Stockholm.

'Concern about radon grows in Britain and America', *New Scientist* (1988), 22 September, p. 24.

Ferrari, L., et al (1988) 'Air quality in Australian homes: results of the first Australian study', paper presented to ANZAAS Centenary Conference, Sydney, 18 May.

Holdsworth, W., & Sealey, A.F. (1992) *Healthy Buildings*, Longman, Harlow UK.

Nero, A. Jr. (1986) 'Controlling indoor air pollution', *Scientific American'*, vol. 258, no. 5, pp. 24–30.

Pierce, F. (1987) 'A deadly gas under the floorboards', *New Scientist,* 5 February.

Schneider, A. (trans. H. Ziehe) (1988) *Building Biology Correspondence Course*, International Institut fur Baubiologie™ und Oikologie, Neubeuern.

Short, Kate (1994) *Quick Poison, Slow Poison*, Envirobook Publishers, St Albans NSW.

Verkerk, R. (1990) *Building out Termites: An Australian Manual for Environmentally Responsible Control*, Pluto Press, Leichhardt NSW.

CHAPTER 11: HEALTHY ECOVILLAGES AND ECTOWNS

Eco-communities (1994) Building Biology and Ecology Institute, Auckland NZ, BBE no. 18, Spring.

Hinsley, H. (1995) 'Sustainable cities? Today's critical issues for designers', *Architecture Australia*, January–February, pp. 68–9.

Hopkins, N. (1992) 'Davis California, village homes,' *Permaculture International Journal*, vol. 42.

Kanuka-Fuchs, R. (1994) *Tui Community, Golden Bay, Nelson*, Building Biology and Ecology Institute NZ, BBE no. 18, Spring.

The PEOPL Group (1994) *Project Concept Document: Ecovillage Proposal, NSW*, The PEOPL Group, Sydney.

CHAPTER 12:
A LIFESTYLE THAT RESPECTS GAIA

Adams, S. (1994) 'Inside science # 75: no way back', *New Scientist*, 22 October, pp. 1–4.

Airola, P. (1987) *How to Get Well*, Health Plus Publishers, Phoenix.

Bate, R. (1976) *Many Happy Returns*, Friends of the Earth, London.

Pedler, K. (1979) *The Quest for Gaia*, Souvenir Press, London.

Vale, B., & Vale, R. (1976) *The Autonomous House: Designing and Planning for Self-sufficiency*, Thames & Hudson, London.

APPENDIX A

Dalton, L. (1991) *Radiation Exposures*, Scribe Publications, Newham, Victoria.

Elmsley, J. (1993) 'Photochemistry: inside science', *New Scientist*, 16 January.

Riley, K. (1995) Tracing EMFs in Building and Grounding, *Magnetic Sciences International*, Tucson, Arizona.

Smith, C.W. & Best, S. (1989) *Electromagnetic Man: Health Hazard in the Electrical Environment*, Dent, London.

APPENDIX C

California Department of Consumer Affairs (1982) *Clean your room: a compendium on indoor pollution*, No E513, February.

Department of Energy, Bonneville Power Administration, United States (1983) *Environment and power: issue backgrounder, the health impacts of home weatherization*, Portland Oregon.

Division of Energy Conservation, Bonneville Power Administration, United States (1981) *Revised Environmental Assessment: Proposed BPA Regionwide Weatherization Program*, Nos A–1 and A–4, September, Portland, Oregon.

Ehrlich, P. & Ehrlich, Anne (1972) *Population Resources Environment: Issues in Human Ecology*, Freeman, San Francisco.

Environmental Protection Agency (1992) *Environmental Almanac: World Resources Institute*, Houghton Mifflin, Boston.

Ferrari, L., & Johnson, D. (1982) 'Air pollution trends in Sydney', in *Environment and Power*, eds J. Carras & G. Johnson.

Ferrari, L., et al (1988) 'Air quality in Australian homes: results of the first Australian study', paper presented to ANZAAS Centenary Conference, Sydney, 18 May.

General Accounting Office (1980) *Indoor Air Pollution: An Emerging Health Problem*, CED-80-111, 24 September.

Gilbert, D. (1992) 'Ensuring a healthy indoor environment', *Geotecture*, vol. 9, no. 1, pp. 13–29.

Holmes, N. (1990) *Painters Hazard Handbook*, Operative Painters and Decorators Union of Australia, Crows Nest NSW.

Kabos, A. (1986) *A–Z of Chemicals in the Home*, Total Environment Centre, Sydney.

Laura, R. S., and Ashton, J. F. (1991) *Hidden Hazards*, Bantam, Moorebank.

Molhave, L. (1990) 'Volatile organic compounds, indoor air quality and health' *Proceedings of Conference on International Indoor Air Quality*, vol. 5, Toronto, Canada.

National Health and Medical Research Council, Australia (1986) *Code of Practice for the Safe Use of Ionizing Radiation in Secondary Schools*, Australian Government Publishing Service, Canberra.

National Health and Medical Research Council, Australia (n/d) *Ambient Air Quality: Goals Recommended by the National Health and Medical Research Council*, EHB2, Air 221, Canberra.

Randolph, T. (1963) *Proceedings, National Conference on Air Pollution*, US Dept of Health, Education & Welfare, US Govt Printer, Washington DC.

Randolph, T. (1979) 'Domiciliary chemical air pollution in the etiology of ecologic mental illness', in *A Physician's Handbook on Orthomolecular Medicine* (R.J Williams & D.K. Kalita, eds), Keats Publishing Inc, New Canaan, Conn, USA.

Samways, L. (1989) *The Chemical Connection*, Greenhouse Publications, Elwood, Vic.

Spedding, D. (1974) *Air Pollution*, Clarendon, Oxford.

van den Bosch, R. (1980) *The Pesticide Conspiracy*, Prism, Dorchester, Dorset.

Spengler, J., & Sexton, K. (1983) 'Indoor air pollution: a public health perspective', *Science*, vol. 221, no. 4605, p. 10.

Standards Association of Australia (1992) *Plastic Materials for Food Contact Use*, A.S. 2070.2, Standards Association of Australia, Sydney.

'Sunday Spotlight: Killer Chemicals' (1992) *Sun Herald*, 19 July.

Turiel, I. (1983) 'The effects of reduced ventilation and indoor health quality', *Atmospheric Environment*, vol. 17, no. 1.

Worksafe Australia (1988) *Synthetic Mineral Fibres* (draft guide and code of practice) No. 6, National Occupational Health and Safety Commission, Australian Government Printing Service, Canberra.

Worksafe Australia (1990) National Standard and National Code of Practice for the Safe Use of Synthetic Mineral Fibres, National Health and Safety Commission, Australian Government Printing Service, Canberra.

World Resources Institute Environmental Protection Agency (1992) *Environmental Almanac*, Houghton Miflin, Boston.

APPENDIX D

Airola, P. (1987) *How to Get Well*, Health Plus Publishers, Phoenix, Arizona.

Greulach, V., & Adams, J. (1962) *Plants. An Introduction to Modern Botany*, Wiley, New York.

Laura, R. S., & Ashton, J. F. (1991) *Hidden Hazards*, Bantam, Moorebank NSW.

Mindell, E. (1985) *The Vitamin Bible*, Arlington Books, London.

APPENDIX E

Baghurst, P., et al (1992) 'Environmental exposure to lead and children's intelligence at the age of 7 years. The Port Pirie Cohort Study', *New England Journal of Medicine* no. 327:8, pp 1279–1284.

Civil Aeromedical Institute, Federal Aviation Authority Administration, United States (n/d) *Neurophysiological and behavioural assessment of pesticide toxicity*, report by A. Revzin, Oklahoma City.

'Guide to low cadmium phosphate supplements', *Farm*, 16 August 1990.

Kostial, K. (1984) 'Effect of age and diet on renal cadmium retention in rats', *Environmental Health Perspectives* 54 pp 51–56.

Onosoka, et al (1984) 'Effects of cadmium and zinc on tissue levels of metallothionein' in *Environmental Health Perspectives*, vol. 54, pp. 67–72.

Short, Kate (1994) *Quick Poison, Slow Poison*, Envirobook Publishers, St Albans NSW.

APPENDIX G

'Pretty but dangerous' (1983) *Choice*, April, vol. 24, no. 4, pp 3–7.

Sutherland, S. (ed.) (1993) *Australia's Dangerous Creatures*, Readers Digest (Australia), Sydney.

APPENDIX H

Anderson, R. (1968) *Trees of New South Wales*, NSW Department of Agriculture, Sydney.

Australian Plant Study Group (1990) *Grow What Where?* Penguin, Sydney.

Blomberg, A. (1972) *What Wildflower is That?*, Hamlyn, Sydney.

Country Fire Service (n.d.) *Woods and Forests: Fire 'resistance' of trees and shrubs*, no. 14, Goodwood, S.A.

Cunningham, G., et al (1981) *Plants of Western New South Wales*, Soil Conservation Service, NSW Govt Printing Office, Sydney.

Forestry and Timber Bureau (1972) *The Use of Trees and Shrubs in the Dry Country of Australia*, Canberra.

Forestry Commission of New South Wales (1980) *Trees and Shrubs for Eastern Australia*, NSW University Press, Sydney.

Francis, R. (1989) 'Design for bushfire', *International Permaculture Journal*, no. 32.

Kreviter, P. and Tardif, R. (eds) (1986) *The Macquarie Dictionary of Trees and Shrubs*, Macquarie Library Pty Ltd, Sydney.

Molnar, I. (ed) (1974) *A Manual of Australian Agriculture*, Heinemann, Melbourne.

Morley, B. & Toelken, H. (1983) *Flowering Plants in Australia*, Rigby, Sydney.

Williams, L. (1966) *Your Australian Garden: Grevilleas*, Stead Wildlife Research Foundation, Sydney

Acknowledgments

We would like to thank all those who generously provided photographs and the following people to whom we are indebted:

DAVID BAGGS: architect and consultant to the authors, for his advice on Chapters 9 and 10, contribution on straw-bale construction, input to the Resources List and for reviewing the manuscript

HERMAN BAUSER: (of Tersia Australia Pty Ltd) for information on polypropylene tubing

LEX BEWLEY: landscape architect, for his advice on Chapter 7 and for reviewing the manuscript

JOHN CARTER: plasterer, for his advice and plaster samples for radiation testing

RONALD FLINT: alternative medical practitioner, for his advice

KIRSTEN GARRETT: ABC Radio, Sydney, for her advice and for providing access to resources

DALE GILBERT: of the Built Environment Unit of the Queensland Administrative Services Dept, for advice and data on pollution levels

PROF. (EMERITUS) PATRICK HORSBRUGH: for his continuous support and encouragement of work relating to the integration of human settlements with nature

REINHARD KANUKA-FUCHS: bioharmonic architect and Director of the Building Biology and Ecology Institute of New Zealand, who has set the standard in healthy house design and construction for the rest of the world to follow

PHILIP KING: Senior Professional Officer of the Australian Bureau of Meteorology, for providing data

HENRY LAI: for checking the information in Chapter 5

PETER McBRIDE: bioelectrician, for checking the electrical information in Chapter 9 and for his help in experimenting with electromagnetic fields and wiring layouts

NEAL MORTENSEN: architect, for his support

DAVID OLIVER AND GRAHAM OSBORNE: architects, for their contribution on rammed-earth construction

CRAIG PATTINSON: architect, for his continuing support and contribution on natural swimming pools and rammed-earth structures

BRUCE PETERSON: engineer, for reviewing the manuscript

BARRY RICHARDSON: scientist, for his valuable input on the effects of moisture content of air and materials in relation to health and for reviewing relevant parts of the manuscript

GRAHAM AND SANDRA ROSS: for assistance with the bushfire resistant vegetation list in Appendix H.

NEENA SCOTT: for her unfailing support and generosity in providing the photograph of the Yango Mountain deva in Chapter 1

CRAIG SMITH: of Northwest Scientific, California, for his ongoing interest and professional advice

DR CYRIL SMITH: of Salford University, UK, for his continuing support, advice and guidance concerning the health aspects of ionising and non-ionising radiation

PROF. (EMERITUS) WILLIAM TILLER: of the Department of Materials Science & Engineering, Stanford University, California, for his inspirational guidance over the years on scientific issues that could still be classified as parascience

DEREK WALTERS: Chinese astrologer and *feng shui* consultant, for his advice and for reviewing parts of the manuscript

JOHN WHITLOCK: Division of Building Construction & Engineering, Commonwealth Scientific and Industrial Research Organisation (Australia), for his advice on materials

IAN WINNETT: for his advice on healthy pipe materials

Index